PULMONARY FUNCTION TESTS AND INTERPRETATION IN HEALTH AND DISEASES

Editor

P. S. Shankar

MD, FRCP(Lond), FAMS
DSc(Gul), DSc(NTR), DSc(RGUHS, DSc(TU), DLitt(Hampi)
Emeritus Professor of Medicine, Rajiv Gandhi University of Health Sciences
based at KBN Institute of Medical Sciences,Kalaburagi

THIRD EDITION

www.nationalbookdepot.com

CBS Publishers & Distributors Pvt Ltd.

First Edition 1998
Reprint 2003
Second Edition 2007
Third Edition 2017

Published by

Vaidehi Shah for

The National Book Depot

Opp. Wadia Children's Hospital, Parel, Mumbai - 400 012.
Tel : (+91-22) 2416 5274 / 2413 1362 / 2413 2411 | Fax : 2413 0877
E-mail: nationalbook55@gmail.com
www.nationalbookdepot.com

and

Satish Kumar Jain for
CBS Publishers & Distributors Pvt Ltd
4819/XI Prahlad Street, 24 Ansari Road, Daryaganj, New Delhi - 110 002.
Ph: 23289259 / 23266861 / 23266867 | Fax: 011-23243014
E-mail: delhi@cbspd.com; cbspubs@airtelmail.in
www.cbspd.com

ISBN : 978-93-80206-86-8

Printed by : Neel Graphics

PREFACE TO FIRST EDITION

Pulmonary Function Tests (PFTs) can determine all components of the process of respiration as classified by Pappenheimer consisting of ventilation, distribution, diffusion, perfusion and compliance, objectively and accurately.

Pulmonary function tests are helpful to the clinician qualitatively to prove or disprove a clinical diagnosis and quantitatively to determine the severity of a particular disorder. In addition they provide objective data on progression or remission of disease and on the effects of therapy. The results of pulmonary function tests give a pattern of abnormalities and they are to be interpreted in the background of the patient's clinical findings. The normal values are based on age, height, gender, and ethnic group.

The pulmonary function laboratory must provide measures of static and dynamic lung volumes, diffusing capacity, flow volume curve, arterial blood gases, Pulmonary mechanics and pulmonary hemodynamic studies.

This monograph is a collective work of various authors from different parts of India. There are 23 chapters. The opening chapters provide basis of respiratory mechanics of breathing and pulmonary function equipment. Subsequently the tests for ventilation, airflow, lung volumes, airway resistance and compliance, distribution and small airways have been described in detail. There are chapters on classification of abnormal patterns of pulmonary functions, beside pulmonary function tests, preoperative assessment of pulmonary function, evaluation of PFT by radiology, regional lung functions, PFT during sleep, arterial blood gases and bronchoprovocation tests.

These tests will help the Practicing Physicians and those with special interest in respiratory disease. I am deeply indebted to various contributors who readily responded to my request to write different chapters for the monograph. The articles have been written in a lucid manner giving an updated account on the subject which I am sure the readers will get benefit.

P. S. Shankar
Editor

PREFACE TO THIRD EDITION

The respiratory system is essentially concerned with exchange of gases between the inspired air and blood in the alveolar capillaries. It provides a surface for transfer of gases through which blood gets rid of carbon dioxide and absorbs oxygen.

The process involves ventilation, concerned with movement of gases along the airways to and out of the alveoli, intrapulmonary distribution of air (V) and adequate perfusion of capillaries (Q) matching ventilation and perfusion, thus diffusion of gases over the wide area of the alveolar-capillary membranes. All these processes are closely integrated.

Pulmonary function tests are helpful in the diagnosis and assessment of functional impairment of different respiratory disorders. The tests are also helpful in determining the responses to the treatment. The diseases due to airway narrowing, hyperinflation, decreased volumes and disruption of gas exchanging structures affect expiratory and inspiratory airflow, lung volumes and gas exchange. It is quantified and compared with normal values after adjusting to the age, sex, and height and ethnicity. Arterial blood gases help in determination of the degree and type of respiratory failure and acid-base balance. They are estimated periodically to determine the response to therapy.

The revised third edition of Pulmonary function tests coming two decades after its initial publication. Many chapters have been revised in light of the developments that have taken place in the recent years. New authors have found place in place of some earlier authors. Attempt has been made to provide all information in a comprehensive manner to the practicing physicians, chest physicians and postgraduates.

My thanks are due to various contributors who readily responded to my request to write/ revise different chapters of the monograph. My thanks are to the publisher Sri Raju Shah for the constant encouragement and support. I thank Sri Viren Shah for the beautiful production of the book.

Mumbai
7th July 2017

P. S. Shankar
Editor

CONTENTS

LIST OF CONTRIBUTORS

Ajit Vigg, Senior Consultant in Chest Diseases, Secretariat Road, Khairatabad, Hyderabad - 500 004, Telangana.

Alladi Mohan, Prof. and Head: Dept of Med. Sri Venkateswara Institute of Medical Sciences, Tirupati - 517 507, Andhra Pradesh.

Amita Nene, Head, Dept. of Pulmonary Med. Bombay Hospital, Marine Lines, Mumbai - 400 020.

Anand Saraf, Senior Registrar : Chest Dept. Nanavati Super-Specialty Hospital, Vile Parle West, Mumbai.

B N B M Prasad, Professor of Medicine, Amrita Institute of Medical Sciences, Ernakulam - 608 204, Kerala.

D Behera, Sr. Prof. & Head, Dept. of Pulmonary Medicine, (WHO Collaborating Centre for Research & Capacity Building in Chronic Respiratory Diseases). Postgraduate Institute of Medical Education & Research, Chandigarh - 160 012.

D D S Kulpati, Chest Specialist, Sir Gangaram Hospital, South Ext. Part II, New Delhi - 110 049.

Dhiman Ganguly, Consultant Chest Physician, Suren Sircar Road, Kolkata - 700 010, West Bengal.

G C Khilnani, Professor of Pulmonary Medicine and Sleep Disorders, All India Institute of Medical Sciences, New Delhi - 110 016.

Harmanjit Singh Hira, Director Professor and Head, Pulmonary Medicine, Maulana Azad Medical College, New Delhi.

J C Suri, Consultant, Prof. and Head, Dept. of Pulmonary, Critical Care and Sleep Medicine, Vardhman Mahavir Medical College & Safdarjung Hospital, New Delhi.

J N Pande, Consultant in Med. and Chest Med., Sitaram Bhartia Institute of Science and Research, New Delhi - 110 016.

KT Prasad, Assistant Prof., Dept. of Pul. Med., Postgraduate Institute of Medical Education & Research, Chandigarh - 160 012.

M. Madhusudhan, Assistant Prof., Dept. of Anaesthesiology and Critical Care Medicine, Sri Venkateswara Institute of Medical Sciences, Tirupati - 517 507, Andhra Pradesh.

Mayur H Patel, Head, Critical Care and Emergency Medicine, Sir. H. N. Reliance Foundation Hospital, Mumbai.

Mohankumar Thekkinkattil, Head of the Department and Sr. Consultant Pulmonologist, Sri Ramakrishna hospital, Coimbatore - 641 044, Tamil Nadu.

Nikhil Sarangdhar, Consultant Chest Physician, Group of TB Hospitals, Sewri, Mumbai.

P S Shankar, Emeritus Professor of Medicine, Rajiv Gandhi University of Health Sciences based at KBN Institute of Medical Sciences, Kalaburagi - 585 103, Karnataka.

Saili Bendre, PFT Department in Charge, Suburban Diagnostics, Andheri West, Mumbai.

Salil Bendre, Head, Pulmonary Medicine, Nanavati Super-Specialty Hospital, Vile Parle West, Mumbai.

Salil Bhargava, Professor and Head: Department of Respiratory Medicine, Bundelkhand Medical College, Sagar, Madhya Pradesh.

S N Gaur, Former Director (Acting) and Professor & Head,; Department of Pulmonary Medicine. Vallabhbhai Patel Chest Institute, Gaur Clinic, 130-A, Patparganj Village, Delhi - 110 091.

Surinder K. Jindal, Emeritus-Professor, Postgraduate Institute of Med Edu & Research. Medical Director, Jindal Clinics, SCO 21, Sector 20 D, Chandigarh - 160 020, India.

Swapnil Kulkarni, Consultant Chest Physician, Mulund/Thane, Mumbai.

Vikas Agrawal, Consultant Chest Physician & Medical Director. South Mumbai Medical Centre, Mumbai.

Virendra Singh, Director Asthma Bhawan, Jaipur - 302 016, Rajasthan.

V K Vijayan, Former Director Vallabhbhai Patil Chest Institute, Delhi, Senior Consultant in Chest Diseases, Baby Memorial Hospital, Kozhikode - 673 004, Kerala.

1
INTRODUCTION

P S SHANKAR

The clinician should know the underlying physiology and pathology of the lungs during health and disease respectively. The study of pulmonary disease involves history, physical examination of the chest and of other systems of the body, radiologic examination and other imaging techniques, sputum and blood examination, allergic skin testing, pulmonary function tests and fine needle aspiration, bronchoscopy, thoracoscopy, bronchoalveolar lavage and biopsy.

The Respiratory Processes

The respiratory system is essentially concerned with exchange of gases between the inspired air in the alveoli, and blood in the alveolar capillaries. It provides a surface for transfer of gases through which blood gets rid of carbon dioxide and absorbs oxygen. In doing so, the pressures of oxygen and carbon dioxide are maintained in the arterial blood at 100 mm Hg and 40 mm Hg respectively while breathing ambient air at sea level. Lung plays an important role in the maintenance of acid-base balance by offerning a surface for elimination of carbon dioxide produced in the body during metabolic processes (1).

The respiratory process involves ventilation concerned with movement of gases in and out of the bronchial passages, intrapulmonary distribution (V) and mixing of respiratory gases, and adequate perfusion of capillaries (Q), matching ventilation and perfusion, thus enabling diffusion of gses over the whole area of alveolar-capillary membrane. These processes are closely integrated. The act of breathing involves movement of gases in and out of the air passages. While doing these movements, work has to be done to overcome the elastic recoil of the lung and chest wall and the frictional resistance offered by the tissues and the airways.

Pulmonary function tests

The clinical significance of pulmonary function has been established exemplifying the statement of Starling 'the physiology of today is the Medicine of tomorrow'.

The pulmonary function tests (PFTs)

1. Provide an objective evidence of the lung function that has been deranged by the disease process involving the bronchial tress and the lung, the pulmonary vasculature and the chest bellows.
2. Help to identify or exclude a respiratory cause of breathlessness
3. Help in preoperative evaluation by quantifying the lung function in patients urdergoing pulmonary resection so as to offer the prognosis on immediate hazard of surgery and also on their ability to lead useful life following operation
4. Help to the assessment of the course of a disease over time such as chronic obstructive pulmonary disease (COPD)
5. Help to monitor the effectiveness of the therapy undertaken such as bronchial asthma, and interstitial lung diseases

6. Help in differntiating the types of respiratory failure
7. Detect airway hyperresponsiveness, and
8. Help in evaluation of the disability.

Limitations

However there are limitations to the pulmonary function tests. Though the pattern of abnormality indicates the type of problem, the tests themselves are seldom specifically diagnostic as they do not provide any anatomic or aetiologic diagnosis (1). A battery of tests are available which together help in the evaluation of different aspects of pulmonary function. It is only on the establishment of the level of function, it is possible to monitor the progression of the disease or the effect of treatment. No single test can evaluate all aspects of pulmonary function (2).

Uses

Pulmonary function tests are undertaken to find out whether the patient has any lung disease. The results of the pulmonary function tests of a given individual are compared with those obtained from a normal population of comparable height, age and gender. The test is considered abnormal if it falls outside the range based on the standard error of the estimate in which 95% of normal lies (3). Predicted values for some of the pulmonary functions differ by race.

Simple spirometry is utilised initially to determine whether the patient has lung disease. The tests undertaken are FVC, FEV1, and FEV,/FVC ratio. If the results are within normal limits, it has to be concluded that the patient has no ventilatory dysfunction. The only exceptions are certain pulmonary vascular diseases and systemic sclerosis. They may exhibit normal spirometry but an abnormal diffusing capacity. Bronchial asthma being episodic, the patients exhibit normal spirometric value when they are freee from symptoms. Such patients can exhibit airway hyperresponsiveness following inhalational challenges tests (4).

If there is any abnormality in the simple spirometry, the dysfunction is categorized as obstructive ventilatory defect, restrictive ventilatory defect and mixed ventilatory defect.

a) ***Obstructive ventilatory defect***: There is decrease in expiratory flow rates with maximum effort. There is an increase in expiratory resistance due to an increse in airway resistance or a decrease in the elastic recoil of the lung. The FEV1/FVC ratio is reduced below 0.75.

b) ***Restrictive ventilatory defect:*** The volumes of lungs are decreased. Vital capacity is reduced below the predicted normal range. It is associated with a reduction in other volume compartments. FEV1/FVC ratios are normal indicating an absence of airway obstruction. There can be reduction of both FVC and FEV1 with spirometry. The values are expressed as percentage of the predicted value.

c) ***Mixed ventilatory defect***: Some patients exhibit both obstrucative and restrictive ventilatory defects. In predominantly restrictive defect, the FVC will be decreased proportionately more than the FRV1. In predominantly obstructive defect, the FEV1 will be decreased proportionately more than the FVC.

Thus some of the pulmonary function tests are simple (spirometry and peak flow) that can be carried out in the office or ward and they help in moniotring the course of a disease. Other tests, which are also equally useful can be carried out in a fully equipped laboratory.

Methods and measurement

The methods and measurements obtained in pulmonary function testing are as follows:

1. ***Airway function:*** The assessment of airway function includes i) Spirometry (vital capacity, VC), forced vital capacity (FVC), forced expiratory volume in one second (FEV1), FEV1/FVC%, tidal volume, ii) flow volume loops, iii) peak expiratory flow rate

(PEFR) estimated by peak flow meter, and iv) airway resistance by body plethysmography.

2. ***Lung volumes***: The following subdivisions of lung volumes are measured by utilising spirometry, gas dilution technique and plethysmography (tidal volume, total lung capacity, TLC), functional residual capacity (FRC) and residual volume (RV).
3. ***Diffusion:*** Diffusion capacity refers to the magnitude of carbon monoxide gas transfer (DVCO) on the volume of the pulmonary capillary bed and the matching between ventilation and perfusion within the lungs. The technique is utilising single breath diffusing capacity.
4. ***Respiratory muscle function***: Breathlessness may be due to muscles to inflate the lungs. Peak inspiratory and expiratory maximal mouth pressures (PImax and PEmax) respectively are the simple tests utilised to evaluate respiratory muscle strength.
5. ***Exercise tests:*** Exercise tests are helpful in demonstration of integrated functions of cardiorespiratory system.

Impairment

Pulmonary function may be impaired due to physiologic and anatomic abnormalities. They are evaluated by pulmonary function tests. American Thoracic Society has recommended to include forced spirometry measurements and testing of single-breath diffusing capacity (5). The tests enable to categorize majority of individuals according to the degree of impairment.

Category	FVC predicted percent	FEV1 predicted percent	FEV1/FVC	DLCO predicted percent
Normal	80	80	0.75	80
Impairment				
Mild	60-79	60-79	0.60-0.74	60-70
Moderate	51-59	41-59	0.41-0.59	41-50
Severe	<50	<40	0.40	<40

The individuals, who demonstrate no impairment or mild impairment while performing the pulmonary function tests, are able to meet the physical demands of most of the jobs. Those exhibiting moderate or severe impairment on the basis of their pulmonary function tests show diminishing ability or ianbility to met the physical demands of most of the jobs respectively. Exercise testing is advocated for those patients with mild or moderate impairment of pulmonary function tests who complain of shortness of breath while working.

Any impairment can lead to disability wherein the patient is unable to or exhibits a limitation in the performance of tasks undertaken.

REFERENCES

1. Shankar PS Respiration in Chest Medicine, 4th edn, New Delhi, IBH & Oxford 1994; 14-49
2. Bass BH Lung function tests. An introduction, 3rd edn, London, HK Lewis 1966: 5
3. Light RW Clinical Pulmonary function testing. Exercise testing and disability evaluation in Chest Medicine, Essentials of pulmonary and critical care Medicine, 3rd edn, Baltimore, Williams & Wilkins, 1995; 151
4. Cockcroft DW, Hargreave FE Airway hyperresponsiveness. Relevance of random population data to clinical usefulness Am Rev Respir Dis 1990; 142: 497-500
5. Medical Section of American Lung Association: Evaluation of impairment, disability secondary to respiratory disease Am Rev Respir Dis 1986; 133: 1205-1209

2
RESPIRATORY MECHANICS OF BREATHING

SAILI BENDRE / SALIL BENDRE

Introduction

Respiration is the primary function of the respiratory system. It contributes to gas exchange between an organism and its environment. Thus the main function of the lung is to take in oxygen and exhale carbon dioxide. Ventilation is the flow of air through the airways and reaching the alveoli. Diffusion is the process by which air crosses across the alveolar basement into pulmonary capillaries.

The secondary role of the lung includes maintenance of acid-base balance through CO2 exchange. Respiratory mechanics concerns to the factors that determine lung volume and includes forces generated by respiratory muscles to inflate and deflate the respiratory system, forces that impede volume changes (resistance and elastance) and determinants of lung volume and its distribution within the lungs.

Respiration includes external respiration and internal respiration. External respiration includes pulmonary ventilation (inflow and outflow of air between atmosphere and lung alveoli, diffusion of oxygen and carbon dioxide between alveoli and blood, transport of these gases in the blood and body fluids to and from the cells, and regulation of respiration. Internal respiration is concerned with intracellular oxygen utilization as a part of metabolic process.

Ventilation of lungs

The volume of air a person breathes in a normal breathe is called tidal volume (TV). Minute volume (VE) is the product of tidal volume and respiratory rate. Usually tidal volume is 5 to 10 ml per kg.

The air in the trachea which does not take part in exchange is called anatomical dead space. In the lungs are some alveoli which are ventilated but not perfusedm and they comprise the physiological dead space .

That part of minute ventilation not taking part in gas exchange is dead space ventilation (VD).... Anatomical plus the physiological dead space.

Alveolar ventilation (VA) is the actual amount of ventilation which takes part in gas exchange.

$$VA = VE - VD = 5 \text{ litres/min}$$

Work of breathing

The respiratory muscles normally work only during inspiration. Normal work of breathing requires 2-3% of resting oxygen consumption. They include.

i. Elastic work- work required to epxand lung against elastic force
ii. Tissue resistance work- work required to overcome viscosity of lung and chest wall
iii. Airway resistance work-work required to overcome airway resistance

Volume changes during respiration

The lung is like a balloon suspended in the thoracic cage. It is tied at the hilum. The lung is encased in thin layer called pleura. The visceral pleura is the inner layer and the parietal pleura is the outer layer.

Ventilation consists of the bulk movement of air from outside the body through air passages into alveoli. The amount of inspired air that reaches the sites of gas exchange is determined by the distensibility of the lung parenchyma and factors governing movement of air through airways. Ventilation therefore depends on the capabilities of the respiratory muscles, and the mechanical properties of the conducting airways and vital respiratory units.

Mechanics of Breathing

Boyle's Law describes the relationship between the pressure (P) and the volume (V) of a gas. The law states that if the volume increases, then the pressure must decrease (or vice versa). This relationship is often written algebraically as PV = constant, or $P_1V_1 = P_2V_2$. Both equations state that the product of the pressure and volume remains the same. (Boyle's Law applies only when the temperature does not change.)

Breathing occurs when the contraction or relaxation of muscles around the lungs changes the total volume of air within the air passages (bronchi, bronchioles) inside the lungs. When there is a change in the volume of the lungs, the pressure of the air in the lungs changes in accordance with Boyle's Law. If the pressure is greater in the lungs than outside the lungs, then air rushes out. If the opposite occurs, then air rushes in. Here is a summary of the process:

1. **Inspiration** occurs when the inspiratory muscles—the diaphragm and the external intercostal muscles—contract. Contraction of the diaphragm leads to an increase in the size of the thoracic cavity, while contraction of the external intercostal muscles elevates the ribs and sternum. Thus, both muscles cause the lungs to expand, increasing the volume of their internal air passages. In response, the air pressure inside the lungs decreases below that of air outside the body. Because gases move from regions of high pressure to low pressure, air rushes into the lungs.
2. **Expiration** occurs when the diaphragm and external intercostal muscles relax. In response, the elastic fibers in lung tissue cause the lungs to recoil to their original volume. The pressure of the air inside the lungs then increases above the air pressure outside the body, and air rushes out. During high rates of ventilation, expiration is facilitated by contraction of the expiratory muscles (the intercostal muscles and the abdominal muscles).

The inspiratory muscles are the diaphragm and the external intercostals muscles. The internal intercostals muscles are the important expiratory muscles.

The external intercostals muscles originate from an upper rib and insert on the next lower rib more anteriorly in a diagonal direction.As the ribs are angled downward, their elevation leads to antero-posterior and lateral expansion of thorax. Hence, there is a certain amount of bucket handle effect.

The accessory muscles include the sternomastoid and other strap muscles of the neck and they originate from the neck and skull. By raising the clavicles and the sternum they elevate the ribs and enlarge the thorax. Activation of these muscles occurs during increased respiratory demand.

Thus, the lungs can be expanded and contracted by downward and upward movement of diaphragm to lengthen or shorten chest cavity and by elevation and depression of ribs to increase and decrease the anteroposterior and lateral diameter of chest cavity.

a) During inspiration, contraction of diaphragm pulls the lower surfaces of the lungs downwards. During expiration the diaphragm simply relaxes and the elastic recoil of the lungs, chest wall and abdominal structures compress the lungs. During heavy breathing, active contraction of abdominal muscles pushes the abdominal contents upwards against the bottom of the diaphragm to give the extra force to empty the lungs.

b) In the natural resting position, the ribs slant downward, allowing the sternum to fall backward towards the spinal column. During inspiration the rib cage is elevated and the ribs now project almost directly forward, moving the sternum forward and away from the spine, resulting in a 20% increase in AP diameter of the chest. Apart from the external intercostal muscles which elevate the chest cage and the sternocleidomastoids which lift the sternum upwards, the anterior serratus which lifts many of the ribs, and the scalene which lifts the first 2 ribs are the other important inspiratory muscles. The internal intercostal muscles give a leverage by pulling the rib cage downward during expiration. The abdominal recti compress the abdominal contents upwards towards the diaphragm and aid expiration considerably. The internal intercostals are placed diagonally between the ribs and cause an opposite leverage during expiration when they contract.

The movements of respiration are called the bucket handle and pump handle movements.

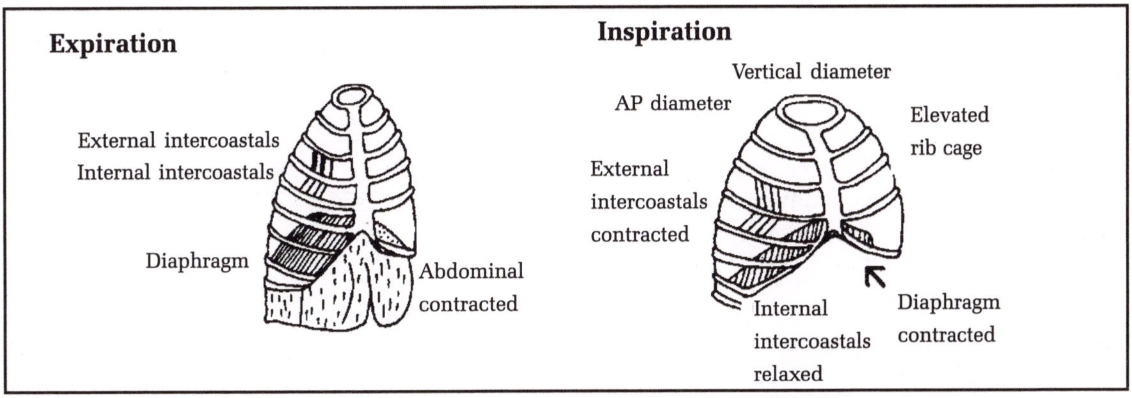

Note: *During inspiration thoracic cavity increases both vertically and anteroposteriorly, The reverse is seen during expiration*

Fig. 1: Expansion and contraction of thoracic cage during respiration

Pressure changes during ventilation

The lung is an elastic structure that can collapse like a balloon to expel air through trachea. the chest wall tends to recoil outwards. Expiration occurs due to passive recoil..

The pleural pressure is slightly negative at the beginning of inspiration (-5 cm of water). During normal inspiration with the expansion of chest cage still more negative pressure is created (-7.5 cm of water) and the lung volume increases by 0.5 litres. During expiration, the events are reversed.

Alveolar pressure is the pressure inside the alveoli which decides the rate of gas flow in or out of the lungs. It is atmospheric (0 cm of water) during equilibrium and drops during normal inspiration (-1 cm of water) allowing 0.5 litre of air to enter into the lungs. During normal expiration, the alveolar pressure rises (+1 cm of water) and expels 0.5 litre of air out of the lungs.

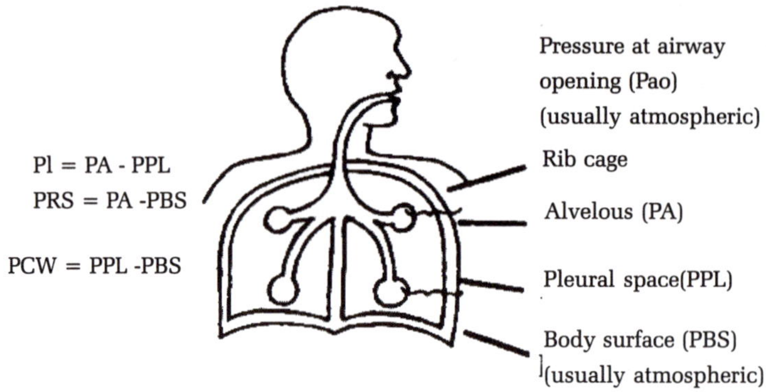

PA - Alvcolar pressure; PPL = Interpleular pressure
PBS - Body surface pressure; PCW - Transthoracic pressure
PRS - Transpiratory pressure (relaxation pressure)
PL - Transpulmonary pressure

Note: The lung volume is determined by its trans-respiratory pressure which is the sum of transpulmonary and transthoracic pressures. It can be also calculated as the difference between alveolar and intrapleural pressures.

Fig 2. Pressures during ventilation.

Transpulmonary pressure is the pressure difference between the alveoli and the pleural space and is a measure of the elastic forces in the lungs that tend to collapse the lungs at each point of expansion (recoil pressure). The lung volume is determined by the transpulmonary pressure, which is 20-30 cm of water at the maximum distension (limiting volume) and 0 cm of water at equilibrium volume (resting volume) without airflow. A positive transpulmonary pressure tends to inflate the lungs, while a negative transpulmonary pressure tends to deflate the lungs.

Compliance

Lung compliance is simply the relationship between how much pressure is required to produce a degree of volume change of the lungs. It is affected by the elastic properties of the lung, which are reduced in emphysema, where lung compliance is high. Lung compliance can be reduced in diseases such as idiopathic pulmonary fibrosis, where the elastic fibres of the lung (elastin) are replaced by stiffer collagen. Patients with decreased lung compliance need to work harder in order to breathe.

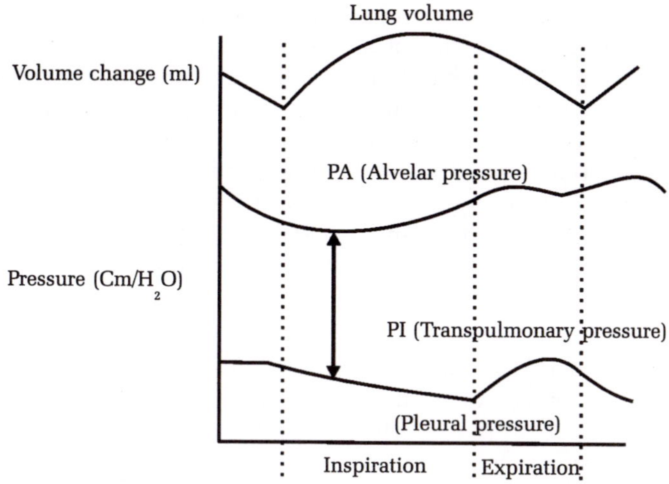

Note: *The lung volume increases by the end of inspiration when transpulmonary pressure is highest*

Fig. 3 Changes in Lung volume and pressure during normal breathing.

Factors affecting lung compliance

Two main factors determine lung compliance. The first is the connective tissue of the lung, which is rich in the protein elastin, which as its name implies is inherently stretchy. This elastic property of the lung allows the lungs to recoil of their own accord during passive expiration.

There are two examples of changes in the elasticity of the lung. Firstly, in fibrotic diseases such as idiopathic pulmonary fibrosis elastin is replaced by collagen, which is not as elastic. This makes the lungs harder to inflate (since it won't stretch as easily) and hence have reduced compliance. By contrast, in emphysema - where the elastin is degraded - the lungs have increased compliance and are very easy to inflate, but have reduced capacity to recoil. A patient with a lung such as this may have to force their expiration in order to get the air out of their lungs.

The second major influence on compliance is easy to forget about because it is only affected in quite specific circumstances (pre-term labour): pulmonary surfactant. If pulmonary surfactant is absent or production is reduced, then the surface tension in the fluid lining the alveoli is so high that they are virtually impossible to inflate at all. As a consequence, lung compliance is decreased enormously.

In disease states where some of the alveoli become filled with fluid, compliance will also decrease. Oedema due to inflammation of the alveoli – sometimes seen in pneumonia – will cause such a decrease but there can be non-inflammatory causes of alveolar oedema as well. For example, in left-sided heart failure, the heart cannot adequately pump the blood from the pulmonary vein to the body. As a result, back pressure accumulates in the lung and water is forced by this hydrostatic pressure into the alveoli. In both cases, compliance is reduced because fluid-filled alveoli cannot be inflated.

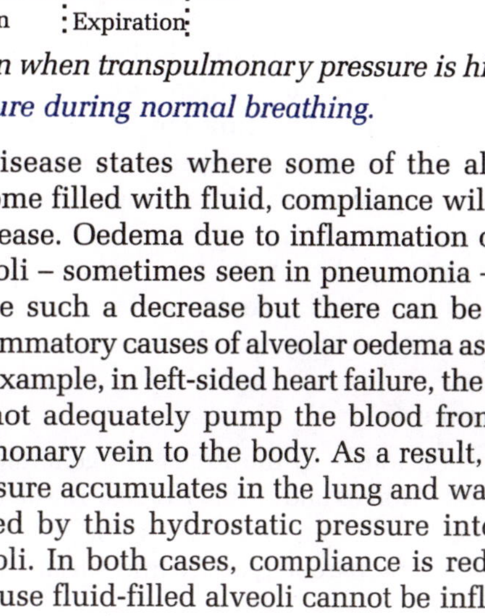

Note. *Maximal inspiratory pressures occur at low lung volumes (optimal length of inspiratory muscles) and maximal expiratory pressure occur at high lung voumes.*

Fig 4: Respiratory system pressure volume curve

The residual volume of the lungs is the amount of air remaining in the lungs at the end of a forced expiration and depends on the strength of the expiratory muscles while functional residual capacity (equilibrium volume) is the amount of air remaining in the lungs at the end of a normal quiet expiration. Total lung capacity is the maximum volume achieved by the lungs and depends on the compliance of the lung and the strength of the inspiratory muscles.

The normal compliance is 0.2 litres/cm H2O. It means for each cm H2O increase in transmural pressure, the gas volume increases by 0.2 litres. To stretch the lungs by 0.5 litres, the transpulmonary pressure must increase by 2.5 cm H2O. Decreased compliance is seen in restrictive lung disease, where greater forces are required to expand the lungs by overcoming the high elastance forces. Compliance also depends on the size of functional lung tissue. Conversely in emphysema, compliance is increased and lungs get overdistended with destruction of alveolar septa and alveolar surface area while recoil forces of lungs are decreased.

Elastance

The recoil forces in the lungs are generated by both tissue forces and surface forces. Tissue forces are due to collagen and elastin and contractile fibres in lung parenchyma, while surface forces are generated at the interface of 2 different phases e.g. liquid-gas. Surface tension forces tend to collapse alveoli and are countered by the normal surfactant produced by type II alveolar cells. Tissue interdependence allows mechanical stabilization of alveoli and neighbouring alveoli, holding back alveoli that tend to collapse. Reduction in surfactant results in respiratory distress syndrome.

Respiratory system pressure-volume curve (relaxation pressure-volume curve) can be recorded by a spirometer. The respiratory system normally functions at the middle of the sigmoid-shaped curve where the system is more distensible. The curve is steepest at the middle and flat at high and low lung volumes. It results from summation of elastic properties of chest wall and lungs.

Resistance

It is a dynamic property created by changing lung volumes due to friction of gas molecules between each other and walls of airways (airway resistance) as well as by friction of tissues with lung volume changes (tissue resistance). Airway resistance forms 80-90% of total resistance force. It is equal to the ratio between pressure during respiration and rate of gas flow in and out of lungs and is measured in cm H_2O / L/ sec.

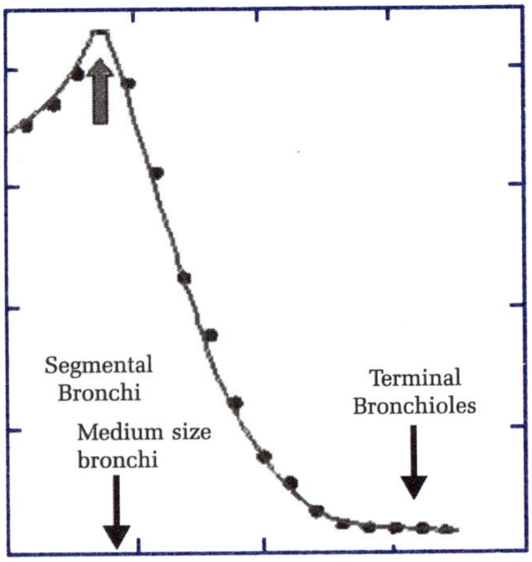

Fig.5. Airway resistance

Rate of gas flow depends on gas velocity and cross sectional area of airways. Velocity depends on pressure gradient between alveoli and mouth, the driving force determining airflow (trans-airway pressure).

Cross sectional area depends on the size of bronchi, the highest resistance being in intermediate size of bronchi. Only 10% of resistance is contributed by peripheral (small) airways <2 mm diameter because of the large number of these airways and large cross sectional area. The smaller the airways, the higher is the resistance. However, as these airways generate only 10% of total airway resistance, an increase in resistance in small airways results in just 15% increase in total airway resistance.

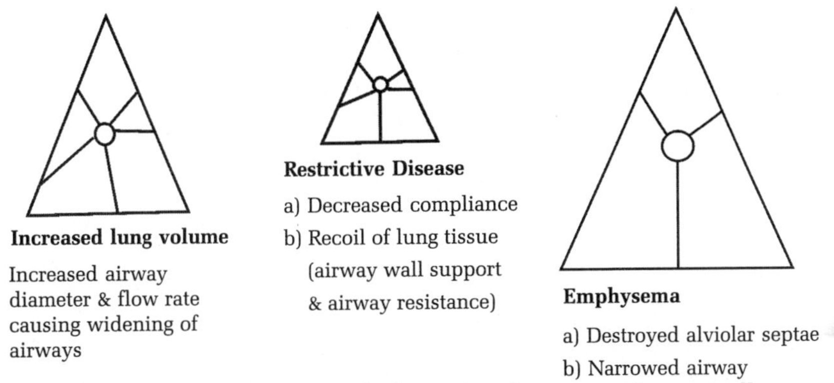

Fig.6. Factors affecting radial traction forces on airway walls

Effort independent flow: During forced expiration when intrapleural pressures are positive and lung volumes are less than 80% of total lung capacity, effort independent flow occurs. Expiratory flow rate remains constant at each lung volume, but intrapleural pressures vary greatly.

Dynamic compression of airways occurs during forced expiration and it limits flow rate during the terminal 80% of expiration. Increase in lung volume causes a radial traction on airways by alveolar septa, resulting in increased airway diameter. Due to optimal muscle length, expiratory muscle force also increases. In restrictive lung disease, radial traction dilates airways allowing relatively high flow rates at smaller lung volumes. Conversely in emphysema, the elastic recoil is decreased, making the airways more easily compressible with a resultant increase in airway resistance. This further reduces the rate of gas flow at any given lung volume and causes a pressure drop in small airways with further narrowing of airways.

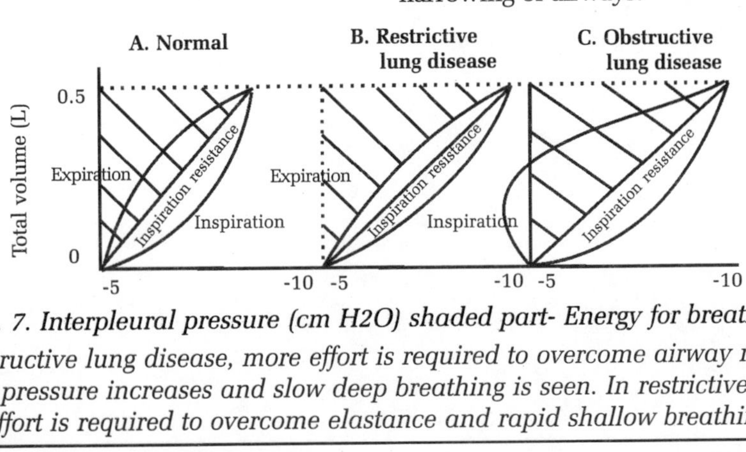

Fig. 7. Interpleural pressure (cm H2O) shaded part- Energy for breathign

Note: In obstructive lung disease, more effort is required to overcome airway resistance and intrapeleural pressure increases and slow deep breathing is seen. In restrictive lung diease, a greater effort is required to overcome elastance and rapid shallow breathing is seen.

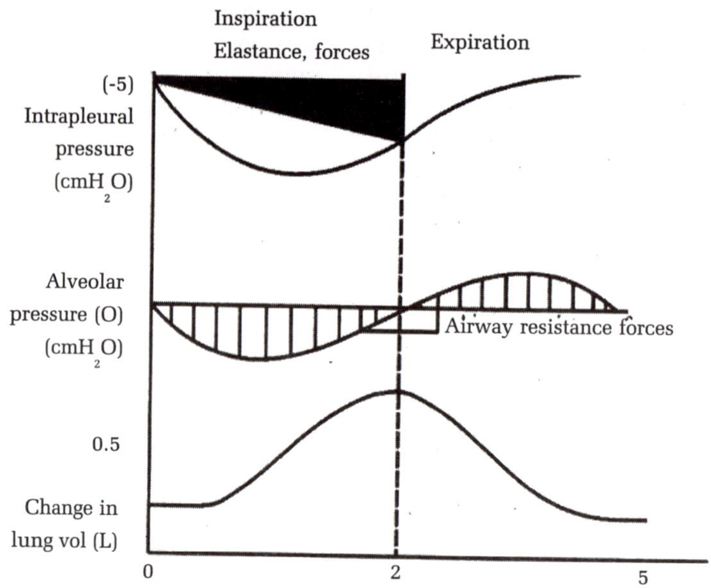

Note. In obstructive lung disease, airway resistance is high and larger gradients are necessary during inspiration and expiration. In restrictive lung disease, elestance is high and more negative intrapleural pressures are required at the end of inspiration.

Fig 8. Events in respiratory cycle according to resistance and elastance forces

Thus, in restrictive lung disease, elastance (recoil) is increased and compliance (distensibility) is decreased requiring a greater force of breathing. This is achieved by rapid shallow breathing which permits adequate ventilation by minimizing elastance work. Conversely, in obstructive lung disease, the resistance is increased and is overcome by a slow, deep breathing which ensures a good tidal volume.

Equal pressure point

The equal pressure point is the point at which pressure inside the airway equals pressure outside (intrapleural pressure). Above the equal pressure point there is a tendency for airway collapse (which is opposed by cartilaginous support in larger airways and traction by alveolar elastic recoil in smaller airways).

During a forced expiration, when intrapleural pressure is positive, the effective driving pressure for airflow is alveolar pressure minus intrapleural pressure, (which equals alveolar elastic recoil pressure).

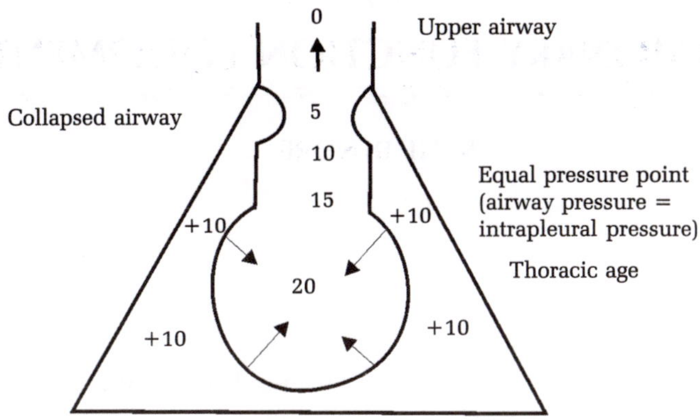

Note. Airway pressures start reducing during expiration in the outflow tract, beyond equal pressure point. Hence they get compressed by the relatively greater intrapleural pressure. During forced expiration intrapleural pressure is greater than airway pressure causing narrowing of airway, increased resistance and limitation of airflow.

Fig. 9: Equal pressure point and intrathoracic pressures

During the course of a forced expiration the equal pressure point moves toward the alveoli and collapsible small airways. The lung volume decreases, leading to smaller alveoli with less alveolar elastic recoil. As elastic recoil decreases, the effective driving pressure for air flow decreases and the traction on the small airways decreases

Density dependence of flow rate

The lower the density of air, the higher is the flow rate achieved during forced expiration. This is because the turbulent flow is improved in central airways due to the lower density of air and is demonstrated by breathing a mixture of helium and oxygen. The laminar flow in the small airways remain unaffected.

Summary

Respiration is a dynamic process. Inspiration is active and exhalation is by passive recoil. The rib cage, the diaphragm, the intra pleural pressure are responsible for lung inflation. Lung compliance and airway resistance control the ventilation volumes and gas exchange. Respiratory mechanics are complex and any abnormality in its ability manifests as dyspnea and hypoxia.

3
PULMONARY FUNCTION EQUIPMENT

SALIL BENDRE

Introduction

Pulmonary function testing is a valuable tool for evaluating the respiratory system. Insight into underlying pathophysiology can often be gained by comparing the measured values for pulmonary function tests obtained on a patient at any particular point with normal values derived from population studies. The *percentage of predicted normal* is used to grade the severity of the abnormality. Pulmonary function testing is often used in clinical medicine for evaluating respiratory symptoms such as dyspnoea and cough, for stratifying preoperative risk, and for diagnosing common diseases such as asthma and chronic obstructive pulmonary disease.

Pulmonary function tests (PFTs) can include simple screening spirometry, formal lung volume measurement, diffusing capacity for carbon monoxide, and arterial blood gases. These studies may collectively be referred to as a *complete pulmonary function survey*.

PEFR Meter

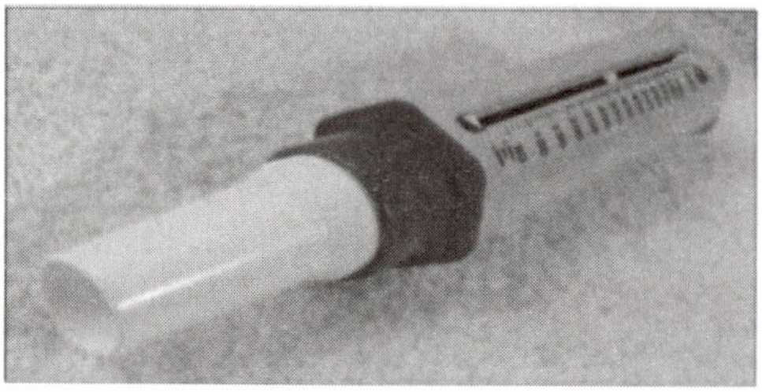

Fig 1. Peak expiratory flow meter

The **peak expiratory flow rate** (**PEFR**) is a person's maximum speed of expiration, as measured with a **peak flow meter**, a small, hand-held device used to monitor a person's ability to breathe out air. It measures the airflow through the bronchi and thus the degree of obstruction in the airways. It is an important aid in the diagnosis and subsequent management of asthma.

Peak flow meters are relatively inexpensive, portable, robust and ideal for patients to use in home settings for day to day objective monitoring of asthma. From changes in recorded values, patients and doctors may determine lung functionality, the severity of asthma symptoms, and treatment. The measurements provide an indirect assessment of airway hyper responsiveness, which correlates closely with the degree of airway inflammation.

One of the most useful roles of peak flow meter is deciding the pharmacotherapy of asthma and judging exacerbation episodes for immediate attention in asthmatics. It is a useful screening tool in the diagnosis of Obstructive Lung Diseases and occupational asthma.

Spirometer

Spirometers can be classified as : a) **Volume-displacing spirometers** and b) **flow-sensing spirometers**.

Volume-displacement spirometer

The conventional **volume-displacement spirometers** provide a direct measure of respired volume from the displacement of a bell (water-sealed), piston (rolling seal), bellows (wedge bellows) or diaphragm. The indices FEV1 and FVC are generally manually calculated from the spirogram.

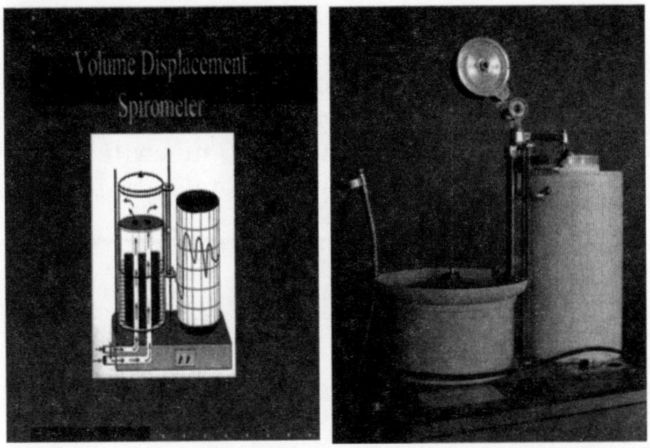

Fig. 2 Spirometer

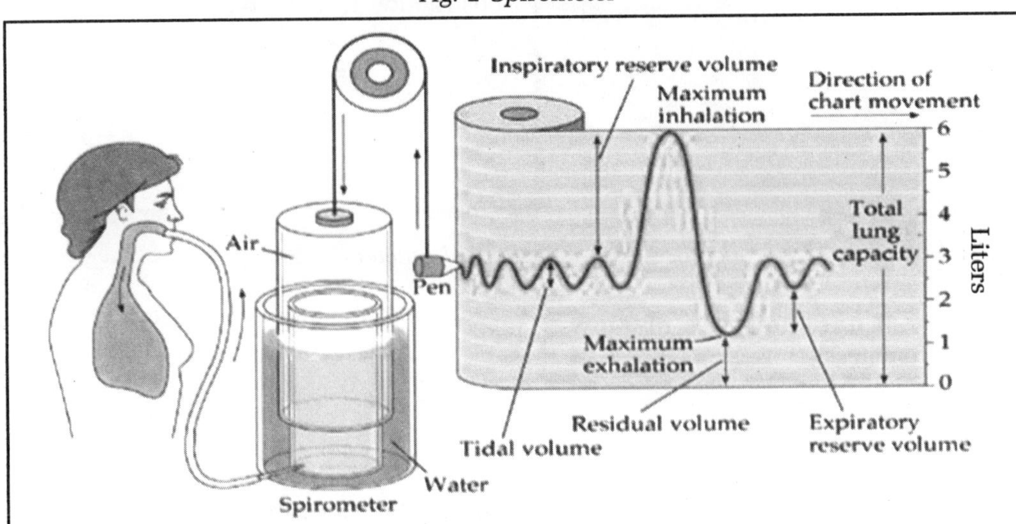

Fig. 3 Spirometry

Summary of Characteristics of Volume-Displacing Spirometers

Pros :

Directly measures volume so more accurate

Low cost,

Ease of operation,

Water-seal spirometer is considered to be a gold standard.

Cons:

Some are very large and bulky – less portable

Time consuming

Water in water-seal devices needs to be changed & levels need frequent checks.

Leaks

Manual calculations are necessary

Infection control issues.

Flow-sensing spirometers

The **flow-sensor based spirometers** utilize a sensor that measures flow as a primary signal and calculates volume by electronic (analogue) or numerical (digital) integration of the flow signal.

The most commonly used flow sensors detect and measure flow from a pressure drop across a known constant resistance (e.g. Pneumotachograph), cooling of one or more heated wires (anemometer), or by electronically counting the rotation of a turbine blade. The recent introduction is of an ultrasonic-flow-sensor based spirometer. The flow-based spirometers are lighter, portable and provide a print out with all the the spirometry indices desired. The appropriateness of the results depends on the use of correct predicted normal values and criteria employed to classify ventilator defects and grade their severity.

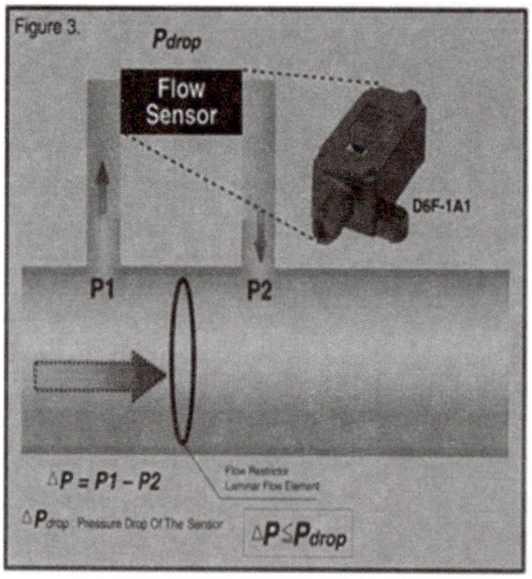

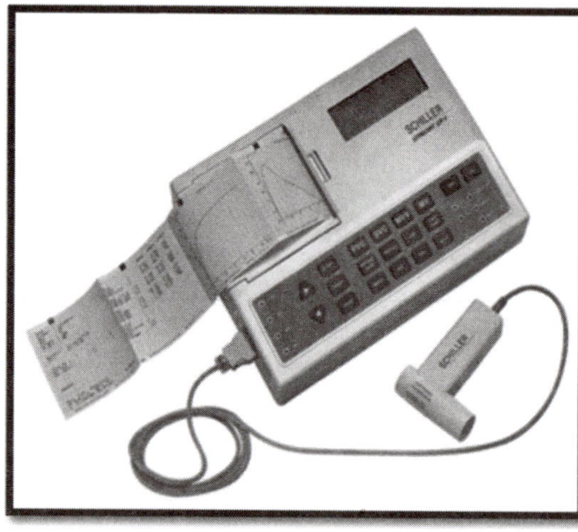

Fig 4. Flow sensing spirometers

Summary of Characteristics of Flow-Sensing Spirometers

Pros :

Smaller and usually more portable

Computerized; so no manual calculations.

Bidirectional devices provide flow-volume loop capability.

Easier infection control with some models.

Cons :

Frequent and careful calibrationchecks needed for some models

Moisture and secretions can cause problems

Gas composition can affect results

May not sense low flows

Static and dynamic spirometry

The terms static and dynamic spirometry simply identify tests that are purely volume-based (Static) and those based on time (Dynamic).

Slow Vital Capacity (Static)

Slow vital capacity was arguably the first ever recorded lung volume. The full excursion of the maneuver gives a measure of the change in volume of gas in the lungs from complete inspiration to complete expiration or vice versa. The recording of volume versus time is called a spirogram. In the example shown, the recording begins with the subject quietly breathing in a steady-state condition followed by a maximal breath-in and a full breath-out. The spirogram of a slow vital capacity maneuver has several key identifying components:

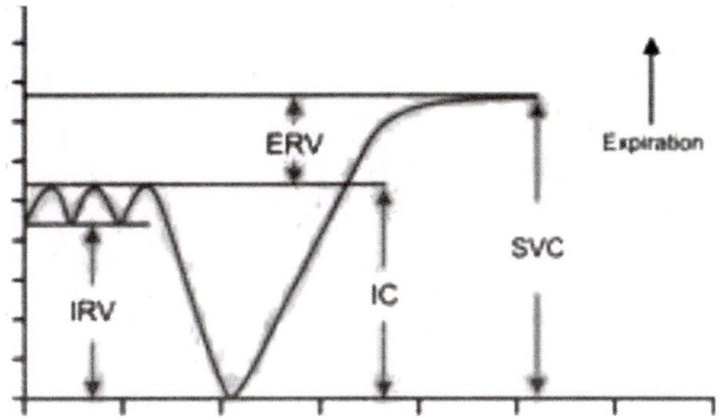

Fig 5. Identifying the Sub-divisions of Slow Vital Capacity

Slow Vital Capacity (SVC) is the maximum volume of air which can be exhaled or inspired in a slow/steady maneuver.

Vital Capacity (VC) is the largest of the volumes from either a forced (FVC) or a slow (SVC) maneuver.

Expiratory Reserve Volume (ERV) is the maximum volume of additional air that can be expired from the end of a normal expiration.

Inspiratory Capacity (IC) is the maximum volume of air that can be inspired from end expiratory position. Called a capacity because it is the sum of 2 lung volumes: IC = IRV+TV

Forced Vital Capacity (Dynamic)

Flow volume loops are perhaps the most recognizable of all pulmonary function tests. The shape of the curves are extremely diagnostic but the very nature of the effort required to reproduce the shape (loop) means that often data is of a poor quality..

In most pulmonary function labs, flow volume loops are usually the first tests gathered from the spirometry testing. By examining the information and shape of the loop, it helps clinicians further understand the way air is moving into and out of the lungs and help identify specific diseases that can otherwise be very hard to diagnose.

From the information gathered with this test certain deductions about what is happening throughout the lung can be made. In particular we comment on obstructive lung disorders and degree of the disease. Obstructive lung disease is simply put, a problem with the airways that do not allow airflow to move smoothly from the alveoli (air sacs of the lungs) and smallest airways out through the trachea (main windpipe) and ultimately out through the mouth when exhaling or inhaling. There are a number of common processes that can lead to this kind of a problem including emphysema, asthma and chronic bronchitis.

The results of dynamic PFT tests place patients in 1 of 3 categories:

- Normal lung function
- Obstructive disease
- Or restrictive disease

In obstructive lung disease, patients have decreased airflow (decreased FEV1/FVC ratio) and usually have normal or above-normal lung volumes.

In restrictive lung disease, patients have decreased lung volumes or TLC with normal airflow (normal FEV1/FVC ratio but with reduced values for both FVC and FEV1 individually).

For many years, the forced expiratory effort was only represented as a plot of volume against time.

Identifying Measurements on the Forced Expiratory Maneuver

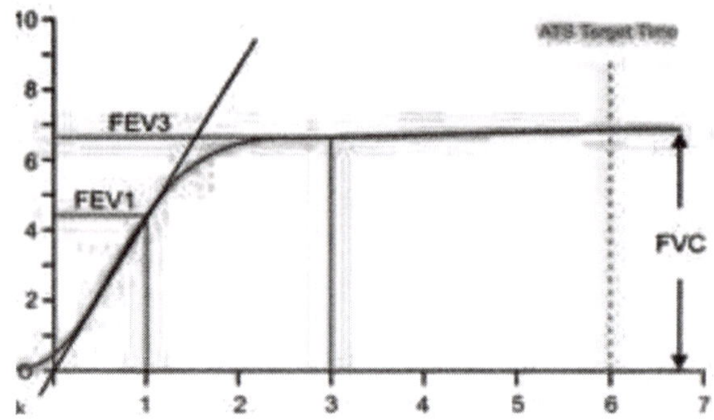

Fig. 6 Measurements on the Forced Expiratory Maneuver.

Forced Vital Capacity (FVC) is the maximum volume of air which can be exhaled or inspired during a forced (FVC) maneuver. For the tests to be of significance, it is recommended that the forced effort be 6 seconds or longer in duration.

In most cases, the SVC is always greater than FVC. As more obstruction is present in the lungs the difference between SVC and FVC is more pronounced.

Forced Expired Volume in one second (**FEV1**) is the volume expired in the first second of maximal expiration after a full inspiration and is a useful measure of how quickly the lungs can be emptied.

FEV1/FVC is the FEV1 expressed as a percentage of the FVC and gives a clinically useful index of airflow limitation.

The forced volume excursion when plotted against flow rate reveals perhaps the most recognizable shape in pulmonary function testing. There are many measurements that can be taken from this single dynamic effort:

Identifying Measurements on the Flow Volume Loop

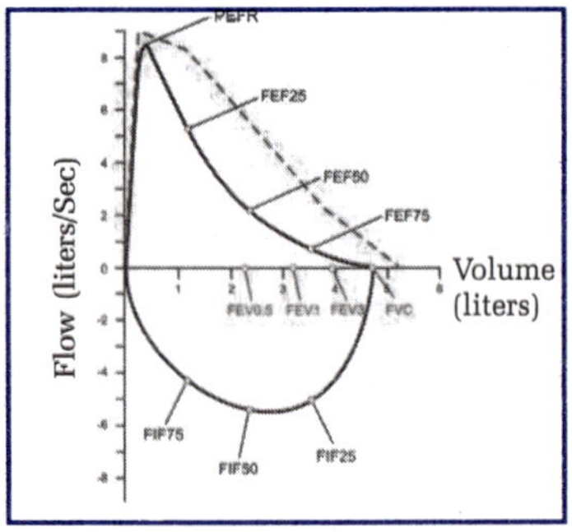

Fig. 7. Measurements on the Flow Volume Loop

Peak Expiratory Flow Rate (PEFR): The first landmark reached is the PEFR. The first blast of air exhaled from the patient reaches this flow rate almost immediately. The flow rate then quickly slows as more air is exhaled. This landmark is very important in judging if the patient is giving maximal effort, overall quality of the test, strength of expiratory muscles, and the condition of the large airways, such as the trachea and main bronchi.

Forced Expiratory Volume after 0.5 seconds (FEV0.5): The FEV0.5 indicates the amount of air exhaled with maximum effort in half a second.

Forced Expiratory Volume after 1 second (FEV1): The FEV1 indicates the amount of air exhaled with maximum effort in the first second. The FEV1 is another very important landmark in assessing the overall status of the patient and quality of the test. This test result is also important in pre- and post-bronchodilator tests in determining the effects of bronchodilators on the airways.

Forced Expiratory Volume after 3 seconds (FEV3): The FEV3 indicates the amount of air exhaled with maximum effort in the first three seconds.

Forced Expiratory Volume after 6 seconds (FEV6): The FEV6 indicate the amount of air exhaled with maximum effort in the first six seconds. This parameter is primarily used to ensure expiratory efforts meet or exceed 6 seconds.

Forced Vital Capacity (FVC): Another important result of a Flow Volume Loop is the FVC. Many of the other results depend on this number. The FVC is the total volume of air exhaled with maximal effort.

Forced Expiratory Flow at 25% of FVC (FEF25%): The FEF25% is the flow rate at the 25% point of the total volume (FVC) exhaled. Assuming maximal effort this flow rate is still indicative of the condition of fairly large to medium size bronchi. This landmark is used in calculations with the FEF75% to give FEF25-75%, the middle half of the FVC, which many physicians look at as not being dependent on patient effort and an indicator for obstruction in the small airways. This value is very dependent on the total volume exhaled (FVC) and tends to be highly variable from test to test.

Forced Expiratory Flow at 50% of FVC (FEF50%): The FEF50% is the flow rate at the 50% point of the total volume (FVC) exhaled. This landmark is at the midpoint of the FVC and indicates the status of medium to small airways, it's sometimes looked at instead of the FEF25-75%.

Forced Expiratory Flow at 75% of FVC (FEF75%): The FEF75% is the flow rate at the 75% point of the total volume (FVC) exhaled. This landmark indicates the status of small airways and is used in the FEF25-75% calculation. The damage done by most chronic pulmonary diseases show up in the smallest airways first and early indications of this damage begin to appear toward the end of the expiratory part of the Flow Volume Loop.

Forced Inspiratory Flow at 25% of FVC (FIF25%) : The FIF25% is the flow rate at the 25% point on the total volume inhaled. The inspiratory flow rates are relatively unimportant in assessing the asthmatic. Abnormalities here are indicators of upper airway obstructions. Areas of the mouth, upper and lower pharynx (back of the throat), larynx (voice box), and vocal-cords impact the inspiratory flow rates.

Peak Inspiratory Flow Rate (PIFR) : The fastest flow rate achieved during inspiration.

Forced Inspiratory Flow at 50% of FVC (FIF50%) : The FIF50% is the flow rate at the 50% point on the total volume inhaled.

Forced Inspiratory Flow at 75% of FVC (FIF75%) : The FIF75% is the flow rate at the 75% point on the total volume inhaled.

Some of the other numbers that can be calculated from the Flow Volume Loop are:

FEV1/FVC%, and FEV3/FVC% - These are ratios calculated by dividing the Forced Expiratory Volume results by the Forced Vital Capacity and expressed as a percentage of the FVC.

Forced Expiratory Time (FET) - The time it takes to exhale as much air as possible. To obtain reliable FVC values, the expiratory effort should be continued for at least 6 seconds. The FET should never be less than 6 seconds unless the patient is severely restricted.

The illustration below shows the variety of flow volume loop shapes that often relate to particular disease. When looked at in relation to the lung volume further clinical information can be revealed.

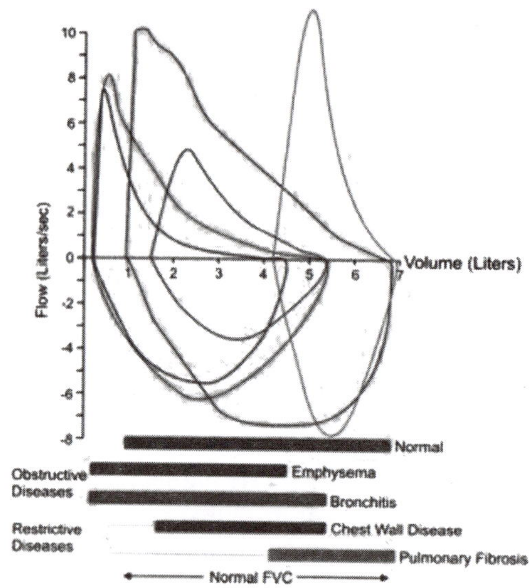

Fig 8. variety of flow volume loop shapes.

CHART SHOWING THE TYPICAL RESULTS OF DISEASE ON SPIROMETRY

Typical Results of Disease on Ventilatory Function

	Obstruction	Restriction
FVC	↔↓	↓↓
FVC_1	↓↓	↔↓
FEF_{25-75}	↓↓	↔↓
MVV	↓↓	↔↓

↔ Normal ↓Reduced ↑Increased

Fig 9.

The volume of gas that can be breathed in 15 seconds when a person breathes as deeply and quickly as possible. Also called *maximum breathing capacity*. The result is extrapolated from 15 seconds to show what could be achieved over one minute. As a general guide, the value should correlate closely to the FEV1 x 35.

This test is usually performed whenever spirometry is done. If people have weakness in the muscle of breathing this test can help identify these difficulties. The MVV is a test of ultimate effort dependency and is often discarded by physicians. Since it has been shown that the FEV1 x 35 is a good indication of MVV, many centers simply report that result. Disability criteria however still require an actual MVV to be done!

Lung volumes

Understanding and identifying the lung volume components is essential in pulmonary function testing.

Measurements of lung volumes are important to confirm or clarify the nature of lung disorders. The flow volume loop may indicate an obstructive or restrictive or obstructive/ restrictive pattern, but a further test of lung volume is often necessary for clarification.

In an obstructive lung disease, airway obstruction causes an increase in resistance. During normal breathing, the pressure volume relationship is no different from a normal lung. However, when breathing rapidly, greater pressure is needed to overcome the resistance to flow, and the volume of each breath gets smaller. The increase in the effort to breathe can cause an overdistention of the lungs.

The flow volume loop may show lower than normal FEV1 and FEF25-75, but it is not until a lung volume has been determined that an increase in TLC, FRC and RV can be confirmed.

Common obstructive diseases include asthma, bronchitis and emphysema.

In a restrictive lung disease, the compliance of the lung is reduced which increases the stiffness of the lung and limits expansion. In these cases, a greater pressure than normal is required to give the same increase in volume.

The flow volume loop may show lower than normal FVC, but the FEV1 and FEF25-75 may only be mildly affected. The lung volume measurement will clearly show a reduction in TLC, FRC and RV.

Common causes of decreased lung compliance are pulmonary fibrosis, pneumonia and pulmonary edema. Patients whose respiratory muscles are unable to perform normally because of a neuromuscular disease or paralysis can show a restrictive pattern.

The total volume contained in the lung at the end of a maximal inspiration is subdivided into volumes and also into capacities.

There are four lung volume subdivisions which:

a) Do not overlap.
b) Can not be further divided.
c) When added together equal total lung capacity (TLC).

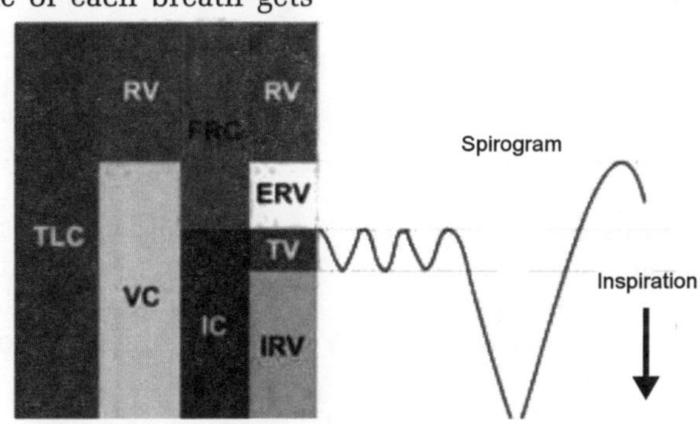

Fig 10. Lung volume subdivisions

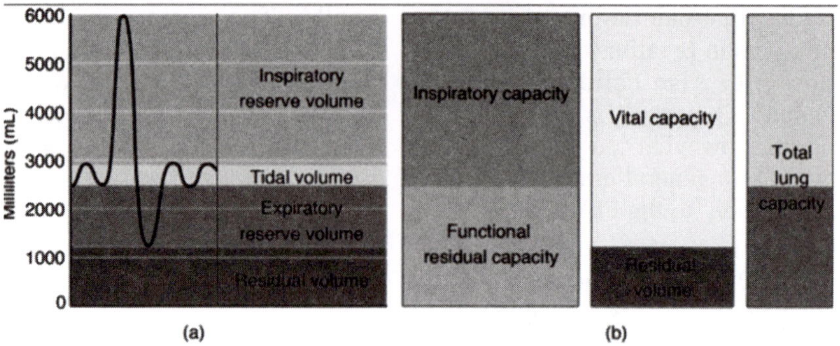

Fig 11.

Identifying the lung volumes

- **Tidal Volume (TV) :** It is the volume of air inhaled and exhaled with each breath during normal breathing.
- **Inspiratory Reserve Volume (IRV) :** It is the maximal volume of air that can be forcibly inhaled after normal inspiration during tidal breathing.
- **Expiratory Reserve Volume (ERV) :** It is the maximal volume of additional air that can be forcibly exhaled from the end of a normal expiration during tidal breathing.
- **Residual Volume (RV) :** It is the volume of air remaining in the lungs at the end of maximal exhalation. It is calculated as the difference between the functional residual capacity and the expiratory reserve volume. It is the only lung volume which cannot be measured with a spirometer.

Identigying the lung capacities

If two or more lung volumes are taken together, it is known as lung capacity.

- **TLC** or **Total Lung Capacity** is the volume of air contained in the lungs at the end of a maximal inspiration. It is the sum of the residual volume (**RV**) and the vital capacity (**VC**). The total lung capacity measures the maximal size of the lung. It is 6000 ml.

  Thus, TLC = RV + VC or TLC = RV + IRV + TV + ERV

- **Vital Capacity** (**VC**) is the maximal volume of air which can be forcefully inhaled after a complete exhalation (inspiratory VC or VCI) or it is the volume of air which can be exhaled from the lungs after a maximal inhalation (expiratory VC or VCE). It is called a capacity because it is the sum of inspiratory reserve volume, tidal volume, and expiratory reserve volume.

  Thus, VC = IRV + TV + ERV = TLC - RV

  Vital Capacity is the largest of the volumes from either a forced (FVC) or a slow (SVC) manoeuvre.

  Since it is not possible to estimate static lung volumes accurately by the expiratory vital capacity in patients with obstructive lung disease, the inspiratory vital capacity is more preferable.

- **Functional Residual Capacity (FRC) :** It is the volume of air remaining in the lungs at the end of a normal exhalation.

  FRC = RV + ERV

  This capacity can be measured only indirectly. In practice, a gas dilution method or body plethysmography is used. In body-plethysmography, the thoracic gas volume at the level of the functional residual capacity is measured. The thoracic gas volume is identical to the functional residual capacity in healthy individuals, but in pathological conditions, differences are observed.

- **Inspiratory Capacity (IC)** : It is the maximum volume of air which can be inhaled from the end expiratory position.

  IC = TV + IRV

Static and dynamic lung volumes

Pulmonary gas transport depends on the degree and speed with which the pulmonary gas volume can change. Static lung volumes are measured by methods in which the velocity of the gas plays no part. The measurements taken during fast breathing movements are described as dynamic volume changes like FEV1, FIV1 and MVV.

Static lung volumes and capacities

In pulmonary function laboratory, the measurement of static lung volumes usually refers to the measurement of total lung capacity (TLC), residual volume (RV), functional residual capacity (FRC), and vital capacity (VC). These measurements are essential for the accurate analysis of lung function besides providing information for further diagnostic process and assessment of treatment.

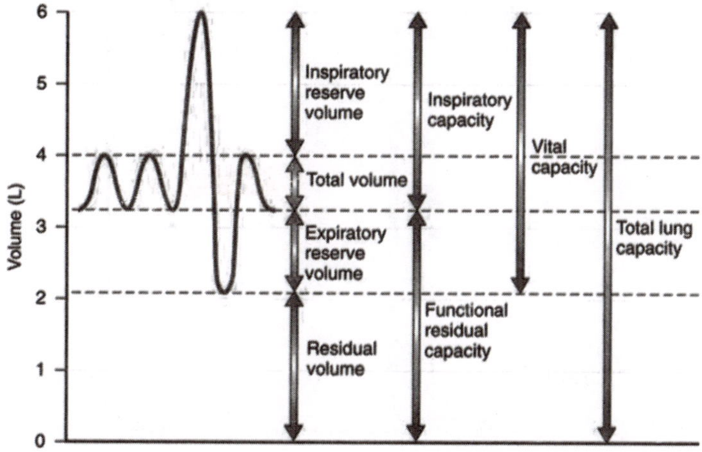

Fig 12. Static lung volumes and capacities

Measuring lung volumes

The two major steps in measuring lung volumes are : a) determining FRC and b) measurement of slow vital capacity (SVC) and its subdivisions.

FRC is most commonly determined with one of three basic techniques : a) Body plethysmography b) multiple-breath closed circuit helium (He) dilution, or c) multiple-breath open circuit nitrogen (N2) washout.

a) Body Plethysmography

Pfluger was the first to apply Boyle's law to measure RV in 1882 by constructing a large metal container called man-box or man-can. However, DuBois and his colleagues are credited with the modern application.

Types of body plethysmograph: a) Constant volume variable pressure b) Constant pressure variable volume c) Mixed.

Principle of working : Boyle's Law – Pressure (P) and Volume (V) are inversely proportional to each other at constant temperature. Product of PV remains constant at constant temperature i.e., P1V1= P2V2= constant .

The body-box is a closed box of a volume of about 600 litres, with rigid walls usually made of metal. The patient sits inside the sealed box, closes lips tightly over the mouthpiece and breathes quietly. During inspiration and expiration there is alternating rise and fall of pressure within the airtight box which can be detected by a manometer or pressure transducer. To measure airway resistance, the patient pants in and out shallowly through a pneumotachograph at a rate of 2 to 3 breaths per second.

Pants induce abduction of the vocal cords allowing equilibrium of pressure at the mouth with that within the lung. A shutter at the mouthpiece is suddenly closed and the patient pants against the closed shutter for 1 to 2 seconds. The mouth pressure which is assumed to be equal to the alveolar pressure, is now noted. With the box pressure and the alveolar pressure,

Resistance = $(P_{alv} / P_{box}) = P_{alv}$ / Flow.

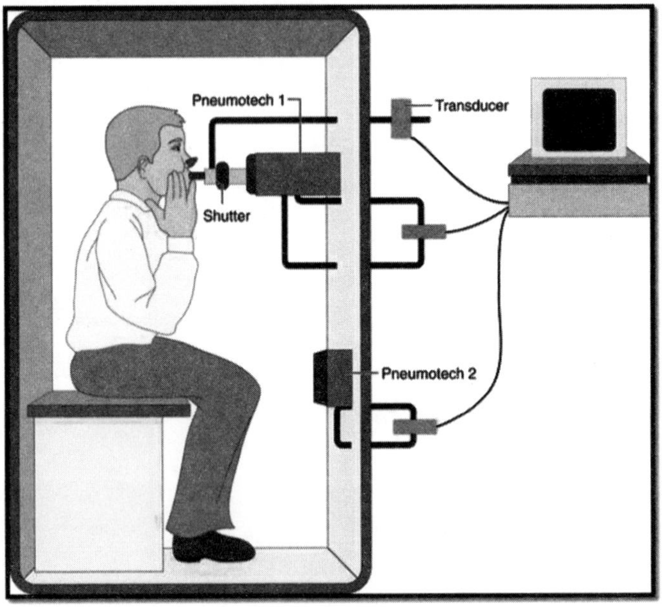

Fig 13. Measurement of airway resistance in body plethysmography

To measure FRC with body plethysmography, the patient sits inside a sealed box and breathes quietly for several breaths and then pants against a closed shutter. The gas volume trapped in the lungs when the shutter is closed can then be measured by applying Boyle's law. This method is the most accurate because it measures the total gas volume in the thoracic cage or the thoracic gas volume (TGV).

The body box is also used to measure airway resistance (Raw). Airway resistance (Raw) is a measure of the resistance (measured in cm h1O) to airflow (measured in L/second) afforded by all anatomical structures between the atmosphere and the lung alveoli, including the mouth, nasopharynx, and the central and peripheral airways. It is used for evaluation of airway responsiveness, provocation testing, characterization of various types of obstructive lung disease, localization of the primary site of flow limitation, and evaluation of localized obstruction.

Volume standardization of the airway resistance may be accomplished by dividing the conductance, SGaw (the reciprocal of the resistance) by the TGV at which the resistance measurement was made.

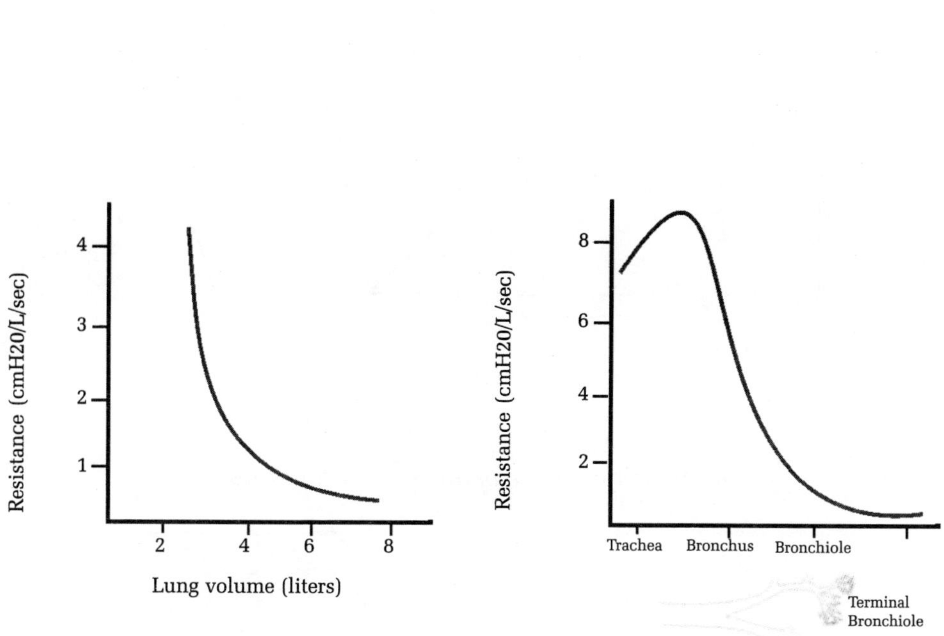

Fig 14. Measurement of airway resistance in body box.

While a single small airway provides more resistance than a single large airway, resistance to air flow depends on the number of parallel pathways present. For this reason, the large and particularly the medium-sized airways actually provide greater resistance to flow than do the more numerous small airways.

Airway resistance decreases as lung volume increases because the airways distend as the lungs inflate, and wider airways have lower resistance.

- Parameters:
  - **Raw** Airways Resistance
  - **SGaw** Specific Conductance
  - **Gaw** Conductance
  - **VTG** Volume of Thoracic Gas

The example below shows a typical airway resistance test performed in the following order:

1. Quiet, regular breathing to establish the end-tidal FRC baseline (FRC 0).
2. The subject is then asked to begin shallow breathing at a slightly faster rate (approximately 1 breath per second) and Flow -v- Box Pressure is recorded.
3. The mouthpiece shutter is closed and Mouth Pressure -v- Box Pressure is recorded. The shutter opens and the test is complete.

The VTG is an important factor when standardizing the airway resistance to the volume at which it was measured. This allows for the reporting of specific conductance (SGaw).

The same panting technique, or quiet breathing technique in some systems, is used but first with the shutter open and then with the shutter closed. Raw is used to assess airflow obstruction rather than lung volumes.

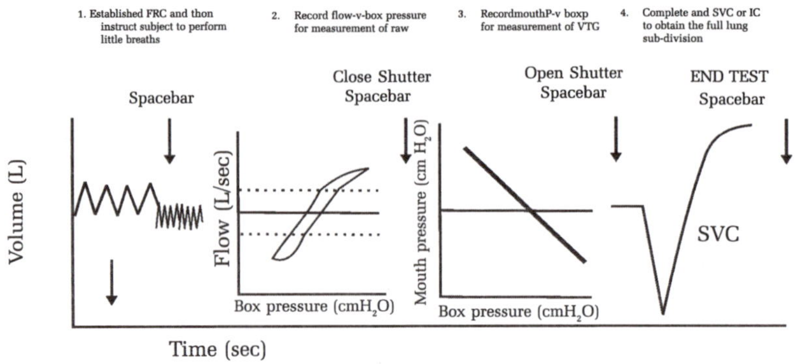

Fig. 15. Performance of airway resistance test

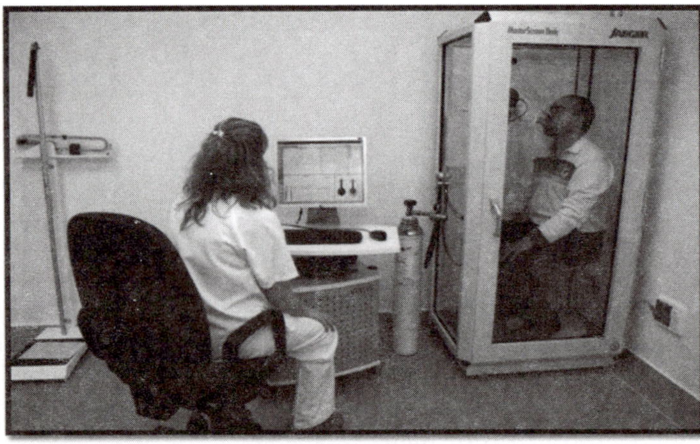

Fig 16. measurement of specific conductance

b) Helium dilution

Helium dilution is a classic method used to measure the lung volume and capacities. The origins of the technique are reputed to date back to Sir Humphrey Davy's book, *"Researches Chemical and Philosophical"*, published in 1799, describes the measurement of his own lung volumes, including the first recorded measurement of the residual volume. He also measured his own rates of oxygen consumption and carbon dioxide production. He is famous for his investigations into nitrous oxide, but he also investigated the effects of breathing nitric oxide and carbon monoxide. He made these observations with a gasometer and analysis of his expired air, and his work anticipated the invention of blood gas analysis.

- Why use helium?

  Helium is an inert (lighter than air), colorless, odorless, tasteless gas and is not toxic. Furthermore, it cannot transfer across the avleolar-capillary membrane and is thus contained when in the lungs.

  Closed circuit helium dilution studies have been a standard method of measuring the 'hidden' residual volume in the lung for many years.

  The method employs the simple principle of gas dilution using helium, an insoluble inert gas that mixes easily in the lungs.

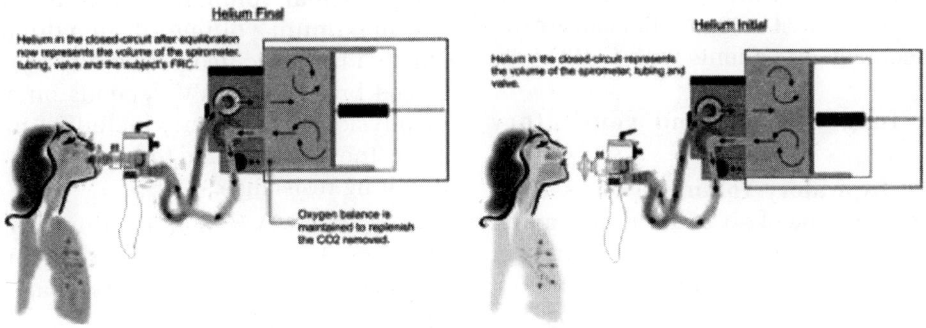

Fig. 17 Helium dilution measurement of lung volumes

During helium dilution measurement of lung volumes, patients breathe from a known volume and concentration of helium gas for a period of typically 4 to 7 minutes. The oxygen concentration in the starting mixture is set at 30% to ensure patients with COPD can remain comfortable during the test. A carbon dioxide absorber is situated in line with expired breath to keep the closed-circuit CO_2 level below 0.5% and avoid discomfort and hyperventilation. Oxygen is added to the system to maintain the starting volume in the spirometer. Since the type of thermal conductivity helium analyzer employed in the SpiroAir can be affected by changes in concentrations of CO_2, O_2 and Water Vapor, a chemical absorber removes the interference of CO_2 and Water Vapor. A simple algorithm corrects the helium signal for changes in oxygen background.

Once connected to the closed-circuit, equilibration between the starting and final helium concentrations should occur within 7 minutes. A state of equilibrium is defined as helium concentration changes of less than 0.02% over a 30 second interval.

The functional residual capacity (FRC) is calculated from the helium concentrations as follows:

FRC = (% helium initial - % helium final) / % helium final x system volume

The dead space of the system (patient valve, filter and mouthpiece) is subtracted from this value.

The FRC can be underestimated with the helium dilution technique in conditions such as bullous emphysema or severe airways obstruction. Trapped lung gas does not communicate with the inhaled helium mixture. Plethysmographic measurement of lung volumes is preferred in these cases.

The FRC can be overestimated or unmeasurable when leaks are present. Leaks may develop in the equipment valves or circuitry, or, more commonly, at the mouthpiece. A system leak is likely to be the cause if the graph of the delivered helium concentration does not flatten, ie, when equilibrium is not reached, within 7 minutes. The ComPAS software will warn of possible leak conditions.

c) Nitrogen washout (recovery)

Nitrogen recovery is another gas dilution technique for measuring lung volumes. Only those instruments that can measure DLCO can offer N2 recovery ability. Since N2 is resident in the lung at all times, it has an infinite time to reach whatever communicating airways it can. During the performance of DLCO, the subject exhales to residual volume (all the way empty) and then breathes-in diffusion gas until completely full (TLC). The new N2 from the DLCO mixture rapidly mixes with the N2 that was in the residual volume and thus TLC can be directly measured. The technique has to assume the partial pressure of CO_2 in the alveolar at the start of the test. For this reason, having a separate measure of PACO2 (alveolar CO2) from an end-tidal CO2 monitor can greatly improve accuracy on patients with COPD.

Dynamic lung volumes and ventilatory capacity

The **Forced Expiratory Volume** in one second **(FEV1)** is the volume of air exhaled during the first second of a maximal forced expiration beginning at the end of complete inspiration. The time interval of one second is arbitrary, but is adequate in most cases. During the onset of forced expiration, the airways begin to be compressed and the flow reaches its maximum value. This is strongly an effort-dependent phase. In the subsequent phase, when about 20% to 30% of the vital capacity has been exhaled, the larger airways are compressed and thus have a flow limiting function. In consequence, this phase is only slightly dependent on the expiratory force. The flow during this phase provides information about the intrathoracic resistance to breathing, especially about the resistance in the small non-compressed airways. It is dependent on the elastic properties of the lung tissue and is of the magnitude of the vital capacity and airway obstruction. But when the vital capacity is affected, this measure may underestimate the extent of flow limitation.

The **Forced Inspiratory Volume** in one second **(FIV1)** is the volume of air inhaled in the first second of maximal forced inspiration beginning from the end of complete exhalation. During this manoeuvre, the intrathoracic pressure is markedly subatmospheric and the large intrathoracic airways are distended maximally. Thus, the FEV1 is also effort-dependent. In extrathoracic narrowing of the airways, the inspiratory flow is limited because the extrathoracic airway below the level of obstruction collapses as a result of the marked subatmospheric pressure. FIV1 expressed as a percentage of the vital capacity is an index of inspiratory airway obstruction.

The **Maximal Voluntary Ventilation (MVV)** is the maximum volume of air which can be exhaled in a specified period during rapid and forced breathing. MVV depends on a number of physiological factors, including movement of the thoracic cage and the respiratory muscles and lung resistance.

Today, the MVV test is most commonly performed as part of the cardio-pulmonary exercise test, where it is used as index of maximum ventilatory capacity.

The test is performed on the same spirometer system used for forced spirometry. The patient encloses his mouth over the mouthpiece and a nose-clip is placed on his nose. When directed, the patient should breathe in and out deeply and rapidly for 12 to 15 seconds. The tidal volume during this manouvre should approximate 50% of the vital capacity with a breathing frequency of approximately 90 breaths /min. The exhaled volume during this short period is extrapolated to 1 minute and reported at BTPS in litres/min.

Relationships between and reference values for lung volumes

Lung volumes and capacities are measured in the upright position (sitting and standing) and are converted to BTPS conditions. The largest value of atleast three technically correct measurements of vital capacity, FEV1 and FIV1 is used. For practical reasons, only one determination of the FRC is carried out by the indicator gas method. In body plethysmography, several measurements of thoracic gas volume are averaged.

Determining factors

Factors which determine :

- **The size of the lung :** Height, age, sex, weight, habits, race, posture and daily activity.
- **Maximal inspiration:** Force of the inspiratory muscles (muscular dystrophy), elasticity of the lungs (lung fibrosis), and elasticity of the thorax (ossification of the cartilage).

- **Maximal expiration :** Obstruction, closure and compression of the small airways (emphysema), the force of the expiratory muscles (muscular paralysis) and deformities of the lungs and thorax (kyphoscoliosis).

Presentation of data

- **Absolute values :** The data is given as a percentage of the reference values (normal values). Derivations from the normal must be considerable before they can be regarded as pathological.
- **Reference values :** The reference values (BTPS) are taken from a research of a population, and applied both to the sitting and standing position. The anthropometric variables are sex, height and age. The equations are based on the observation that the total lung capacity (TLC) depends on the height and sex of the subject, and that the subdivisions of the TLC in smaller lung volumes is most exclusively age-dependent.

The absolute value for a single lung volume is thus dependent on age, height and sex.

Diffusion of gases

The process of diffusion is defined as the flow of particles from an area of higher concentration to an area of lower concentration. The measurement of diffusion, as performed in pulmonary functions laboratories, provides information about the transfer of gas between the alveoli and the pulmonary blood capillary and is referred to as the diffusing capacity. The term diffusing capacity of the lung for carbon monoxide (DLCO) is used in this context.

Lung Diffusing Capacity

This test is used to evaluate how well oxygen moves into and out of the lungs. Certain diseases will lead to difficulties in getting oxygen from in the alveoli (air sac in the lung) into the blood where it is carried to the rest of the body.

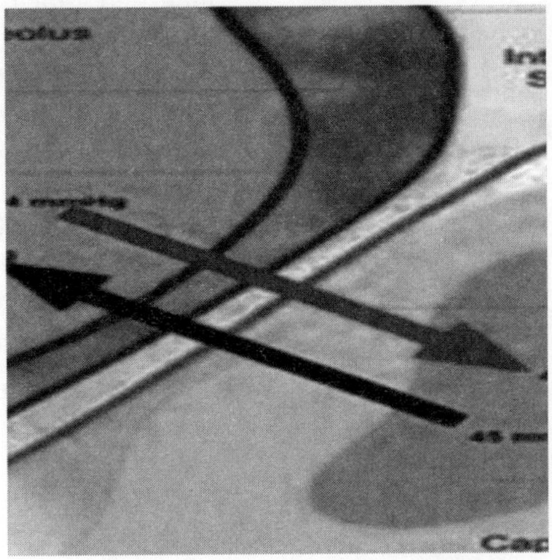

Fig 18. Lung diffusion capacity.

In many ways, DLCO is a general measure of the complete 'efficiency' of the lungs because it is influenced by three key components: The surface area of the lung with contact to diffusing alveoli (VA - Alveolar Volume), the thickness of the alveolar-capillary membrane (Dm - Membrane Diffusion) and the volume of blood available in the capillary bed of the lung (Vc - Capillary Blood Volume).

- DLCO may be abnormal in conjunction with obstructive, restrictive, or normal spirometry.
- Increased DLCO is rarely important but may occur with polycythemia or lung hemorrhage.
- DLCO can help distinguish emphysema from chronic bronchitis.
- Asthma produces a normal and sometimes increased DLCO.
- A reduced DLCO with a reduced TLC is indicative of parenchymal disease (eg, interstitial fibrosis), which impairs the diffusion of oxygen from the alveoli to the capillaries.
- Normal DLCO with reduced TLC: The lung parenchyma is not damaged and the restriction is extrapulmonary.
- Decreased DLCO with normal spirometry and lung volumes: decreased oxygen-carrying capacity.
- Reduced DLCO infers interstitial disease suspected by history and physical examination. Obtain chest CT.
- Pulmonary vascular disease may present with decreased DLCO with normal spirometry and lung volumes. Occlusion of part of the pulmonary vascular bed reduces blood flow and decreases diffusion capability.

In this test we use a special gas mixture containing 0.300% CO, 10.0% Helium, 21,0% O_2 and balance N2. The CO is used to trace the diffusion in place of O_2 because it is a one-way transfer across the alveolar-capillary membrane for combination with Hb. The helium in the mixture is used to obtain a measure of the alveolar volume.

The challenge of Single Breath Diffusion testing is to obtain a representative sample of gas from an area of the lungs where diffusion is taking place. The patient first breathes all the way out to residual volume and is then connected to the test gas. They breathe all the way in to TLC and are then instructed to hold their breath for approximately 10 seconds. After having held your breath for ten seconds, the first amount of gas that leaves your lips when you breathe out, has been resident in the physiological dead-space (mouth, trachea and two main bronchi) and must therefore be discarded before collecting a valid gas sample.

- Parameters:
  - **DLCO** Single Breath Diffusing Capacity
  - **VA** Alveolar Volume
  - **DL/VA** Diffusion per unit area of Lung Volume

Bronchial provocation (Challenge) testing

When the physician assessing a patient is concerned that they might have asthma, first spirometry is performed. If no obstruction is identified further testing is sometimes required. A medication called methacholine is used to 'provoke' airway response.

When the airways of people with asthma are exposed to this medication, it will stimulate a response, which can be measured. If there is a positive response, asthma can be clearly identified and treated appropriately.

In most cases, methacholine challenge testing involves repeated FEV1 efforts at increasing levels of the drug. The sooner the patient reacts by a 20% reduction in their FEV1 compared to room air (normal) conditions the more likely their prevalence to asthma.

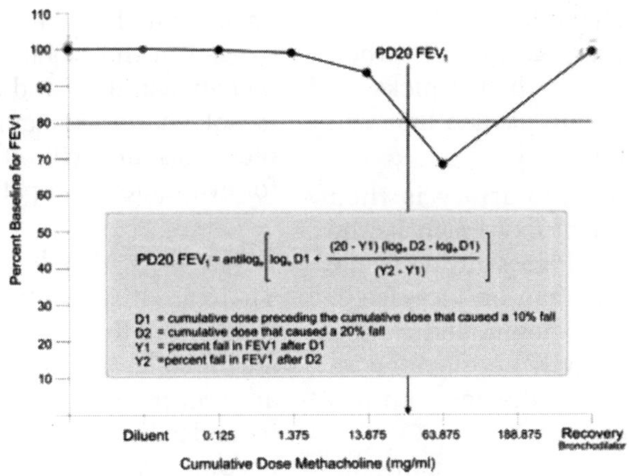

Fig. 19. Methacholine challenge test

Challenge testing determines presence of airway hyper reactivity. After initial spirometry, patient inhales a specific concentration of methacholine chloride and spirometry is repeated. A reduction in FEV1 20% below the prior test indicates asthma.

Impulse Oscillometry

Impulse Oscillometry (IOS) allows a differentiation between restrictive and obstructive pulmonary function impairments by means of a combined determination of volume and frequency – dependence of parameters related to mechanics of breathing.

Pulmonary distribution disturbances as the most frequent lung function impairments in humans can be detected very rapidly. The lung function parameter recorded via pulse oscillometry allow a better diagnostic differentiation as far as the early detection of COPD is concerned.

Impulse oscillometry test can be performed quickly and easily and is especially useful in preliminary diagnostics in daily routine, for clinical trend observations as well as for epidemiologic studies. Since, very minimal patient co-operation is required, it is also suitable for paediatric studies.

Test: Respiratory flow is overlayed by short time test pulses with different frequencies via amplifiers. On the basis of the applicated flow signal the pressure-pulse response of the pulmothoracic system allows the signals to be analyzed with the help of a lung model. Thus, a differential diagnosis for different lung function impairments is possible thanks to the characteristic differences in amplitude spectra of respiratory impedence. For a scientific approach detailed information can be obtained from the time trends and amplitude spectra of the individual pulses.

Benefits of impulse oscillometry:

- Fast, non-invasive test conducted with minimal expenditure of time for both, patient and doctor.
- Detection of unaltered tidal breathing without the additional strains of forced breathing manoeuvres.

Further Pulmonary function tests

The following tests are commonly performed in the pulmonary function laboratory.

Arterial Blood Gases

Most blood tests performed use blood drawn from veins in the arms. An arterial blood gas is a blood test, which requires taking a sample of blood from the artery, usually in the wrist. Blood from the artery comes straight from the heart, after it has been oxygenated (blood which travel through the heart and lungs gets rid of carbon dioxide which is a waste product it picks up from the body, and picks up oxygen that will be delivered to the body).

The blood sample from the artery is then analyzed for the amount of oxygen in it, the amount of carbon dioxide (there is always some, and in some diseases this can be increased). The pH of the blood, hemoglobin, and carbon monoxide level (which will be elevated in people smoking) and several other tests are also run on the blood sample.

The information gained by this test will help determine if a person might require oxygen or help explain other possible processes occurring.

Pulse Oximetry

Pulse oximetry is a tool to again look at the oxygen levels in people. Oxygen saturation tells us how much of the hemoglobin is loaded with oxygen in the blood stream. Most people will be between 92% and 99% saturated. This test is not nearly as accurate as doing an arterial blood gas, but will often be more than enough for evaluation of a patient's oxygen level.

Respiratory Muscle Strength (MIP MEP)

There are diseases that can affect the muscles throughout the body. The muscles of breathing are the same as those in the leg or the arm. There are groups of muscles used to inhale (breath in) and exhale (breath out). When these muscles become weak, it can lead to problems with difficulty breathing. This test is designed to evaluate those muscles of breathing. The test is often called MIP/MEP - maximum inspiratory and expiratory pressure.

REFERENCES

1. Wanger J. Pulmonary Function Testing, 3rd edn. Jones & Bartlett Learning, 2012.
2. American Thoracic Society. Lung Function Testing: selection of reference values and interpretative strategies. Am. Rev. Respir Dis 1991; 144:202.
3. Cotes JE. Lung Function, 5th edition. Oxford: Blackwell Scientific, 1993.

4

TESTS FOR VENTILATORY FUNCTION

VIRENDRA SINGH

Introduction

The basic function of respiratory system is to provide oxygen into blood and to remove carbon dioxide from the blood. Movement of atmospheric air during inspiration delivers oxygen into alveoli and movement of air from the lungs into atmosphere during expiration removes alveolar carbon dioxide. This process of movement of air in-and-out of lungs during respiration is called ventilation.

Unobstructed airways and good capacity of alveoli for ventilatory air are important lung factors for ventilation. Various clinical and laboratory tests have been described to assess ventilatory functions. Clinical tests suggesting these abnormalities include forced expiratory time (FEV) longer than 6 seconds, blowing of a lighted match at 15cm distance in Snider match test, reduction of length of trachea palpable above sternal notch, tracheal descent with inspiration, inspiratory excavation of supraclavicular and suprasternal fossae, and paradoxical inward movement of lower ribs during inspiration (1). Clinical tests are good to detect qualitative abnormalities but lack the precision of quantitative measurement.

Evaluation of various ventilatory parameters such as lung volumes, capacities, distribution of ventilation, dead space and exercise ventilation can detect abnormal ventilatory functions. Capacities, ventilatory flows and timed lung volume can be measured by spirometer and peak flow meter. Total lung capacity (TLC) is measured by spirometer and peak flow meter. Total lung capacity, residual volume (RV) and functional residual capacity (FRC) can be measured by body plethysmography and closed circuit helium dilution method. TLC as determined by helium dilution method is lower in comparison to plethysmographic method and the difference indicates the amount of trapped air. Nitrogen wash out test is carried out to assess uniform distribution of ventilation. Exercise testing helps to detect ventilatory abnormalities during exercise.

Spirometer testing

In the diseases of lungs and heart a skiagram of the chest provides information about anatomical abnormalities but not of functions. To detect abnormal heart beat electrocardiogram (ECG) is needed and skiagram is not helpful. Similarly to evaluate lung functions spirometry is important. In other words spirometry is like EGC of the lungs.

Indications for Spirometry

Inspite of importance of spirometry, it is still a grossly under-utilized test. In the following clinical situations spirometric tests are indicated:

1. **Detection of COPD in smokers:** Every smoker is a potential patient of chronic obstructive pulmonary disease (COPD). Since COPD is a progressive and potentially fatal disease, early detection and treatment are very important. The early symptoms of patient of COPD are cough and sputum

production. Unfortunately most of the smokers take them as a normal phenomenon of "smokers cough" and do not seek medical consultation. Usually a smoker consults a doctor when he starts having dyspnoea which is a late symptom of COPD and initially manifest only at the time of chest infection (2). Even at this stage with therapy of chest infection the smoker gets a partial relief and lie forgets the disease.

Ideally, spirometry should be done in every smoker and should be repeated annually in patients with abnormal report and every 3 years in a patient with normal report. Progressive reduction in FEV_I is the earliest indication of COPD in smokers. Spirometry assisted counseling is an excellent tool for encouraging patients to stop smoking with quit rate as high as 40% (3-5).

2. **Bronchial asthma:** By demonstrating more than 12% and 200 ml improvement in FEV1 after administration of bronchodilators, bronchial asthma is diagnosed. Values of FEV_I also help in monitoring severity of bronchial asthma.

3. **Detection of lung disease due to domestic fuel pollution:** Majority of housewives in rural areas of our country use smoky fuels for cooking such as firewood, dried dung, crop residues and agricultural wastes. Burning such fuel in a traditional *chula* without proper chimney and ventilation results into lot of smoke consisting of a large number of pollutants. A housewife spends around 6 hours a day in such an environment (6). Large number of studies in our country have shown that exposure to such pollution leads to restrictive and obstructive respiratory diseases (7-11). 5 to 44% of the non-smoker women using "*Chula*" were having evidence of respiratory disease as reported by various workers. Regular spirometric evaluation can make early detection of respiratory disease in housewives exposed to indoor pollution.

4. **People exposed to pollution on roads:** Vehicular pollution has been found to be an important cause of respiratory symptoms in people in metropolitan cities (12).

5. **Workers in various types of occupations:** Workers in different occupations such as fertilizer plants, plastic plants, smoldering, stone cutting and carving and at places where working environment is dusty and smoky are at a higher risk of developing respiratory problem (13-15). Regular spirometric evaluation can identify persons at higher risk and detect respiratory disease early. Annual spirometry test is advised in people working in an environment with dust, smoke and fumes (16).

6. **Pre-surgical screening:** Patients with airflow obstruction are at increased risk of developing post-surgery complications such pneumonia and atelectasis. Therefore, spirometry is indicated in pre-surgical check-up before thoracic and upper abdominal surgery and in patients with history of smoking, cough, wheezing or pulmonary disease. Since obese persons are at higher risk of developing post surgical respiratory problems spirometry test should be done in all obese persons during pre-surgical check-up. Presence of mild obstruction carries a low risk but moderate to severe airway obstruction puts a patient in high risk category (17). Restrictive disorders are not a contraindication to surgery. Though FVC is reduced yet such patients have good flow rates and therefore do not feel difficulty in cough and expectoration after surgery. Hence patients with restrictive diseases can be operated safely if they have FVC above 1L.

Contraindications for spirometry

Spirometry should be avoided during specified period as mentioned in the table 1. Though spirometry is quite safe procedure yet it is contraindicated in the situations given in table 2.

Table 1 Spirometry should be avoided for specified activity

Activity	Avoidance Period
1 Heavy meals	2 hours
2 Alcohol	4 hours
3 Vigorous exercise	30 minutes
4 Smoking	1 hour
5 Short acting beta agonist	4 hours
6 Long acting beta agonist	24 hours

Table 2: Spirometry is contraindicated in following situations

1	Hemoptysis
2	Recent Myocardial infarction
3	Recent eye surgery
4	Recent Abdominal surgery
5	Thoracic/abdominal aneurysm
6	Pneumothorax

Methods of spirometry

Spirometry is an easy test to perform but at the same time it is very easy to get a wrong report. Since FVC maneouvre is effort dependent, it can give wrong results if effort is inadequate. Therefore proper guidelines should be followed. Before starting the tests, technician should ascertain that the subject has understood the instructions and observes following precautions:

- Unobstructed mouth piece: remove prosthetic dentures if loose, put mouth piece over tongue so that tongue does not obstruct the mouthpiece
- Sit straight in a arm chair without crossing the legs
- Maximum inspiration
- Good start
- Smooth continuous expiration with maximal effort

The patient is seated comfortably with nose clip on. He is asked to take a maximal deep breath-in to fill the lungs and hold the mouth piece firmly in the mouth. Then he is asked to blow out all the air as rapidly, forcibly and completely as possible. At least three tracings of reasonably good effort are taken.

Spirometric parameters are taken from these tracings. A recommended approach is to record maximal readings of forced expiratory volume in one second (FEV_1) and forced vital capacity (FVC) whether or not they are from the same tracing (18,19). Other measures of flows are taken from the single "best test" curve. The "best test" curve is one which gives the largest sum of FEV_1 and FVC (20).

Interpretation of spirometry tracings:

Similar to ECG spirometer also generates curves and values. Spirometers generate two types of curves volume-time and flow-volume curves. Curves are helpful in detecting inadequate patient effort and indices help in diagnosis of both obstructive and restrictive type of ventilatory defects. Spirometry measures three variables such as flow, volume and time.

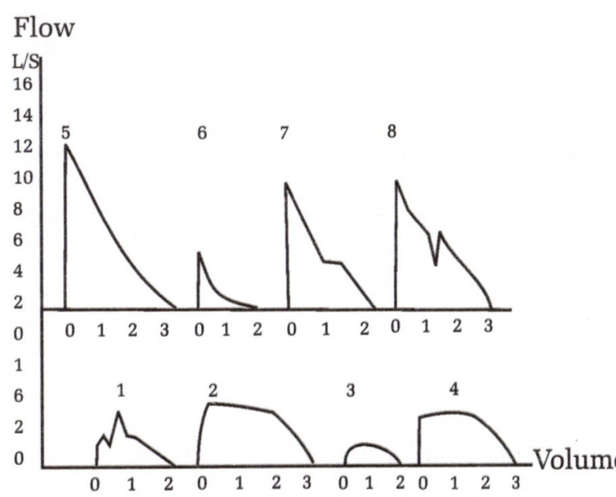

Fig. 1 Flow-volume curve.

A) **Flow-volume curve** (Fig 1, no 5):

Normally as a patient exhales, the curve moves up rapidly from zero scale to attain the peak. It occupies one third part of the curve. In next 2/3rd part of the curve flow rate falls and tracing moves downward smoothly to meet the volume axis and is termed as slope of the curve. Slope displays an upward concavity more marked in the later part.

a) ***Abnormal pattern in peak:***

- Blunt peak (Sand mound, Fig. 1, no 3): Such appearance indi-cates inadequate effort and test should be repeated. Reduced flow rate along with expiratory plateau indicates upper airway obstruction. Peak expiratory flow rate (PEFR) values will be disproportionately less in comparison to FEV_I in such situations.
- Notch (Fig 1, no 1): A notch in the initial part indicates either a cough or hesitant start. After initial flow first peak appears and then glottis is closed leading to a notch. Flow restarts making second peak. Test should be repeated.
- Delayed peak (Fig. 1, no 2) : Sometimes curve starts from zero but peak is delayed. This pattern indicates defective start and test should be repeated.
- Steep curve: In restrictive lung diseases such as interstitial lung disease the curve is more steep and straight. Upward concavity is reduced.
- Rat tail appearance (Fig 1, no 6): In airway obstruction airflow starts with sharp peak but flow rapidly due to airway collapse resulting in shift of upward concavity proximally and subsequent long plateau. This appearance is described as rat's tail appearance and is characteristically present in airflow obstruction.

b) ***Abnormal patterns on the slope:***

- Notch on the slope (Fig 1, no 8): Sometimes descending slope has undulations and these are because of coughing. Notches in proximal part indicate repetition of the test since it can give a falsely reduced FEV_1. Coughing in later of the slope can be overlooked.
- Abrupt termination of the slope (Fig 1, no 7): Instead of slow and smooth pattern tracing abruptly falls on volume axis after peak. During the test when patient stops expiration before complete exhalation, this pattern appears. Such tests should be repeated. In such a situation spirometric parameters will show typical restrictive defect with FEV_1/ FVC ratio as high as 100%.
- Knee on the slope: Sometimes a hump appears on the descending slope specially in young persons. It is described as knee and does not have any clinical significance.

B) **Volume-time curve** (Fig 2, no 5):

As a patient exhales tracing starts from zero and takes a steep upward course rapidly indicating high flow. Then a plateau reaches which continues for rest of expiratory duration. Normally steepness of the slope is reduced after first second.

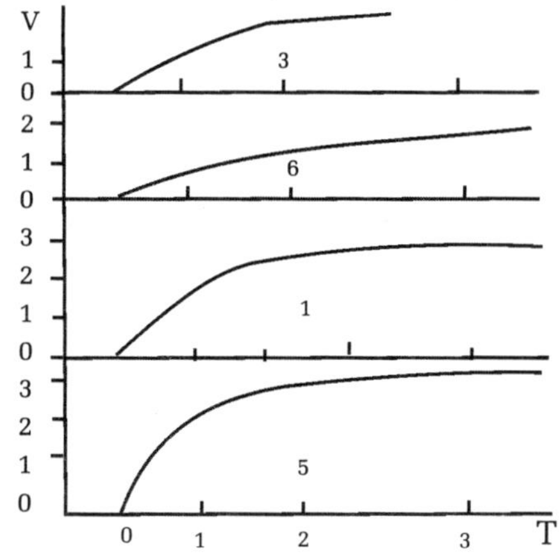

Fig. 2. Volume-time curve

Abnormal patterns:

- Steep ascent: Steep ascent with reduction in expiratory duration is characteristic of restrictive defect.
- Shallow ascent (Fig 2, no.6) : In airflow obstruction instead of steep, slope is shallow due to low flow rate. The duration of expiration is prolonged.

- Ledges on the slope (Fig 2, no I) : Because of coughing ascending slope shows small ledges. If these appear in the first sec-ond the test should be repeated. Cough in later part does not affect results.

  A quick method of assessing good effort in a spirometry is to observe following two criteria:

- Peak of flow-volume should be sharp. Peak expiratory flow rate (PEFR) is best non-invasive test of expiratory effort and should be proportional to FEV_1 (21).
- Expiratory effort lasts for more than 6 seconds in volume-time curve.

Interpretation of spirometric data:

Though spirometric indices do not make exact diagnosis yet they accurately define the functional pulmonary abnormalities. For the purpose of diagnosis most commonly used indices are FVC, FEV_1 and FEV_1/FVC ratio. Other parameters are used as additional supporting evidence.

Spirometric parameters depend on height, age, sex and race (22). Some studies also indicate that socio-economic status has major effect on pulmonary functions. When Chinese and Japanese, change to Western diet and attitude, their pulmonary functions increased to values similar to white (23, 24). In India, variations in values of spirometry, has been reported depending upon height, age, sex and socio-economic status. Higher values have been reported in North Indians in comparison to central India (25-29). Normal values in Indian population are lower in comparison to Western people.

Spirometric parameters have a wide normal range and therefore instead of a cut off limit a range is described to assess normal-abnormal. Therefore assessment of a relative change in a parameter in comparison to previous test reports is more valuable and used frequently in follow-up monitoring of diseases. FEV_1 in obstructive and FVC in restrictive diseases are the best parameters for monitoring the progression of these diseases. Various variables of spirometry data can be described in following group.

A) Forced expiratory volumes:

a) **FVC:** The volume of the air a person exhales with forceful expiration after maximal inspiration. Normally it is reached within 3-4 seconds. Airway obstruction prolongs this time.

b) **Timed volumes**: During FVC maneouvre volume obtained in 0.5, 1 and 3 seconds are displayed in the printout data of commonly available spirometers. These are reduced both in obstructive and restrictive lung diseases. FEV_1 is the most commonly used parameter.

c) **FEV_1/FVC ratio**: Since timed volumes are dependent on vital capacity and body size, therefore shows variations. By expressing timed volume as a ratio of vital capacity, reduces the variability. This ratio is an useful index of assessing magnitude of airway obstruction.

B) Forced expiratory flows:

Expiratory flows averaged over pre-selected segments of spirogram are used in assessment of airway functions. Average flow during first 200 to 1200m1 vital capacity is called forced expiratory flow 200-1200 (FEF 200-1200). Average flow during 25 to 75% of vital capacity is called forced expiratory flow 25-75 (FEF 25-75) and during 75 to 85% of vital capacity is called forced expiratory flow 75-85% (FEF75-85).

FEF 200-1200 gives information about large airways. FEF 25-75 is a sensitive index of airway obstruction present in most of clinical conditions such as asthma and COPD (30). It is also called maximal mid-expiratory flow rate (MMEFR). FEF 75-85 is an indicator of small airway dysfunction (31). It is also called maximal end expiratory flow rate. The information gathered from flows is similar to timed volumes.

C) **Maximum voluntary ventilation (MVV) :**

Largest minute ventilation achieved with effort is called maximum voluntary ventilation. The subject is asked to breathe in and out as hard and as fast as possible. The ventilation is continued for 12 seconds and amount of volume when multiplied by five would give MVV. MVV can also be calculated by multiplying FEV_1 by 35. MVV is effort dependent and therefore depends on strength of diaphragm and chest muscles on one hand and pulmonary compliance and airway patency on the other hand. It is a useful screening test before upper abdomen and thoracic surgery.

Abnormal Spirometric patterns

1. **Restrictive defects:** A group of diseases give a restrictive pattern in spirometry. Restrictive pattern is characterized by lower value of FVC with normal ratio of FEV_1/FVC. FVC is reduced in all restrictive defects because of reduction of intra-thoracic gas volume. FVC is less than 40% of the predicted is categorized as severe restriction while 40 to 60% is moderate and 60 to 80% is mild restriction.

   Airways in lungs are kept open by traction of alveolar septas. In interstitial lung diseases due to fibrous matter in the parenchyma traction pull increases and airways are widened in dimensions. This results in relatively supernormal PEFR in interstitial lung disease but not in restrictive diseases due to causes outside lung. Following three types of disorders can give rise to restrictive defects in spirometry:

   - **Intrinsic lung diseases:** Inflammation or fibrosis of lung parenchyma (interstitial lung diseases, post tubercular parenchymal fibrosis), alveolar filling by fluid or exudate (pneumonia, pulmonary oedema), or removal of part of lung (pneumonectomy).
   - **Mechanical factors compressing lungs:** Obesity, kyphoscoliosis, pleural effusion and fibrosis, pregnancy, ascites, pain during inhalation as in rib fracture and poor effort due to tight clothing.
   - **Neuromuscular disorders resulting in reduced effort:** General weakness (malnutrition), diaphragmatic paralysis, steroid induced and other myopathies and neuropathies. Functional residual capacity and residual volume are reduced in all types of restrictive defects except when caused by neuromuscular disorders and ankylosing spondylitis.

2. **Airway obstruction:** Spirometric patterns in airway obstruction typi-cally shows reduced FEV_1/FVC ratio. It is a sensitive index of air-flow obstruction. With age normal values decline. Young persons have 85% but it declines with age and becomes 65% at the age of 80 years. Once a diagnosis of airflow obstruction is made, absolute values of FEV are more useful for follow-up of asthma and COPD patients and in evaluation of bronchodilator response.

   Similar to restriction airway obstruction is also described as mild, moderate and severe on the basis of FEV_1. FEV_1 less than 75% of the predicted is mild, less than 60% of predicted is moderate and less than 40% is severe. If obstruction is associated with restriction then FEV, can not be taken as a criteria because it is also reduced in restriction. In such a situation FEV_1/FVC% should be employed. FEV /FVC% between 60 and 70 is mild, between 40 and 60 moderate and less than 40 severe airflow obstruction. Timed flows are also abnormal in airway obstruction but adtl little to FEV_1.

   - **Upper airway obstruction:** Ratio of FEV_1 (FEV0.5) in patient with upper airway obstruction is greater than 1.5. This is because FEV0.5 is more reduced in comparison to FEV_1 in patients with upper airway obstruction.

- **Small airway obstruction:** Normally small airways contribute only 20% in airway resistance. But in smokers small airway obstruction is an early manifestation of lung disease and it leads to increased resistance at the level of small airways. Spirometric evidence of small airway disease is characterized by reduced FEF25- 75% with a normal FEF200-1200, a normal FEV_1, and normal FEV_1\FVC ratio.

3. **Obstruction with reduced FVC:** Normally in airway obstruction FVC is not reduced. But in many cases residual volume increased leading to reduction in FVC. Other possibility is a coexisting restrictive disorder. Taking a slow vital capacity and recording spirogram after administration of bronchodilator improves FVC in many of patients with obstruction but not in restriction. If confusion still persists skiagram of the chest is examined. Hyperinflation will be present in obstruction and small lungs characterize restrictive disorder.

Calibration of spirometer:

- ***Syringe calibration***: With time, accuracy of spirometer may change therefore regular calibration of spirometer is very important. It can be done with help of a 3L calibration syringe. Volumes can be checked at 1,2 and 3L levels. Flow rates can be checked by using a calibration syringe provided with tinier.
- ***Biological calibration:*** Any healthy person working in laboratory can check his readings on the spirometer. Normally variations in FEVI and FVC is less than 10%. Periodic checks of the same person ensure spirometric calibration.

Cleaning of spirometer:

Though chances of frequent cross infection with spirometric use is rare in West but may not be uncommon in our country where prevalence of infective respiratory disease is high. Reports of positive bacterial and AFB cultures from spirometric tubes emphasises the need for taking proper measures of prevention of infection (32-34). Apart from pyogenic and bacterial infections hepatitis B has also been shown to spread through saliva. Following are important in checking spread of infection in spirometers (35).

- Avoid testing of the patients having evidence infections such as pneu-monia, bronchiactasis, lung abscess, tuberculosis, hepatitis and AIDS.
- Maximum chances of infection are with MVV and inspiratory manoeuvres. Therefore clean the tubings and mouth piece of spirometers before and after doing these tests. Most of the respira-tory diseases require only expiratory spirograms therefore avoid doing inspiratory spirograms, in such patients.
- Use a segregation chamber while using a volume spirometer (36).
- Use a low resistance disposable bacterial filter.
- Tubing of spirometer should be cleaned daily by immersing it in the disinfectant solution.
- Use disposable cardboard mouthpieces.

Peak flow meter testing

A peak flow meter is a handy tool to measure airflow obstruction. Similar to a thermometer measurement of fever or glucometer measuring diabetes a peak flow meter measures severity of asthma. These diseases have a uniform normal and abnormal cut value but peak flow value varies depending on age, height and sex. Therefore it is important find normal value of individual person.

Normal values of PEFR

Various studies have come out with nomograms of PEFR values. These values depend on age, sex and height of the patient (37, 38). Since there are wide individual variations in PEFR in general population for self monitoring "personal best PEFR" or individual base line value is a better index (39). The highest value form the PEFR, recorded several times in a day for many asymptomatic days is called "personal best PEFR" and is used as normal for that particular person.

Utility of peak flow meters in bronchial asthma:

- **Diagnosis:** Asthma is a disease which is characterized by variable airflow obstruction. Since clinical examination lacks sensitivity, therefore, a minimal requirement for diagnosis of asthma is documentation of positive reversibility test. After baseline measurement of PEF 400 ug Salbutamol is administered to a patient and PEF is again taken after 15 minutes. Twenty percent increase in PEFR is diagnostic of asthma. If reversibility test is negative, a peak flow charting is done twice a day for atleast one week. In adults more than 10% and in children more than 13% variation in diurnal PEF is diagnostic of variability and suggestive of asthma.
- **Identification of trigger factors:** Regular PEFR recording can identify trigger factors of asthma. Morning and evening PEFR is recorded and finding of a reduced PEFR is correlated with exposure to potential triggers factors in the preceding hours. Repeated reduction and exposure to same trigger confirms the provocating factor.
- **Monitoring severity:** Asthma is a disease characterized by worsening of breathing symptoms in night-time and improvement in day-time. Majority of patients consult a doctor in day-time therefore assessment during night-time severity is based on patient's history only. It leads to under-estimation of the severity of asthma.

  PEFR reading is useful for measurement of airflow obstruction at that time. PEFR is said to be reduced if it is less than 80% of the predicted or personal best. Sometimes due to diurnal variability it may not be accurate measure of asthma severity. Diurnal variability in PEFR is an excellent index correlating closely with airway hyper responsiveness. Diurnal variability can be measured by taking two measurements first at the time of morning awakening (6AM) and second at 6PM(40). Reddle and his colleagues have shown that in stable asthmatic subjects PEFR measurement taken at first morning awakening is also a very good index of severity measurement since it correlates with airway hyper-responsiveness (41) .
- **Therapy of asthma:** Treatment based on PEFR improves patient compliance, reduces the chances of under and over treatment. Now we know that asthma is a progressive and potentially fatal dis-ease, if untreated or undertreated.
- **Self management programs:** Based on relative change in PEFR in comparison to personal best are the zone criteria of asthma severity. These zone criteria were proved to have distinct benefits in asthma management.

  Green zone: Reading in green zone signifies 80 to 100% of personal best. This zone suggest that treatment plan is working one should continue this strategy.

  Yellow Zone: PEFR values between 50 to 80% are in yellow zone. It is a zone of caution and asthmatic patients with their PEFR in this zone should be cautious and therefore make adjustment of daily activities and dose of the drugs.

  Red Zone: PEFR values below 50% of the personal best signify dan-ger zone and suggest immediate medical attention.
- **Therapy of asymptomatic airway obstruction:** Presence of inflammation and fibrosis in biopsies of airway mucosa has shown that asthma is a continuous and progressive disease similar to hyper-tension and diabetes. It has also been shown that

untreated or undertreated asthma can lead to progressive and irreversible airflow obstruction even in mild asthma patients (42, 43). Airway obstruc-tion has been demonstrated in patients even in remission (44). Treat-ment in such cases can check the progressive deterioration of lung functions in such cases (45).

Therefore, the current view is to treat asymptomatic asthmatic patients as we treat asymptomatic patients of hypertension or diabe-tes. Values of PEFR and its variability are taken as important criteria in asthma as blood sugar in diabetes or blood pressure reading in hypertension.

- **Therapy in emergency room:** PEFR values taken 15 to 30 minutes after nebulization is an important criteria in dealing acute attack of asthma. If post important bronchodilator value is less than 33% of predicted or the best then asthma is categorized as life threatening and patient should be hospitalized. If post bronchodilator values are less than 50% of the predicted or the best, asthma is categorized as severe and patient is given oral steroids. Patients with PEFR 50-75% of predicted or the best are observed closely with continuing therapy. Patient is discharged from emergency room when post bronchodilator PEFR is more than 75%, (46, 47).

Conclusion

In hospitals patients suffering from respiratory diseases constitute a sizeable group. For diagnosis and monitoring the progression of the disease a doctor depends on clinical examination with stethoscope. However, subjective data and clinical examination with stethoscope are poor guide of severity assessment and detection of both obstructive and restrictive type of respiratory diseases. Proper ventilatory functions are needed for diagnosis and monitoring of patients with respiratory diseases. Spirometry provides accurate measurement of ventilatory functions and is quite useful in clinical practice. Peak flow meters are important equipment in management of asthma and evaluation of dyspnoea both in clinic and in emergency room.

REFERENCES

1. Campbel EJM, Howell JBL. Physical signs of diffuse airways obstruction and lung distension Thorax 1962; 24:1.
2. Dosman J, Bode F, Ghezzep RH et al. The relationship between symptoms and functional abnormalities in clinically healthy cigarette smokers. Am Rev Respir Dis 1976; 114: 297-304.
3. Ockene JK, Hymowitz N, Sexton M, et al. Composition of patterns of smoking behaviour change among smokers in the Multiple Risk Factor Intervention Trial (MRFIT) . Prey Med 1982; 11:881-890.
4. Petty TL, Pierson ill, Dick NP, et al. Follow-up evaluation of a prevalence study for chronic bronchitis and chronic airflow obstruction. Am Rev Respir Dis 1980; 121:881-890.
5. Hepper NG, Drage CW, Davies SF,et al. Chronic obstructive pulmonary disease; A community oriented program including professional education and screening by a voluntary health agency. Am Rev Respir Dis 1980;121: 97-104.
6. Behera D; Health effects of Indoor air pollution due to domestic cooking fuels. Indian J Chest Dis and All Sci 1995; 37:227- 238.
7. Behera D, Jindal SK. Respirtory symptoms in Indian women using domestic cooking fuels. Chest 1991;100: 385-388.
8. Padmavati S, Joshi B. Incidence and aetiology of chronic cor pulmonale in Delhi: A necropsy study. Dis Chest 1964;46:457-464.
9. Behera D, Jindal SK, Malhotra H. Ventilatory function in nonsmoking rural Indian Women using different cooking fuels. Respiration 1994;61:89-92.
10. Dhar SN, Pathania AGS . Bronchitis due to biomass fuel burning in North India: "Gujjar Lung": An extreme effect. Semin Respir Med 1991 ; 12 : 69-74.
11. Mavalankar DV. Indoor air pollution in developing countries. Lancet 1991; 337: 358-359.
12. Kamat SR, Doshi VB, Patade VD, et al. Third year analysis on regularly followed samples of Bombay air pollution study population and correlation with other factors. In Kamat SR ed Bombay Air Pollution Health Study 1984: 111.
13. Sharma VK, Garg VK, Parihar HL et al. Respiratory morbdity and pulmonary fuction impairment in "Solderers": An occupational hazard in Modern electronics. Lung India 1993; 11: 143-46.
14. McFadden ER Jr. Kiser oR, deGroot WJ.Acute bronchial asthma: relations between clinical and physiologic manifestations. N Engl J Med 1973;288: 221-5.
15. Bhargava WJ, Khurana SB, Mahajan R. Effect of FEV1 of workers exposed to low doses of noxious gases in a fertilizer plant. Lung India 1994;12:117-121.
16. Brooks SM(Chairman), Task Group on Screening for Respiratory Disease in Occupational Settings. Official ATS Statement. Am Rev Respir Dis126;952-956,1982.
17. Brooks SM(Chairman), Task group on screenng for respriatory disease in occupational settings. Official ATS Statement. Am Rev Respir Dis 1-2;126:952-956.
18. Nathan SP, Lebowitx MD, Knudson RJ. Spirometric testing: Number of tests required and selection data. Chest 1979;76: 384.
19. Garden RM(Chairman). Snowbird workshop on standardization of spirometry.ATS Statement. Am Rev Respir Dis .1979;119:831.
20. Garden RM, Hanknson JL, Clausen JL. ATS Statement on standardization of spirometry. Am Rev Respir Dis 1987; 136: 1285-1298._

21. Enright PL, Johnson LR, Connet JE et al. Spirometry in lung health study. Methods and quality control. Am. Rev. Respir. Dis. 1991;143: 1215-1223.
22. Clausen JL.Prediction of normal values in pulmonary function testing. Pulmonary function testing: Clinics in Chest Medicine 1989;10:157.
23. Knudson RJ, Lebowitz MD, Holberg CJ et al. Changes in normal maximal expiratory flow volume curve with growth aging. Am Rev Respir Dis 1983; 127: 725-734.
24. Gardner RM, Capro RO Nelson SB . Spirometry and flow-volume curves. Clinics in Chest Medicine 1989; 10; 145-154.
25. Kamat SR, Sharma BS, Raju VRK, et al. Indian norms of pulmonary function: Observed values, prediction equations., and intercorrelations. JAPI 1987; 36:491-196.
26. Udwadia PE, Sunawala JD, Shetya V M. Lung function studies in healthy Indian subjects. JAPI 1987; 36:491-496.
27. Jain SK, Ramiah TJ. Normal standards of pulmonary function tests for healthy Indian men 15-40 years old. Comparison of different regression equations (Prediction formulae). Ind J Med Res 1969; 57: /453-66.
28. Jain SK Gupta CK. Age, Height and body weight as determinants of ventilatory norms in healthy men above forty years age. Ind J Med Res 1967;55: 599-611.
29. Purohit SD, Srivastava AB, Gupta PR, et al. Spirometric norms in healthy adults of Rajasthan: Lung India .1989; 7: 15-25.
30. Leueallen EC, Fowler WS. Maximal Mid Expiratory Flow. Am Rev Tuberc 1955; 72:783.
31. McFadden ER, Linden RA. A reduction in maximal and expiratory flow rate. A spirographic manifestation of small airway disease. Am J Med 1972; 52:725.
32. Tisi GM. Stat, of the art: Preoperative evaluation of pulmonary function. Validity, indication and benefits. Am Rev Resp Dis 1979; 119: 293-310.
33. Renfrow DP, Thomann CA, Rutala WA. Infection risk associated with spirometry 12th annual educational conference for practitioners in infection control. 1985 ; 12: 161.
34. Houston L, Parry P, Smith AD., Have you looked into your spirometer? Breath 1981; 12 : 10-12.
35. Enright PL, Hyatt RE. Spirometer evaluation in office spirometry. Enright. PL , Hyatt RE eds. 1987; 93.
36. Singh V, Arya A Mathur US. Bacteriology of spirometer tubing and evaluation of methodolgy to prevent transmission of infection. JAPI 1993; 41: 193-194.
37. Singh V, Mathur US, Bhandari VM et al. Peak expiratory and peak inspiratory flow rates: Comparative study of pink city flow met with Wright peak flow meter. Lung India 1987;4:171-174.
38. Gregg I, Nunn AJ. BMJ 1989;298: 1068-70.
39. Kashyap S, Malik SK. Peak expiratory flow rate in healthy school boys from Himachal Pradesh (North India) Indian J. Chest Dis and All Sci I987;29:216-218.
40. National Heart, lung and blood Institute: Guidelines for diagnosis and management of asthma. National asthma education program. Expert panel report. J Allergy Clin Immuno11991;88:477-492.
41. Reddel HK, Salome CM, Peat JK. Which index of peak expiratory flow is most useful in the management of stable asthma? Am J Respir Crit Care Med 1995;151: 1320-1325.
42. Gibson PG. Wlodarczyk J, Hensley MJ et al. Using quality control analysis of peak expiratory flow recordings to guide therapy for asthma. Ann Intern Med 1995; 123:488-492.

43. Ulrik CS, Lange P. Decline of lung function in adults with bronchial asthma. Am J Respir Crit Care Med 1994; 150:629-634.
44. Godden DJ, Ross R, Abdulla M, et al. Outcome of wheeze in childhood: symptoms and pulmonary function 25 years later. Am J Respir Crit Care Med 1994; 149: 106-112.
45. Boulet LP, Turcotte H, Brochu A et al Persistence of airway obstruction and hyperresponsiveness in subjects with asthma remission. Chest. 1994;331: 700-705.
46. Haahtela T, Jarivan M, Kava T et al Effect of reducing or discontinuing inhaled budesonide in patient with mild asthma. N Eng J Med 1994; 331: 1024-31.
47. British Society Guidelines on the management of asthma. Thorax 1997; 52:81-824.

5
LUNG VOLUME TESTS

JN PANDE, GC KHILNANI

Aim of lungs

The ultimate aim of the lungs is to achieve normal oxygenation (arteralization) of the mixed venous blood perfusing the pulmonary capillaries. For this the lungs have to be properly ventilated and its numerous alveoli adequately perfused. Further, there should be an efficient process of alveolo-capillary gas exchange. It is important that the ventilation of individual alveolar units matches their perfusion. Ventilation of the lungs is a mechanical process which results in alternate increase and decrease of the intrathoracic volume. Enhanced lung volume following deep inhalation is accommodated mainly in the alveoli which increase in size. In order to ensure uniform distribution of the inspired air to different regions of the lung, it is essential that these regions have uniform mechanical characteristics, e.g compliance and airway resistance. Also each one of these gas exchange units should be adequately perfused by the mixed venous blood. The exchanging surface of the alveolar-capillary membrane should be structurally and functionally normal to permit rapid exchange of respiratory gases. Many of these functions may be disturbed in disease states resulting in abnormalities of gas exchange.

Lung volume

The lung volumes are altered in many diseases of the lung, pleura, diaphragm and chest wall, hence, have a definite place as diagnostic tool in the investigation of a variety of diseases. For ideal interpretation of lung volumes in disease the normal value for that particular person in health should be known. However, since this information is almost never available, the normal values are calculated according to the tables drawn by studies in healthy population. Age, gender, height, body weight and ethnicity is taken into account for calculating predicted values of lung volume of a person. On the whole the lung volumes are smaller in famale and short persons. Life-long residents of high altitude living in hypoxic environments have relatively larger lung volumes. There is a significant variation in the lung volumes of populations living in various parts of globe. On the whole, people from India have significantly lower lung volumes as compared to the Western population. This may be due to genetic, environmental or nutritional factors. In most reports, North Indians seem to have relatively larger lung volumes as compared to the South Indians. North Indians also have larger lung volumes as compared to New Guineans, Chinese and Africans. In view of these variations in lung volumes in different populations, it is necessary to have normal standards for the population in an ethnic alteration produced by disease. After an age of 20-30 years, most of the lung advancing age, an opposite trend is seen to increase with advancing age.

Definitions

Total lung capacity: The total volume of air contained in the lung after a maximal voluntary inspiration, is termed as total lung capacity (TLC). This volume of air can be subdivided into four fractions (Fig. 1).

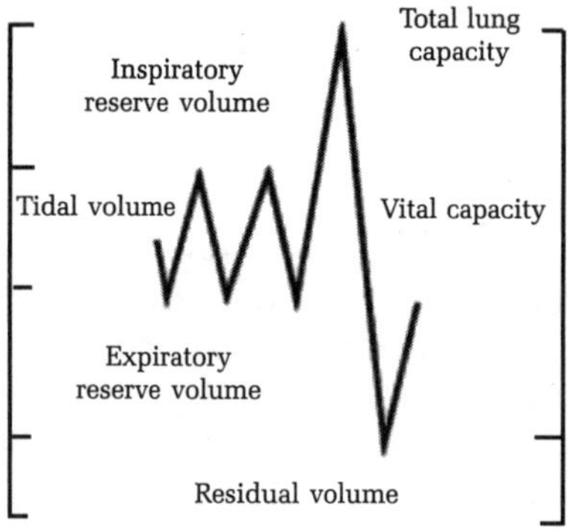

Fig. 1: Subdivisions of total lung capacity

a) **Tidal volume (VT):** The volume of air inhaled or exhaled with each breath during resting, quiet respiration is termed as tidal volume.

b) **Inspiratory reserve volume (IRV):** This is the volume of air that can be inspired by maximum voluntary effort starting from resting and inspiratory position.

c) **Expiratory reserve volume (ERV):** This is the volume of air that can be inspired by maximum voluntary effort starting from the resting end-expiratory position.

d) **Residual volume (RV):** This is the volume of air present in the lungs (in airways) following a maximal voluntary expiration.

So, TLC = VT + IRV + RV

It is customary to measure a combination of some of these lung volumes as lung capacities as given belwo:

Inspiratory capacity (IC): It is the volume of air that can be inspired by maximum inspiratory effort starting from end inspiratory position. It is a sum of VT and IRV.

Vital capacity (VC): It is the maximum volume of air that can be exhaled or inhaled following a maximum inspiratory or expiratory effort respectively. It is equal to the sum of IC and ERV.

The ventilatory function of the lungs is concerned with the delivery of an adequate volume of inspired air into the alveoli over a given time. This is possible only if the dimensions and elasticity of the lung and the thoracic cage, the respiratory passages, the bellows mechanism of the thorax and the respiratory drive are normal. Any abnormality in any one or more of these components may lead to ventilatory impairment. It is possible to assess the ventilatory function of the lungs with the help of a variety of measurements and parameters which estimate several static or dynamic characteristics of lung mechanics. Many of these parameters are routinely measured in clinical respiratory laboratories.

Measurements of lung volumes

Spirometry

Various lung volumes and capacities which do not include residual volume (such as vital capacity, inspiratory and expiratory reserve volume and tidal volume) can be measured by simple spirometry. This is the most frequently performed measurement inmost of the clinical respiratory laboratories. Volume tracings against time are usually recorded using conventional water –filled spirometers. A large variety of dry (waterless) spirometers are also available. They include the rolling seal spirometer and the electronic spirometers. The latter are smaller in size, portable and easy to use, but need to be calibrated frequently against standard volumetric devices. The American Thoracic Society (995) has given detailed recommendations regarding the minimum requirements of a spirometer, its use and calibration. All lung volumes are usually expressed under BTPS conditions i.e body temperature and pressure when saturated with water. They are compared with predicted values for the given population and expressed as percent of the predicted value. Generally any value beyond the range of 80-120% predicted is considered abnormal although there is no scientific basis for this clinical practice.

Measurement of resident gas volume in the lungs

The total volume of gas present in the lungs at a given state of lung inflation cannot be estimated by simple spirometry. The following two approaches are generally used for estimating lung volumes which include resident air (e.g TLC,FRC, RV, etc)

Inert gas dilution methods

1. ***Closed circuit method:*** Rebreathing into a bag containing a known quantity of an inert gase such as helium or argon and estimating the gas concentration at the end of the lung-bag equilibration (usually achieved after 3-5 minutes in normal subjects) permits the calculation of resident air in the lungs by the dilution principle. It is necessary to incorporate a CO_2 absorption canister (soda lime) to the circuit to prevent build up of CO_2 concentration during rebreathing. In patients with chronic obstructive lung disease rebreathing for a longer period is required to achieve complete equilibration of gas concentrations in the bag and the lungs.

2. ***Open circuit method***: In this method the subject breathes 100% oxygen through a one-way valve. The expired gases are collected in a large Tissue spirometer. At the end of 7 minutes of oxygen breathing it is assumed that the nitrogen in the air contained in the lungs at the time of starting the washout procedure has now been transferred into expired air collected. The amount of nitrogen thus recovered from the lungs can be estimated. By assuming that the nitrogen would have been present in the lungs at a concentration of 80% appropriate lung volume can be estimated. Rebreathing or nitrogen washout procedures are usually initiated at the resting end-expiratory point so that volumes measured by these procedures would represent FRC.

Plethysmographic method

The body plethysmographic method permits rapid estimation of the volume of air in the thorax generally referred to as thoracic gas volume (TGV). The subject is seated inside a constant volume total body plethysmograph. He breathes through a mouth piece into a tube fitted with an electronically or pneumatically controlled shutter. If the shutter is closed and the subject works his respiratory muscles to alternately compress and expand the air in his thorax, then with the use of the intrathoracic pressure (or mouth pressure) inside the body plethysmograph (box pressure) and the volume of air in the plethysmograph (box volume minus the body volume) permits calculation of TGV by application of Boyle's law, assuming the volume changes to be isotheramal. This manoeuver also permits the computation of alveolar pressure from box pressure which is useful for the calculation of airway resistance.

Plethysmographic TGV is usually obtained during panting against a closed shutter. The volume thus obtained is comparable to FRC in normal subjects. In patients with chronic obstructive lung disease, the TGV is usually higher than FRC obtained by the inert gas methods. This is because of incomplete washout of the resident gas or incomplete equilibration during rebreathing due to the existence of very slowly ventilated air spaces in the lungs of these patients. The difference between the two measurements may be considerable in the presence of non-comunicating bullae or air cysts in the lung.

FRC, airway conductance (Gaw) increases linearly with lung volume. Their ratio, termed specific airway conductance (SGaw) remains fairly constant. But below FRC, SGaw falls disproportionately due to the airway closure in the basal parts of the lung, and in normal subjects SGaw at RV is 30 to 65% less than SGaw at FRC.

In smokers with smoking history of 5 pack years or more, the fall in SGaw at RV is invariably more than 70%. In very heavy smokers it reaches 100%,i.e, airway closure is almost complete at RV and no airflow occurs during early inspiratory effort after slow expiration to RV, Similar observations have been made in patients with asthma and bronchitis, who also show small airways obstruction. In fact, a recent study on patients with perennial bronchitis showed abnormal fall in Gaw at RV in almost all cases.

Thus, the sensitivity of this technique in detecting small airway obstruction seems much higher than even the so called gold standard 'frequency dependence of dynamic compliance'. This is probably due to the fact the value of SGaw at FRC serves as its own control.

Dynamic functions

The lung volumes and capacities mentioned so far assess only the static dimensions of the lungs. It is equally important, however, that the lungs be capableof filling and emptying, air at a reasonably fast rate in order to be able to meet the ventilatory demands of the body in accordance with the oxygen requirements. This is possible only if the air conducting passages from oro-nasopharynx down to the terminal bronchioles are normally patient and free of disease. Several physiologic parameters may be measured in order to assess the normal patency of the airways. Some of these physiologic parameters are routinely measured in most clinical respiratory laboratories, excepting those that require more sophisticated equipment.

Most of the parameters are derived from an analysis of a single maximal forced expiration. The subject inhales to TLC and then breathes out with maximal voluntary effort to RV. The volume thus expired is called forced vital capacity (FVC). It is almost equal to VC in normal subjects, but may be significantly less in patients with obstructive airway diseases. The following information is obtained from this manoeuvre using appropriate measuring devices.

Forced expiratory volume in first second (FEV1)

The forced expired volume is defined as the volume expired in the first second during forced vital capacity exhalation. This is measured from the analysis of the forced expiratory spirogram. It may be expressed as absolute volume in litres at BTPS, or as percent of the forced vital capacity. In normal subjects, FEV1 is more than 80% of FVC. Values of FEV1 are reduced in both central and peripheral airways obstruction. In patients with reduced lung volumes (restrictive ventilatory defect), FEV1 expressed as % FVC may be suprnormal (>90%).

Peak Expiratory Flow Rate (PEFR)

This is defined as the maximum expiratory flow rate sustained for at least 20 milliseconds during the forced expiratory manoeuvre. It is measured with the help of specially designed instruments (e.g. Wright peak flow meter), which are small handy and portable and give the reading of the peak flow rate on a dial or a liner scale. Patients may be asked to monitor the peak expiratory flow rate at frequent intervals at home to assess the response to treatment. Peak flow rate is influenced to a greater extent by narrowing of the large airways. It may be completely normal in patients with moderately severe peripheral airway disease resulting from chronic bronchitis or emphysema.

Maximum Mid-expiratory flow rate (MMFR, FEFm25-75%)

MMFRis defined as the mean flow rate during the exhalation of the middle 50% of the forced vital capacity breath. It can be easily obtained by analysis of the forced expiratory spirogram. It is influenced by both central and peripheral airways obstruction and is reduced to restrictive lung diseses where FVC is reduced even though there may be no airway narrowing.

Flow volume curves

Flow volume curves are obtained by displaying volume changes on the abscissa and the flow changes on the ordinate of an x-y recorder during a forced maximal expiratory and inspiratory manoeuvre (Fig. 2).

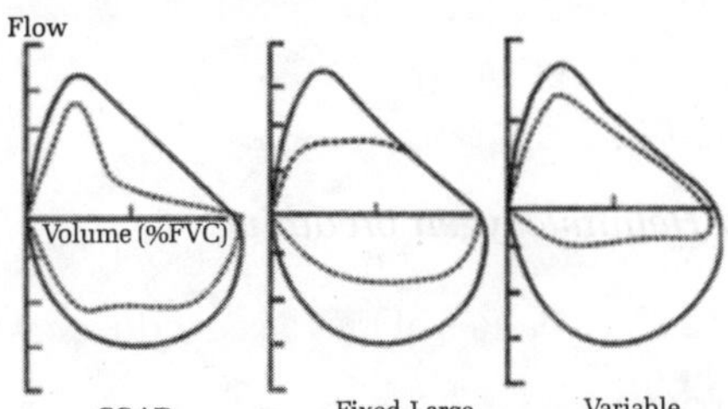

Fig. 2: Flow volume curves: The dark line depicts the normal predicted curve and the dotted line depicts curve in diseases

Flow rate is obtained with the help of a pneumotachograph whereas the volume changes may be obtained by (i) electronically integrating the flow signal, (ii) breathing into a spirometer, or (iii) recording the volume changes in a constant pressure body plethysmograph. The last method gives change in thoracic gas volume, which differs from those in the expired volume due to intrathoracic gas composition.

Forced expiratory flow volume curves give information on the site of airflow obstruction. Thus patients with predominantly peripheral airways obstruction exhibit a decrease in flow rates at low lung volumes whereas their initial peak flow is affected only to a smaller extent. This results in the characteristic curvilinear maximum expiratory flow volume curve. In patients with large airway obstruction (e.g, tracheal compression by a tumour) , the sharp peak in the early phase of maximum expiration is replaced by a plateau, while the terminal flow rates at low lung volumes are affected to a smaller extent. Typical alterations in flow volume curves in subjects with different types of airways obstruction are show in Fig.2.

The information contained in the maximum expiratory flow volume curves may be summarized in the form of parametric numbers, e/g/ the peak expiratory flow rate and the maximal expiratory flow rates obtained when only 50% or 25% of teh FVC remains to be exhaled (V50 and V25 respectively). Visual inspection of a curve, however, brings out the abnormalities much more clearly. Though, there is a large inter-individual variation in maximum expiratory flow rates, particularly at low lung volumes, in a given individual, however, the flow volume curves are effort independent over the latter two-thirds of the forced expiration which means that maximum flow rates are achieved even with moderate expiratory effort, and more strenuous effort does not increase the flow rate further. The peak expiratory flow rate, which is recorded during early expiration, is effort dependent in most subjects. The physiological mechanisms underlying expiratory flow limitation will be discussed later.

Inspiratory flow volume curves are effort dependent over the entire vital capacity range. The curve has a plateau-like appearance, so that the flow rates are not affected by the lung volume. A marked reduction in inspiratory flow rate is characteristic of extrathoracic large airway narrowing, e.g due to bilateral vocal cord paralysis.

Flow volume curves may also be recorded with the subject breathing in 80% helium 20% oxygen mixture. In normal subjects his results in a marked increase in maximum expiratory flow rates at large lung volumes due to lower gas density. At low lung volumes however, the density-dependent rise disappears. The flow rate may be even less than that observed during air breathing due to high viscosity of the He/O2 mxture. The largest lung volume at which the maximum expiratory flow rates on breathing He/O2 mixture or air are identical and it is referred to as the volume of isoflow. In patients with peripheral airways obstruction the increase in flow rate of large lung volumes while breathing He/O2 mixture is less remarkable and the volume of isoflow is increased (Fig. 3).

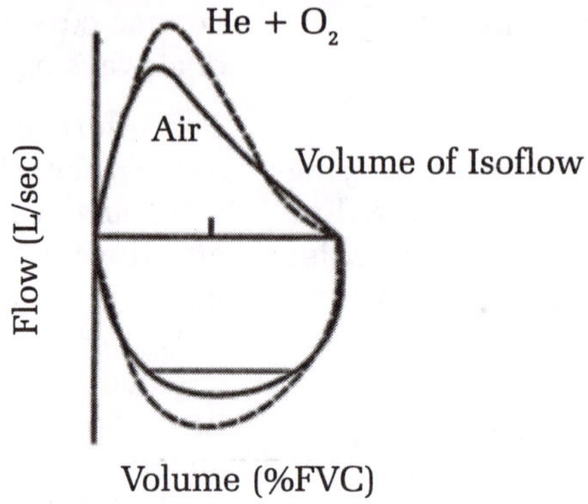

Fig. 3: Flow-volume curve as recorded by Helium/oxygen breathing

REFERENCES

1. Desman J, Bode F, Urbanetti J, Martin R, Macklem PT The use of a helium oxygen mixture during maximum expiratory flow to demonstrate obsstruction in small airways in smokers J Clin Invest 1975; 55: 1090-99

2. DuBios AB, Botelho SY, Comroe JH Jr, A new method for measuring airway resistance in man using a body plethysmography. Value in normal subjects and in patients with respiratory disease. J Clin Invest 1956; 35: 327-35

3. Handbook of Physiology Section 3. The respiratory system Vol iii Mechanics of breathing. eds Macklem PT, Mead J Bethesda, Amer Physiol Soc 1986

4. Handbook of Physiology Section 3 The respiratory system Vol iv Gas exchange eds Farhi LE, Tenney SM, Bethesda, Amer Physiol Soce 1987

5. Standardization of spirometry 1994 Update, 1995 Amer J Respir Crit Care Med 1993; 152: 1107-36

6
AIRWAY RESISTANCE AND COMPLIANCE

HARMANJIT SINGH HIRA

Supplementary tests

The pulmonary function tests to measure airway resistance and compliance are classified as supplementary because they do not constitute standard clinical spirometry. Supplementary pulmonary function testing provides additional information sometimes necessary to define a patient's pulmonary disease process to a better way.[1]

Airway Resistance (Raw) is the driving pressure necessary to move a volume of gas in a specific period of time. Mathematically, it is the ratio of the driving pressure to the flow and is expressed in cm of water per litre per sec (cm H_2O/L/s).

Compliance (C) is a measure of the distensibility of the chest and/or lungs. It refers to the volume change in the lung per unit of pressure change and is expressed in litres per centimeter of water (L/cm H_2O).

Airway resistance

Airway resistance is determined by body plethysmography. Airway resistance is the ratio of the driving pressure of the airflow and can be represented with the following formula: AP.

$$Raw = \frac{AP}{V}$$

Where Raw is airway resistance; AP is driving pressure; and V is airflow.

The driving pressure (AP) is equal to the airway pressure (PaO2) minus the alveolar pressure (Palv). To measure the driving pressure, the body plethysmograph is used. The patient is placed in a scaled plethysmograph (Fig 1). Volume changes in the thorax will create volume changes in the chamber, which in turn is reflected by changes in the chamber pressure. During inspiration, the lung increases in size. This creates a subatrmospheric pressure in the alveoli, and air moves into the lung because of the pressure gradient. At the same time, the increased size of the thorax is compressing the gas in the chamber, and a reciprocal increase in chamber pressure results (Boyle's law). During exhalation the reverse occurs. Recording the pressure in the plethysmograph (Pp) during this time provides a value for one variable in the formula used to calculate the airway resistance.

In the absence of airflow, airway pressure at the mouth is equal to the alveolar pressure (Palv). While the patient is breathing, an electronic shutter momentarily closes (Fig1). This creates a no-flow situation, and the alveolar pressure can be determined. During this time, if one measures the airflow (V) with a pneumotachometer, the airway pressure can be calculated by the following formula[2]:

$$Raw = \frac{Palv/Pp}{V/Pp}$$

Where Raw is airway resistance; Palv is alveolar pressure; Pp is plethysmograph pressure and V is airflow.

The formula describes the relationship between two sets of ratios (1) changes in the alveolar pressure and pressure in the plethysmograph (Palv/Pp) and (2) changes between flow and pressure in the plethysmograph (V/Pp). For the test, the patient is usually instructed to pant at VT of approximately 100 to 200 ml at high rates, usually greater than 100 breaths per minute. Panting reduces many of the artifacts that would otherwise interfere with the test results.[3]

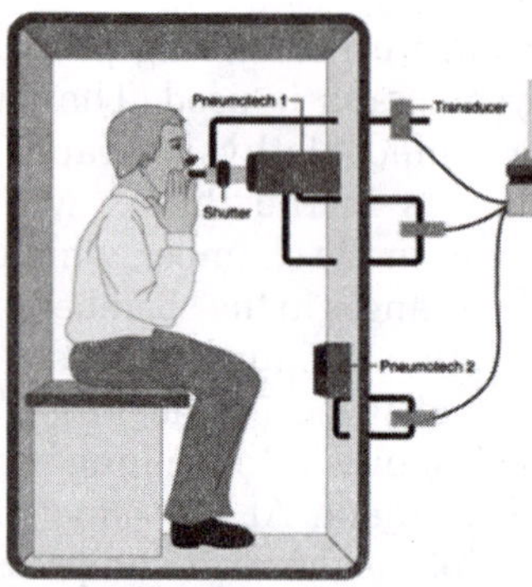

Fig. 1: Showing working of airway resistance in the body plethysmograph (source: pgdoc.blogspot.com)

Airway resistance is normally between 0.5 and 2.5 cm H2O/L/s measured at the standardized flow of 0.5 L/s. It is lower during inspiration and higher during exhalation. In addition, airway resistance decreases with increasing lung volumes, primarily because of the increasing airway calibre. Any factor that reduces the calibre of the airway will cause an increase in airway resistance. Such factors include edema, bronchial secretions, bronchoconstriction, and vascular congestion (inflammation). A loss of lung elastance (increased compliance) will also cause an increase in airway resistance because of the loss of parenchymal support surrounding the small airways. Therefore, disorders such as asthma, emphysema, and bronchitis will cause an increase in airway resistance.

When patient is being mechanically ventilated, airway resistance to gas flow is measured in the clinical setting with the following physiologic formula.[3]

$$\text{Raw} = \frac{\text{Peak pressure} - \text{Plateau pressure}}{\text{Flow}}$$

Airway resistance is driving pressure divided by flow rate. Driving pressure is the difference in the pressure between the beginning of the circuit i.e. the (Peak pressure) and the end of the circuit, the alveoli (plateau pressure).

High airway resistance may be caused either by patient factors or by the factors related to ventilator circuitry. Examples of patient related factors include bronchoconstriction, secretions in the airway, or bronchial mucosal edema, as in thermal injury. Examples of ventilator circuit factors are as follows: 'biting' or kinking of the endotracheal tube, kinking of the ventilator tubing between the bed rail and the mattress, and water in the ventilator tubing. In all these conditions that cause increased resistance, gas flow into the lungs is decreased if the pressure getting the air into the lungs is not increased. Increased airway resistance therefore decreases the patient's tidal volume and alveolar ventilation. It also increases the amount of pressure required to get air into the lungs. Finally the distribution of ventilation becomes uneven. The areas of the lung that have the least resistance are ventilated better than high-resistance area.

Compliance

Compliance is a measure of the dispensability of the lungs (C), the thorax (Cr or both CLT). In essence, it measures the case with which the lung volume is changed. It is expressed in litres per centimeter of water (L/cm H_2O). Increased compliance means a greater increase in lung volume per cm of water pressure; likewise, a reduced compliance means a smaller change in lung volume per centimetre of water (Fig 2). Fig 3 shows tracings as slope drawn from the beginning point dividing expiratory and inspiratory limb. A shift of slope towards the pressure axis indicates a decrease in compliance seen in patient of emphysema. While a shift towards the volume axis indicates an increase in compliance in case of ARDS.

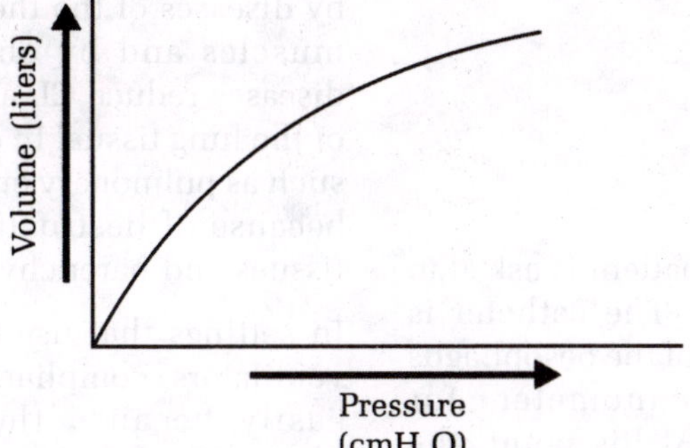

Fig.2: Normal tracings of pressure-volume demonstrating compliance.

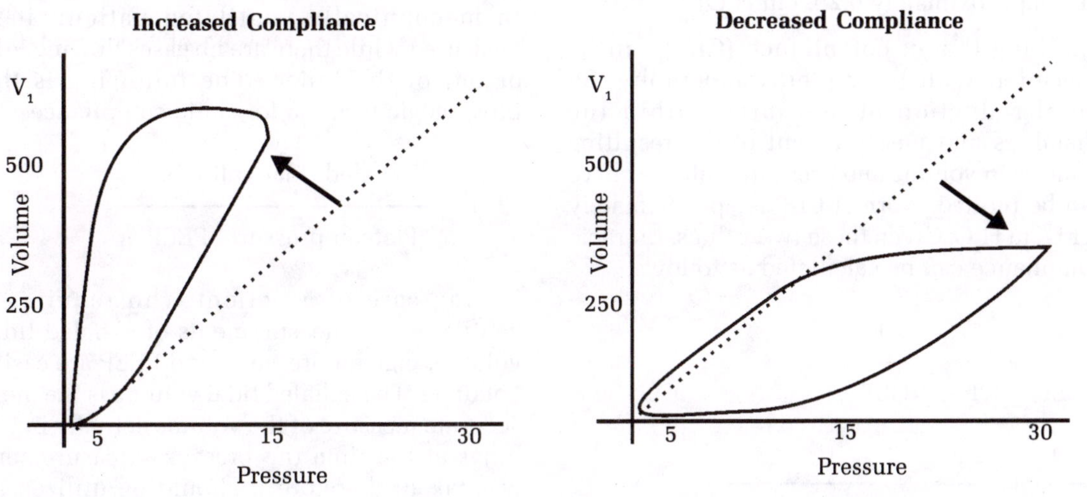

Fig 3: A slope drawn from the beginning point dividing expiratory and inspiratory limb. A shift of slope towards the pressure axis indicates a decrease in compliance (emphysema). While a shift towards the volume axis indicates an increase in compliance (ARDS).

When one is determining the CLT, it is necessary to know the transpulmonary pressure and the specific lung volumes at each pressure in doing this, a pressure-volume curve is generated (Fig, 2). The transpulmonary pressure (PL) is the difference between the intrapleural pressure (Ppl) and the alveolar pressure (Palv): PL=Ppl-Palv. When compliance is measured under static conditions (static compliance), the alveolar pressure is equal to the atmospheric pressure (Patm).[3] In this case, the atmospheric pressure is assumed to be equal to zero by standard; therefore the transpulmonary pressure is equal to the intrapleural pressure: P1= Ppl

The formula for calculating static lung compliance (CLst) is

$$CL = \frac{AV}{AP}$$

where AP is the pressure gradient or PL, since PL= Ppl

Therefore

$$Cl = \frac{AV}{AP}$$

For measurement of CL, the patient is asked to swallow a balloon catheter. The catheter is positioned in the lower third of the oesophagus and connected to a manometer for measurement of pressure. At his point, the esophageal pressure is equal to the intrapleural pressure. Pressure changes can be plotted against various lung volumes (Fig. 2). Normal CL is approximately 0.2 L/cm H_2O).

The lung-thorax compliance (CLT) can be measured with body plethysmography. By serial reduction of pressures within the chambers and measurement of the resulting changes in volume and pressure-volume curve can be plotted. Normal CLT is approximately 0.1 L/cm H_2O. Given these two values, thoracic compliance can be calculated as follows:

$$\frac{1}{CL} + \frac{1}{CT} = \frac{1}{CLT}$$

$$\frac{1}{0.2} + \frac{1}{0.2} = \frac{1}{0.1\text{L/cm } H_2O}$$

The total CLT is about one half of either the lung or thorax compliance. This is a result of the opposing forces of the lung and thorax.

When compliance measurements are made during the breathing cycle, dynamic compliance is measured. In the normal lung, the dynamic compliance (Cdyn) is equal to the lung compliance because of the opposing forces between the lungs and the thorax.

Changes in lung and chest wall compliance occur in the several disease processes. CL is most affected by bronchopulmonary diseases, whereas chest wall compliance is most affected by diseases of the thoracic nerves, joints, and muscles and by obesity. Restrictive lung diseases reduce CL as a result of the stiffness of the lung tissue. In obstructive lung diseases such as pulmonary emphysema, the CL is high because of destruction of the lung support tissues and parenchyma.

In settings that use the new microprocessor ventilators, compliance can be obtained very easily because the ventilator performs measurements of respiratory mechanics after the operator inputs only a few simple commands. Static compliance is the true measure of the compliance of the lung tissue. In mechanically ventilated patient, it is measured while there are no gases flowing into or out of the lungs.[3] The following is the physiologic formula for static compliance.

$$CLst = \frac{\text{Exhaled tidal volume}}{\text{Plateau pressure- PEEP}}$$

During care of a patient who requires a ventilator, the measurements of exhaled tidal volume, plateau pressure, and PEEP are easily obtained. The exhaled tidal volume is the most accurate measure of the volume actually in the lungs at the time the pressure measurement was taken; therefore it should be utilized as the volume measurement. The plateau pressure is obtained by instituting a 2-second inspiratory pause at the peak of inspiration. The pause creates the condition of no gas flowing into the lungs. At the point where no gases are flowing, and with the glottis open, the pressure within the alveoli is obtainable in the form of the plateau pressure, reflects pressure due to the elastic recoil forces of the lung tissue alone, on the volume of gas in the lungs. No pressure resulting from the flow of gases is measured. When the calculation is performed, any artificial pressure placed in the airway such as

PEEP, must be subtracted from the plateau pressure. When a patient does not have an endotracheal tube in place, measurement of static compliance is still possible. This is achieved by measuring pleural pressure, which reflects alveolar pressure, with an oesophageal balloon.

Dynamic compliance (Clyde) is not a pure measurement of lung compliance. The following is the physiologic formula for dynamic compliance in the mechanically ventilated patient.[4]

$$\text{CLdyn} = \frac{\text{Exhaled tidal volume}}{\text{Peak inspiratory pressure - PEEP}}$$

Again, the exhaled tidal volume should be used as the numerator because it is the most accurate measurement of the volume actually in the lungs at the time the pressure measurements are taken. The pressure in the airway at the peak of inspiration then divides the exhaled tidal volume. At this point, gases are still flowing in the lungs, and some pressure increased will be due to the movement of the gas particles (resistance). Any artificial pressure, such as PEEP, must be subtracted from the pressure measurement when the calculation is performed.

The normal value of dynamic compliance is 50 to 80 ml/cm H_2O. Dynamic compliance measures are always smaller than static compliance because peak airway pressure is always greater than plateau pressure. A decrease in dynamic compliance may indicate a decrease in lung compliance or an increase in airway resistance.[5]

REFERENCES

1. Bates DV Basic pulmonary physiology *in* Bates DV ed Respiratory function in disease, 3rd edn, Philadelphia, WB Saunders 1989; 23-66.
2. Hyde WR, Mayeewski RJ Measurement of non-elastic resistance to airflow in Chusid EL ed The selective and comprehensive testing of adult pulmonary function, 4th end, New York, Future Publishing 1983; 115-134.
3. Mayewski RJ, Hyde RW Measurement of static pressure-volume relationships of the lung and thorax. *in* Chusid EL, ed The selective and comprehensive testing of adult pulmonary function, 4th end, New York, Future Publishing 1983; 79-113.
4. Pierce LNB Practical physiology of the pulmonary system *in* Pierce LNB ed Guide to Mechanical Ventilation and Intensive respiratory care 1st edn, Philadelphia, WB Saunders 1993; 24-56.
5. Youtsey JW Basic pulmonary function measurements in Scanlan CL Spearman CB, Sheldon RL eds Egan's Fundamentals of Respiratory Care 5th end, St Louis, CV Mosby 1990; 374-95.

7

TESTS FOR DISTRIBUTION OF VENTILATION

D D S KULPATI

The distribution of ventilation and the movement of the air or gas into and out of the thorax depend upon the structural and mechanical properties of the lung and chest wall. The gas must flow along the numerous airways before it reaches the alveolar capillary membrane for gas exchange.

The distribution of ventilation can be considered in terms of :

1. Distribution of the tidal volume
2. The rate at which different alveoli fill and empty
3. The relation of distribution of ventilation to pulmonary blood flow differentiating between the ventilation of the unperfused alveoli at one extreme and the failure of ventilation of perfused alveoli at the other, and
4. Spatial distribution in relation to anatomical structures

1. Distribution of tidal volume

Distribution of tidal volume can be divided into 'conducting' and 'gas-exchange' type. The conducting airways include the nose, mouth, pharynx, trachea and bronchi to the level of terminal bronchioles. The conducting airways provide a conduit to the gas exchanging regions and do not participate in oxygen and carbon dioxide exchange. The gas- exchange regions include the respiratory bronchioles, alveolar ducts, alveolar sacs and alveoli.

The amount of gas inspired with each breath is the tidal volume (VT) and its distribution to conducting airways and gas exchanging areas depends upon their relative volumes (Fig. 1). The volume of gas entering or leaving the respiratory system per minute is the minute ventilation (VE) and is calculated as the product of VT and respiratory frequency (f). The expired ventilation is denoted by the 'E' in the symbol for minute ventilation. For an adult of average size VT is 0.5 to 0.71: fess 10 to 12 breaths/min. The inspired gas occupying the conducting airspace do not participate in gas exchange and are 'dead' as far as the carbon dioxide elimination is concerned. Thus, the anatomic dead space is the volume of the gas in the airways, not involved in alveolar gas exchange. The mixing of gases in the terminal airways and the alveoli mainly takes place by diffusion, thus the dead space measured is less than the volume of airways from the mouth to the respiratory bronchioles. The alveolar dead space is the volume of the ventilated alveolar space not involved in the gas exchange across the alveolar capillary membrane. The physiological dead space is the volume of that part of the respiratory tract which is nto involved in the exchange of gases and is, thus, the sum of the anatomic and alveolar dead space (Fig. 2).Under normal conditions, the alveolar dead space is very small. As a rule, anatomic dead space, expressed in milllitre is approximately equal to ideal body weight, expresed in pounds (1-3).

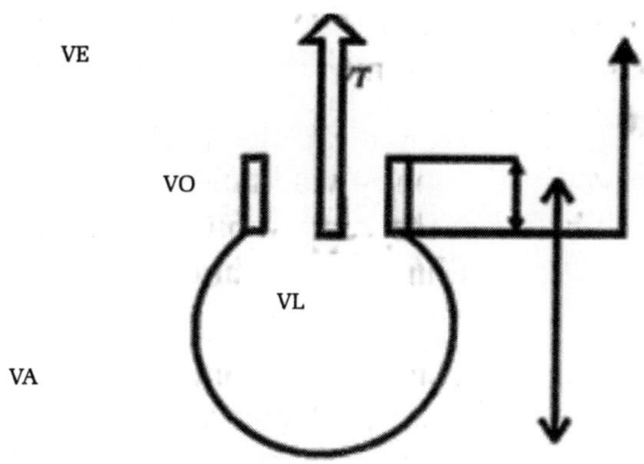

Fig. 1: Distribution of tidal volume. The volume of the lung (VT) is the sum of the alveolar ventilation (VA) and dead space volume (VD). Tidal volume (TV) is the expiratory breathing volume (VE) or the inspiratory breathing volume (VI)

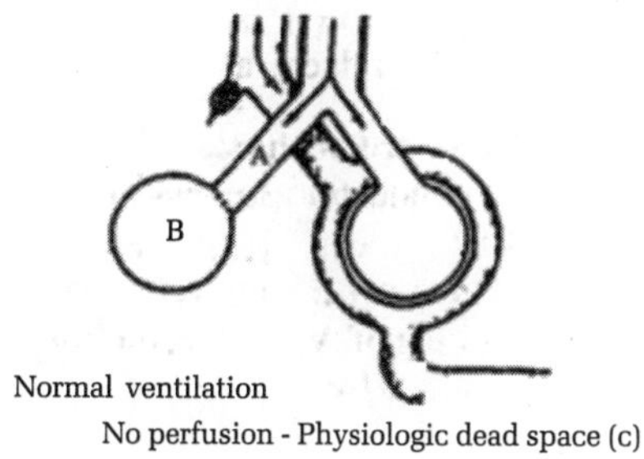

Fig. 2; Anatomic dead space (A) is the area where gas exchange does not take place. Alveolar dead space (B) is the alveolar area which though ventilated normally but does not take part in gas exchange. Physiologic dead space(C) is the sum of the anatomic dead space(A) and alveolar dead space (B) not involved in gas exchange

Anatomic dead space is not constant and is influenced by body weight (1 pound=4.5 kg), posture (more in sitting than supine), position of the neck and jaw (more on extension than flexion of the neck), age (increase by age), lung volume at the end of inspiration, tracheal intubation or tracheostomy (by pass extrathoracic anatomic dead space), pneumonectomy and hypoventilation.

Alveolar dead space may be increased by pulmonary hypotension, severe haemorrhage, anaesthesia with hypotension, embolism, ventilation of nonvascular spae (emphysema) and constriction of precapillary pulmonary vessels or obstruction of pulmonary circulation by external forces.

The 'alveolar volume' is the reminder of the tidal volume (VT-VD) and is distributed to alveoli and related gas-exchanging structures.

Thus,

VE = VT.f

where

VE = Minute ventilation

VT = Tidal volume

f = Respiratory frequency

Substitution of the sum of the alveolar volume (VA) and dead space volume (VD) for VT, yields the following expression:

VE = (VA+VD) f

or

VE = (VA.f)+(VD.f)

The term (VA.f) represents minute alveolar ventilation (VA) and the term (VD.f) represents minute dead space ventilation (VD).

Calculation of physiologic dead space

Carbon dioxide in the expired gas come totally from the alveoli where it is unloaded by pulmonary circulation, as the inspired air contains only negligible amount of this gas. During expiration, carbon dioxide (CO2) in the alveoli, gets diluted in the physiological dead space producing a drop in CO2 concentration in the expired gas relative to its alveolar concentration. The total amount of CO2 in the respiratory system at any instance of the time is the product of initial volume in which the CO2 is contained i.e alveolar volume, and the concentration of CO2 in the alveoli. Alveolar CO2 concentration is calculated as the partial pressure of alveolar CO2 divided by the sum of partial pressures of the gases and water vapour in the alveoli. Because, the sum of partial pressures in the alveoli equals barometric pressure, alveolar CO2 content can be shown as below:

Alveolar CO2 content= VA. PACO2/ PB

The total amount of CO2 remains the same when the alveolar CO2 is mixed with dead space volume. Thus, the amount of CO2 excreted with each tidal volume can be expressed as below:

VT. PECO2/ PB= VA PACO2/PB,

where PECO2 is the mean partial rpessure of CO2 in the mixed expired gas.

Simplifying the above equation, we get
VTPECO2 – VAPACO2

This indicates that the amount of CO2 exhaled with each breath (VT.PECO2) is equal to the amount of CO2 in the alveoli (VA.PACO2). CO2 is neither lost nor added to the gas evolved into the alveoli from the pulmonary circulation i.e the CO2 is just diluted to a new partial pressure (PECO2) by the addition of the physiologic dead space.

VT equals to VD + VA, so the above equation can be rearranged as below:
(VD+VA).PECO2 – VA.PACO2 and by substitution of (VT-VD) for VA.

$$VD = \frac{VT.PACO2 - PECO2}{PACO2} \quad \text{or}$$

$$VD/VT = \frac{PACO2 - PECO2}{PACO2}$$

This is known as ‘ Bohr-mixing equation’ and indicates that the ratio of dead space to tidal volume can be calculated as the difference between the PCO2 of alveolar gas and expired gas divided by the alveolar PCO2. As the alveolar PCO2, closely approximates arterial PaCO2 due to high speed diffusion. VD/VT can be estimated by measuring the PaCO2 (arterial blood)and PCO2 of the expired gas, simultaneously.

In the normal subject, the minute ventilation will be 6L/min, which is the product of the tidal volume of 0.6 L and respiratory rate of 10 breaths/ min. If the PaCO2 is 40 mm Hg and PECO2 is 28 mm Hg, the VD/VT can be estimated by measuring the PaCO2 (arterial blood) and PCO2 at the expired gas, simultaneously.

In the normal subject, the minute ventilation will be 6L/min, which is the product of the tidal volume of 0.6L and respiratory rate of 10 breaths/min. If the PaCO2 is 40 mm Hg and PECO2 is 28 mm Hg, the VD/VR ratio will be equal to 40-28/0.30. Thus VD is (o.30 x 600) equal to 180 ml and VA (600-180 ml) equals to 420 ml. In an average healthy adult VD/VT is approximately 0.30 to 0.35.

Effect of ventilatory pattern on VD/VT

Alveolar ventilation is a critical determinant of the rate of CO2 elimination. Minute ventilation may remain the same, but alveolar ventilation may change depending upon VD/VT (Fig. 3).

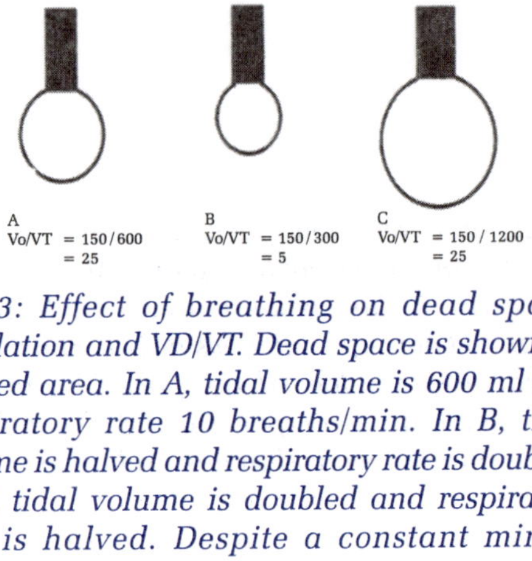

Fig. 3: Effect of breathing on dead space, ventilation and VD/VT. Dead space is shown by crossed area. In A, tidal volume is 600 ml and respiratory rate 10 breaths/min. In B, tidal volume is halved and respiratory rate is doubled. In C, tidal volume is doubled and respiratory rate is halved. Despite a constant minute ventilation, the ratio of dead space to tidal volume varies markedly.

In a healthy young adult, VE is 6L min; f=10 breaths/min, VD = 150 ml. Then, VA is 4500 ml (450 x 10) and VD/VT is 150/600=.25 (Fig, 3A).

If the respiratory rate is increased to 20/min and VE maintained at 6L,VT will be 300 ml. VD= 3000 ml (20 x 150) and VA will be 3000 ml/min. VD/VT is increased to 150/300 = 0.5. The rapid shallow breathing is insufficient with respect to CO2 elimination (Fig. 3B).

Finally, if VT is 1200 ml and RR decreased to 5 /min, VD maintained to 6L/min, the VD will be 750 ml/min and VA will be 5250 ml/min. VD/VT is decreased to 150/1200 or 0.125 and CO2 elimination will be efficient (Fig. 3C).

Physiological dead space is influenced by age (VD increase slightly less than 1 ml per year), body size (VD= 17 ml increase for every 10 cm increase in height), posture (decrease in supine), duration of inspiration and breath holding (VD reduces by prolongation of inspiration by allowing better gas mixing between dead space and alveolar gas), smoking (VD increased) pulmonary disease (pulmonary embolism, emphysema) and during connection to breathing apparatus (apparatus dead space).

The relationship between alveolar ventilation and rte of CO2 production

The rate of CO2 production (VCO2) in young healthy adult is 200 ml/min and PaCO2 is 40 mm Hg. The rate of CO2 elimination equals the rate with which it is produced. Under steady state conditions this can be shown as:

VA= K.VCO2/PaCO2, where K, a constant equals to 0.863 when VA is expressed at BTPS and VCO2 at STPD. This also indicates that at a constant rate of CO2 production, PaCO2 varies inversely with alveolar ventilation. The magnitude of the effect of a change in minute ventilation on alveolar PCO2 depends upon the relationship between dead space ventilation and total ventilation. The higher the VD/VT the greater is the change in VE necessary to produce changes in VAand PaCO2.

Further, the effects of an increase in VD can be counteracted by corresponding increase in the respiratory minute volume. If for example, the minute volume is 10L/min, and VD/VT ratio 30 per cent, the alveolar ventilation will be 7L/min. If the patient is then subjected to pulmonary embolism resulting in an increase of the VD/VT ratio to 50 percent, the minute volume will need to be increased to 14L/min to maintain alveolar ventilation of 7L/min. Should the VD/VT increases to 80 percent, the minute volume would need to be increased to 35L/min and so on.

Relationship between alveolar ventilation and alveolar PO2 and alveolar PCO2

Alveolar PO2 (PAO2) depends upon the uptake of O2 across the alveolar-capillary membrane and alveolar ventilation (Fig. 4, 5). As the partial pressures of the other gases and water vapour

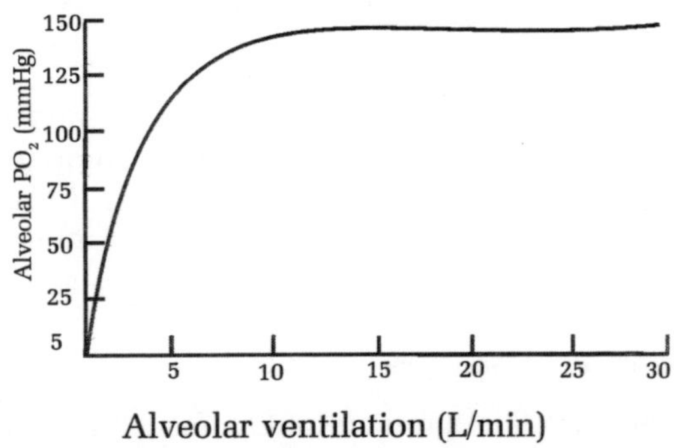

Fig. 4: Relationship between alveolar ventilation and alveolar PO2 rises with increases in alveolar ventilation up to a point and then reaches a plateau

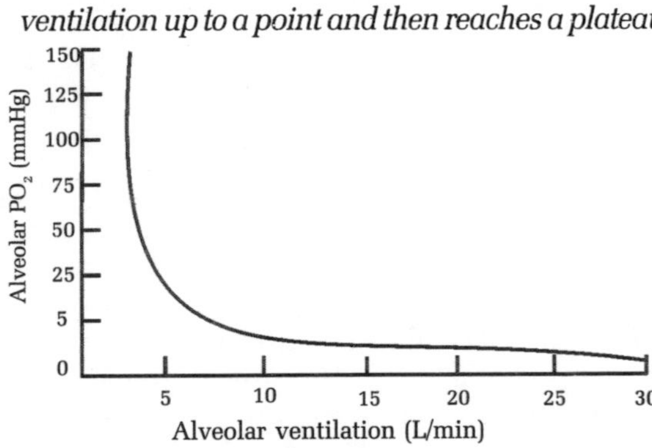

Fig. 5: Relationship between alveolar ventilation and alveolar PCO2, alveolar PCO2 varies inversely with alveolar ventilation. The relationship is plotted for a person of average size who has a normal stable rate of CO2 production (about 200ml/min).

in the alveoli are constant, $PACO_2$ and PAO_2 vary reciprocally as alveolar ventilation is altered. Alveolar PO_2 rises with increase in ventilation up to a pont and then reaches a plateau.

According to alveolar gas equation, the PAO_2 can be calculated, if the partial rpessure of the others are known.

$$PACO2 = \frac{PIO2 - PACO2(FiO2 + 1\text{-}FiO2)}{R}$$

where PIO_2= Partial pressure of O_2 in inspired air; FiO_2 = Fractional concentration of O_2 in inspired air; R = Respiratory exchange ratio.

Under steady stage conditions, the respiratory exchange ratio equals the respiratory quotient (RQ) which denotes the ratio of CO_2, production to O_2, consumption at the cellular level. The CO_2 production is increased by relatively larger contribution of carbohydrates as the fuel resources.

Alveolar partial pressure of O_2 (PAO_2) can be calculated by subtracting from PIO_2 a product of $PACO_2$ and a factor that takes into account the change in total gas volume, if O_2 uptake differs from CO_2 output (FiO_2 + 1- FiO_2/R). In a healthy-resting adult of average size, VO_2 is about 250 ml/min, VCO_2 approximately 200 ml/min. R is therefore, 200-250 or 0.8, This factor reduces to 1.2 when FiO_2 is equal to 0.21, and to 1.0 when FiO_2 is 1.0.

Assuming the barometric pressure of 760 mm Hg and water vapour pressure of 47 mm Hg, PIO_2 can be calculated as the product of total partial pressure of the dry gases in the alveoli and fractional concentration of 0.2. Thus

$$PIO2 = (760\text{-}47)\ 0.21 \text{ and the}$$

$$PAO2 = (760\text{-}47)\ 21\text{-}\ 40\ \frac{(.21+1.21)}{0.8}$$

$$= 149\text{-}48 = 101 \text{ mm Hg}$$

II. Distribution of inspired gas in relation to the rate of alveolar filling

The rate of inflation of the lung as a whole is a function of inflation pressure, compliance and airway resistance. The product of the compliance and resistance equals to time-constant which is the time required for inflation of the lungs, if the initial gas flow rate were maintained throughout inflation. If the inflation pressure is sustained indefinitely, the volume that can get in different units of lungs will solely depend upon their regional compliance. If their time constants are equal the build-up pressure in the different units will be identical at all times during inflation. Thus, the distribution of gas will be independent of the rate, duration or frequency of inspiration; dynamic compliane will not be affected by changes in frequency and if inspiration is checked by closure of the upper airway, there will be no redistribution of gas within the lungs. If, however, the time-constants of different units are different, the distribution of inspired gas will be dependent on the rate, duration and frequency of inspiration; dynamic compliance will be decreased as respiratory frequencies increase and if inspiration is checked by closure of the upper airway, gas will be redistributed within the lungs.

In a healthy subject, the variations in time-constants for different parts of the lung can be demonstrated by the effect on ventilation of fast and slow inspirations. An increase in scatter of time constants in disease can be demonstrated by an increase in 'frequency dependence of compliance' (refer also N_2 washout curve).

Regional distribution of tidal volume

The lung is heterogeneous with regard ot mechanical properties of the airways and parenchyma. It is this heterogeneity which accounts for the differences in the distribution of each breath. Normally, in the upright position, a pleural pressure gradient exists between the apex and the base of the lung. The pleural pressure is greatest (most negative) at the apex with a gradient of about 0.25 cm H2O for each centimeter of vertical height. The pleural pressure is least (least negative) at the bottom with the pressure difference of 8 cm between apex and base of the lung.

As the transpulmonary pressure is the difference between the intra-alveolar and intrapleural pressure, the transpulmonary pressure is greater at the lung apex than at the base. The larger transpulmonary pressure will result in greater alveolar distension at the apex in comparison to the base (Fig. 6). Therefore, application of an inflation pressure produces a greater change in lung volume (LV) at the base than at the apex. This denotes that static lung compliance is higher in the base and, consequently, more of each tidal volume will be distributed to the base. Even if the ventilation is adjusted and normalised for regional lung volume, it is greater at base than at apex. The preferential basal distribution of ventilation is maintained. This will also be predominant at the base.

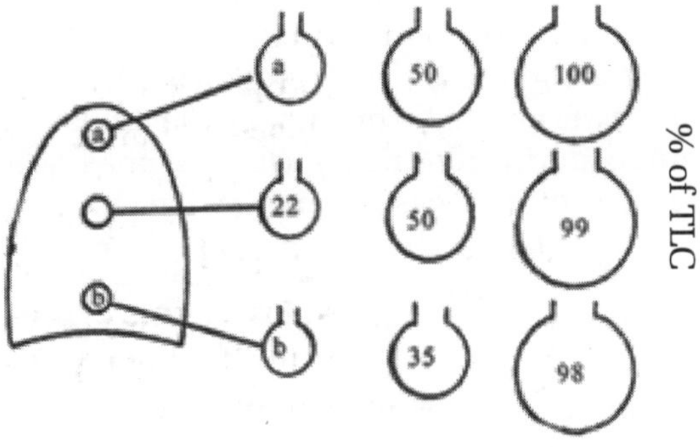

Fig. 6: Schematic of apical and basal alveolar size. Apical alveoli (a) are larger than basal (b)

In disease, intrapleural pressure may exceed alveolar pressure (eg. due to loss of elasticity in emphysema), airways may become compressed at the end of the expiration. If the blood flow in the base persists as before, gas exchange will be impaired resulting in ventilation-perfusion (V/Q) inequality. The factors responsible for the pleural pressure gradient include the weight of the suspended upright lung pulling on the lung apex and the tethering of the lung centrally at the hilum.

III Relation of Ventilation to Perfusion

The distribution of ventilation may depend upon the time constants. This may simply be viewed as changes localised or generalised in resistance or elasticity (reciprocal of compliance). In chronic obstructive lung disease, bronchial asthma characterised by increased airway resistance, most of the inspired volume goes to the non-obstructed alveoli. The net effect will depend upon the extent to which blood is redistributed from the obstructed to the normally ventilated alveoli.

Similarly, in diseases like emphysema (decreased elasticity) and pulmonary fibrosis (increased elasticity) uneven distribution of ventilation occurs. On repeated respiration, areas with increased elasticity will receive a greater proportion of the inspired volume. In some disorders, a combination of altered regional compliance and resistance may occur. The increased airway resistance may be 'dynamic' occurring with expiration resulting in non-uniformity of ventilation. Sometimes, airway resistance and lung elasticity are normal but regional limitation to expansion results in maldistribution of ventilation e.g. lung compression by a pleural effusion, and limited expansion of one hemithorax due to unilateral diaphragmatic paralysis.

IV Spatial and anatomical distribution of ventilation

Distribution between the two lungs depends upon the posture and the manner of ventilation. In the normal subject, right lung has slightly greater ventilation than the left lung in both supine and upright positions. In the lateral position, the lower lung is better ventilated regardless of the side on which the subject is lying. The diminished volume of the dependent lung is associated with the lower diaphragm lying higher in the chest and, thereby, more sharply curved. It will, therefore, contract more efficiently during inspiration. The perfusion of the lower lung is also increased and therefore ventilation-perfusion rations of the two lungs are not altered significantly. The difference in ventilation between the two lungs may be assessed clinically by inspection and auscultation and by chest radiography and screening, and bronchospiroemtry. Spatial distribution in relation to the external anatomy of the trunk can be determined by the expansion of rib cage and abdomen. These can be assessed by magnometry impedence plethysmography, optical contouring and computerized tomography.

Distribution to horizontal slices of the lung studied by using a radioactive isotope of oxygen, showed threefold increase in ventilation at the bottom compared with the top of the lung, at flow rates below 1.5 L/s, starting from FRC. Normal inspiratory flow rate is much less than 1.5L/s.

Postures also affect the distribution of ventilation as the vertical height of the lung is reduced by 30 percent in supine position. The gravitational force generating maldistribution is reduced. During supine position, there is a slight preferential ventilation of the posterior slices compared with the anterior slices. The inequality is not greatly different from that found in upright position. Distribution to zones of the lung can be studied with gamma camera by using Xenon133. This technique is useful for defining pathological conditions resulting in failure of regional ventilation and can also be related to scans which indicate perfusion.

Tests for Distribution of Ventilation

There are number of tests for assessing the overall distribution of ventilation as well as the regional disturbances in ventilation (Table.1). The alterations in the relationship of ventilation to perfusion may result in V/Q mismatch and disturb the gaseous exchange.

Table 1: Tests for assessing distribution and matching of ventilation to perfusion

Physiological variables	Tests
I Overall distribution of ventilation	Multi-breath N2 washout Single breath N2 test Helium-mixing time
II Localised distribution of	Xe131 ventilation scan Lateral position test Bronchospirometry
III Relationship of ventilation to perform CO2 test	Physiological dead space Single breath CO2 test for physiological shunt

I. Multi-breath N2-washout Open circuit

Normally, inspired gas is distributed rapidly to all regions of the lung and the alveoli are filled promptly with the inspired gas. Similarly a tracer gas in the alveoli is eliminated ('washed out' of the alveoli by the process of ventilation) rapidly during repeated inhalations of a tracer-free gas in the lungs having slowly ventilating regions for an extended period of time. An 'overall index' of the efficacy of 'gas-distribution' to the alveoli can be obtained from an analysis of the washout curve of a tracer gas. At the alveoli concentration of nitrogen while breathing air (about 80%), the resident nitrogen is used as the tracer gas in the multi-breath nitrogen elimination (or washout) test. The testing method is possible because N2 is inert and is in equilibrium with the blood and diffuses only very slowly from the blood across the alveolar-capillary membrane. Alveolar concentration is estimated by measuring end-tidal N2-concentration. The alveolar N2 is washed out using O2 as the inspired gas and an open breathing system. This washout is demonstrated by a mono-alveolar model, assuming that the indicator gas at any moment is distributed homogeneously over the alveolar space and the tidal volume and breathing frequency are constant.

During O2 breathing, the alveolar gas is diluted with each breath. The nitrogen fraction of the gas at the mouth is plotted against the number of breaths. The resulting graph consists of the logarithm of N2 concentration on the Y-axis of the plot and the cumulative expired volume on the X-axis. The end-tidal points, identified as the maximal N2 concentration of each breath, are connected by a curve. This curve approximates the decline in the mean alveolar nitrogen concentration. Subjects with normal lungs breathing with a normal respiratory pattern can reduce alveolar N2 concentration to less than 2.5%by breathing oxygen for 7 minutes. Young subjects often reduce the concentration to under 1.5% in this time interval. An end-tidal N2 concentration greater than 2.5% after 7 min is considered abnormal, and is an inhomogeneity of distribution of ventilation (4-7).

The index is dependent on the pattern of breathing as well as ventilation inhomogeneity because increases in tidal volume and raising of the TV/FRC ratio, increased dilution of FRC, resulting in quieter elimination of N2 from the alveoli. Thus the 7 min N2 concentration is not a sensitive index of distribution inhomogeneities, but is most commonly used because of its simplicity. Becklake index and the lung clearance index (LCI), Mixing ratio, Index of deficiency, five breath index (FBI), moment analysis and index of uniformity are more sensitive to gas distribution abnormalities and are relatively independent of patient variables, but their time consuming calculation and less extensive evaluations have not led to acceptance of routine use.

Single breath N2- elimination

In the upright position, the subject is asked to make a full expiration of residual volume and inhale a full vital capacity with oxygen. Without breath holding, the subject then exhales fully to residual volume at a slow, constant rate of about 0.5 liter/sec, while N2 concentration in the expired gas is continuously monitored with the N2 analyser. The N2 concentration is plotted against the volume exhaled.

The inhalation of full breath of O2 from residual volume permits distribution of O2to all regions of the lung. The first gas distributed to alveoli is the anatomic dead space gas, followed b inhaled oxygen. Ventilation may become inhomogeneous in (a) small airway disease which slows ventilation to some alveolar groups, (2) in partial atelectasis and surfactant deficiencies, which after the relative degrees of expansion of some alveoli. Inspired oxygen in these cases, result in varying concentrations of alveolar oxygen, with poorly filling alveoli having lower concentrations of oxygen and greater nitrogen concentrations.

During expiration, 4 phases of 'N2 washout' curve is obtained. During early expiration gas from the upper airways and anatomic dead space is exhaled. Because this region contains pur oxygen from prior inspiration, the nitrogen concentration is zero (phase I_. Phase II represents the transition from the dead space to alveolar, and the nitrogen concentration rises rapidly. Phase III of the expiration exclusively concerns to the alveolar gas. In healthy subjects, with minimal inhomogeneity of ventilation, this phase of the curve (Phase III) is flat and is known as 'alveolar plateau'.

In a variety of parenchymal and airway diseases phase III is not flat and its slope is a measure of inhomogeneity of ventilation and is measured as the best fitting line through the alveolar plateau to begin when 70% of the vital capacity is still to be exhaled. The slope is expressed as %N2 per litre expired gas. The poorly ventilated alveoli receive little of the inspired oxygen and will have a high alveolar N2 concentration during phase III. There is an abrupt rise in N2 concentration in the expired gas (phase II) after the alveolar plateau. This is due to closure of the small airways at the lung bases at low lung volumes. Gravity gives rise to a vertical gradient in the alveolar volume and alveolar ventilation. On a maximum inspiration, O2 flows mainly to result in a vertical N2-gradient, with the highest fractional concentration in the upper part of the lung. During the subsequent expiration the contribution of the lower parts of the lungs, where the N2 contribution decreases, until the lower airways are closed by compression and the flow of the expired gas comes exclusively from the upper parts of the lung, where N2-concentrations are highest. This moment is marked by an abrupt rise in the expired nitrogen fraction and marks the start of Phase IV.

In normal young persons, expiratory airway closure occurs about at the level of the residual volume. It rises with age to the level of the functional residual capacity due to decreasing elasticity of the lungs. Under pathophysiological conditions the closing capacity can even be greater than FRC (trapped gas) and is often associated with abnormalities of the arterial blood gases. It is disputable whether phase IV is determined by airway closure alone (static) or also by flow limitation due to a dynamic compression. Oscillations in Phase II indicate regional differences in N2-concentration and are the result of variation in the rate of gas replacement in different areas of the lung due to movements of the heart and great vessels.

The volume above the residual volume (RV) when small airways closure begins is called the 'closing volume'. This is the portion of vital capacity remaining at the onset of phase IV of the N2 washed-out curve and the sum of 'closing volume' and residual volume is called the 'closing capacity'. In healthy young subjects, airway closure occurs at about 10% of the vital capacity above residual volume. In the elderly, airway closure may occur up to 35 to 40% of the vital capacity above residual volume.

Anatomic Dead Space

The volume of anatomic dead-space (VDanat) is obtained from the graph by measuring the volume between the initiation of the test and phase II. Since phase II is not a perfect transition, its midpoint is used as the limiting value. 'VDanat" is therefore the volume of phase I and one-half of the volume phase II. Its predicted value for a given subject is the weight of the subject in pounds i.e 150 ml in the average adult. It is measured in any disease producing dilatation of non-respiratory tracheobronchial tree, such as bronchiectasis, and it is decreased by loss of bronchial volume, such as plugging of the airways. The slope of the alveolar-plateau (of phase III) is an index of ventilation inhomogeneity. The change in N2-concentration over 1 liter of the plateau is the Phase III slope (DN2 litre). It is normally under 1% /litre in healthy young adult and may increase to 1.5 to 2%/litre with normal ageing. In chronic obstructive pulmonary disease (COPD) values up to 20% /litre may be seen due to ventilation inhomogeneity (Fig. 7).

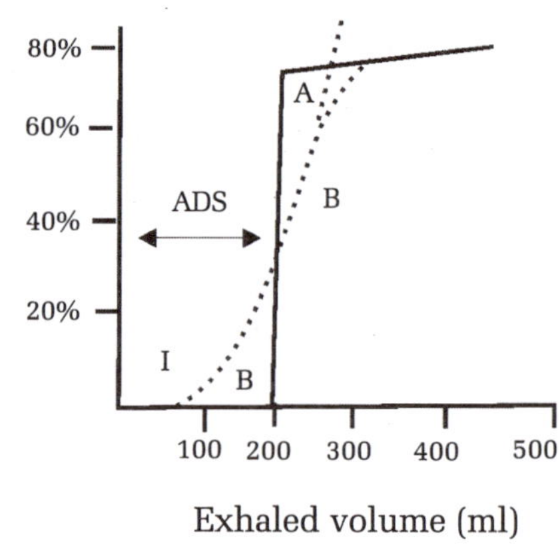

Fig. 7: Measurement of anatomic dead space from the single breath Nitrogen washout curve. Phase II is divided into two segments at a point in which triangle A has an area equal to triangle B. The volume of phase I plus the volume of the initial portion of phase II up to the point of division is the anatomic dead space.

Localised distribution of ventilation

These tests provide specific anatomic information about the distribution of pulmonary ventilation. Bronchospirometry requires selective intubation of the bronchi, but its use has been largely replaced by radionucleide imaging and the use of simpler although, less sensistive tests, such as the lateral position test.

1. Radionucleide ventilation imaging

Radio-isotopes introduced into the lung *via* the ventilation, emit gamma rays which can be measured by four scintillation counters on the dorsum of the thorax, in four lung fields: right and left, apical and basal. This permits static and dynamic imaging for the distribution of ventilation in the lungs on a regional basis, with image resolution at the level of the bronchopulmonary segments. Dynamic studies permit wash-in and wash-out analysis on a regional basis as well (9, 10).

In order to study ventilation, the subject is connected to spirometer filled with 10 liters of oxygen containing the radioactive tracer Xe133. The subject exhales to residual volume, then inhales a breath of the Xe133 mixture containing 5 mCi of radionucleide per liter and holds his breath. During the breath-hold, an initial scan is made-'single breath image'. Each image requires at least 50,000 oscillation counts. The subject then rebreathes the Xe133 gas mixture in a closed system to permit equilibrium of ventilation. After 3 to 6 min a second scan is made-'equilibrium image'. The subject then begins breathing environmental air and Xenon is gone. This series of scans constitute the 'elimination or washout image' phase. The first phase gives the information on areas readily ventilated. The second phase allows more time for rebreathing to allow more time for slowly ventilating areas to appear. The final phase permits dynamic viewing of gas elimination to demonstrate areas of trapping and slow ventilation. This is the most useful phase.

II. Lateral-position test

A simple non-invasive means of assessing relative ventilatory function of each lung is 'lateral position test'. The test estimates the relative contribution of each lung to total ventilation and correlates well with oxygen consumption. It also correlates favorably with radionucleide ventilation scanning.

The test is based on the relative changes in FRC produced by changing from the supine to each of the lateral positions. The subjects begin rebreathing in the supine position from oxygen filled closed circuit spirometer system with a CO2 absorber. After a stable decreasing baseline is reached, the subject is turned on to one side, and rebreathing continues for several breaths. The supine position is repeated, then the subject is turned on to other side, and the test is repeated again. The subject then turns again to supine position to complete the test. The relative distance from the baseline represents the relative degree of function (11).

III. Bronchospirometry

When accurate assessment of ventilation and gas exchange of the individual lungs is required, bronchospirometry can be used. It requires intubation under local anaesthesia and this test is not carried out while the subject is taking tranquillsers or narcotics. It is unpleasant to patient because breathing through the catheter offers great resistance to airflow. Depending upon the purpose of investigation intubation lasts 10 to 40 minutes: longer periods are undesirable (12).

The test is carried out by selective intubation of bronchi with a double-lumen, double-cuff tube (Carlen's catheter). Ventilation and other indices of pulmonary functions, such as O2 consumption (indicative of V/Q mismatching) and CO diffusion, can be made from each lung through the mainstream bronchi.

Complete information about individual lung function can be obtained by radionucleide imaging or non-invasive tests, such as lateral position test. Bronchospirometry, therefore is rarely indicated. Other tests are more complicated to perform and are not carried out routinely for achieving for distribution of ventilation.

For achieving adequate alveolar ventilation for proper gas exchange, the inspired volume of gas must be 'distributed' to the alveoli with a high degree of efficiency and homogeneity. There may be slight variation in ventilation-perfusion relationship between different regions of the lung but within each region distribution to alveoli must be fairly uniform to permit maximal utilisation of the alveolar capillary membrane surface. The assessment of alveolar gas distribution is useful in supporting diagnosis suggested by other tests and in defining degree of impairment. The tests described above provide an index of overall homogeneity of alveolar gas distribution as well as delineate abnormalities of distribution on a regional or lobar basis.

REFERENCES

1. Hlastala M Ventilation *in* Crystal RG, West JB eds The Lung, New York, Scientific Foundations 1991; 1209-14
2. West JB Ventilation *in* Respiratory Physiology. The essentials 4th edn, Baltimore, Williams and Wilkins 1990; 11-20
3. Grippi MA Distribution of ventilation in pulmonary pathophysiology, Philadelphia, JB Lippincott 1995; 41-5
4. Collins JV, Clarke IJH, McHardy S, Sochranee GM, Grawley J Closing volume in healthy smokers. Br J Dis Chest 1973; 67: 19-24
5. McCartty D, Milic Emili J Closing volume in asymptomatic asthma Am Rev Respir Dis 1973; 107: 559-70
6. Vollmer WM, McCamant LE, Johnson LR, Buist AS Long term reproducibility of tests of small airways function, comparison with spirometry Chest 1990; 98: 303-7
7. Hutcheon M, Griffin P, Levison H, Zamel N Volume of isoflow-A new test in detection of mild abnormalities of lung mechanics Am Rev Respir Dis 1974; 110: 458-65
8. Kulpati DDS, Sharma RK, Chauhan MR A study of small airways function by closing volume and density dependent flow volume curves Ind J Chest Dis Allied Sci 1983; 25: 4-9
9. Gold JG, Aberle DR Functional imaging of the airways J Thoracic Imaging 1979; 29: 29-37
10. Ball WC Jr, Stewart PBM, Newsham LGS, Bates DV Regional pulmonary function studied with Xenon J Clin Invest 1963; 51: 41-47
11. Marion JM, Alderson PO, LeFarak SS, et al Unilateral lung function: Comparison of the lateral position test with radionucleide ventilation-perfusion studies Chest 1976; 69: 5-9
12. Svanberg L Bronchospirometry in the study of regional lung function Scand J Respir Dis 1966; Suppl:62;91-96

8
TESTS FOR GAS EXCHANGE FUNCTION

MOHANKUMAR THEKKINKATTIL

Introduction

The functions of the lungs can be divided into two main groups. The bellows function, concerned with the movement of gas in and out of the alveoli, and the gas exchange function, concerned with the transfer of gas between the alveoli and the capillary blood.

Diffusing Capacity for Carbon Monoxide

The diffusing capacity for carbon monoxide (DLco) is a measure of the ability of gas to transfer from the alveoli across the alveolar epithelium and the capillary endothelium to the RBCs. The DLco depends not only on the area and thickness of the blood-gas barrier but also on the volume of blood in the pulmonary capillaries. The distribution of alveolar volume and ventilation also affects the measurement.

Diffusion capacity measurements

DLco is measured by sampling end-expiratory gas for carbon monoxide (CO) after patients inspire a small amount of CO, hold their breath, and exhale. Measured DLco should be adjusted for alveolar volume (which is estimated from dilution of helium) and the patient's Hct. DLco is reported as mL/min/mm Hg and as a percentage of a predicted value.

Conditions that decrease DLco

Conditions that primarily affect the pulmonary vasculature, such as primary pulmonary hypertension and pulmonary embolism, decrease DLco. Conditions that affect the lung diffusely, such as emphysema and pulmonary fibrosis, decrease both DLco and alveolar ventilation (VA). Reduced DLco also occurs in patients with previous lung resection because total lung volume is smaller, but DLco corrects to or even exceeds normal when adjusted for VA because increased additional vascular surface area is recruited in the remaining lung. Anemic patients have lower DLco values that correct when adjusted for Hb.

Conditions that increase DLco

DLco may be higher than predicted in patients with heart failure, presumably because the increased pulmonary venous and arterial pressure recruits additional pulmonary microvessels. DLco is also increased in patients with erythrocythemia, in part because of increased Hct and because of the vascular recruitment that occurs with increased pulmonary pressures due to increased viscosity. DLco is increased in patients with alveolar hemorrhage because RBCs in the alveolar space can also bind CO. DLco is also increased in patients with asthma. Although this increase is attributed to presumed vascular recruitment, some data suggest it may also be due to growth factor–stimulated neovascularization.

Diffusing Capacity for Oxygen

The measurement of the diffusing capacity (DL) of oxygen (DLO2) is technically so complex that, we have to rely on carbon monoxide to provide an approximation of pulmonary gas diffusion. It is extremely important to stress that the measurement of the diffusing capacity of carbon monoxide (DLco) is not synonymous with the actual pulmonary "diffusing capacity", since DLco is altered by several factors, only one of which is the pulmonary has diffusion from alveolus to blood capillary. The carbon monoxide diffusing capacity can be measured by **steady state technique, or a single breath technique, or re-breathing techniques.**

The basic method consists of having the subject inhale a gas mixture containing 0.3% CO and 2.5% helium in air. The expired gas in analysed, and the time during which the inhaled mixture is in the alveoli is calculated. Thus the rate of uptake of CO is measured, as well as the lung volume at which the uptake takes place. In steady state technique the subject breathes the gas mixture for a variable period of several minutes. In single breath for about 10 sec and then exhales. In the rebreathing technique, the subject rebreathes the gas mixture at a rapid respiratory rate form a bag for about 45 sec. When carefully performed, all the three techniques provide comparable results at similar lung volumes. In clinical practice, the single breath method is simplest to perform and quite reproducible. The steady state method is easier to perform in that little or no co-operation is needed from the subject, and is of special value in patients who are severely breathless and cannot hold the breath. In addition, the method can be applied at any lung volume and during exercise. However, due to difficulties in accurately estimating the alveolar carbon monoxide tension, this method is not often employed.

In normal adult subjects, the DLco at rest is about 30 mL/min/mm Hg with a reproducibility of + 2 ml/min/mm Hg with the single - breath technique. DLco may be altered by a wide variety of physiologic and pathologic changes. It is important to note and stress that an abnormal DLco is not synonymous with a defect in gas diffusion at the alveolar capillary level.

Since the DLco will obviously be affected by the alveolar volume (VA) in which the inhaled gas is distributed, it is useful to express it in terms of the VA, i.e., DLco/VA which is synonymous with KCO, or Krogh's constant for CO. in addition, since the DLco is affected by the amount of haemoglobin in the capillary blood, the DLco should be adjusted for the Hb. an approximate relationship between the diffusing capacity for CO and O2 (DLO2) is given by the relationship: DLo2 = DLco X 1.23.

Selection of a gas dilution method: A laboratory may limit its gas dilution studies to one gas, usually helium or nitrogen. When helium is used, FRC is usually measured by the constant volume equilibrium technique. The advantages of helium are that it is available and the instrumentation needed is not expensive as that for faster nitrogen analyzer. Its disadvantages are that dynamic washout studies are not possible and helium must be supplied in tanks. Nitrogen studies, which can be performed with the same instrumentation, are complementary and provide more information. As the atmosphere is source of nitrogen, there is need for its supply.

Source of error in Gas dilution Methods:

There are five main sources of error in gas dilution studies have been identified:

1. Incomplete mixing of gases in the lungs and spirometer will result in over or under-estimation of equilibrium gas concentration, depending on the method used. This can be partially compensated for by extending the time for equilibrium in patients with obstrucion, or by continuously observing the tracer gas concentration during the test.
2. Technical errors in measuring gas concentrations can reduce accuracy, but careful calibration and maintenance reduce this source of error.
3. Diffusion of gases between the lung and blood can produce an error. This error can be partially controlled by adding correction factors to the calculation.

4. Switching the subject to system must occur at the resting end expiratory level or the valves measured will not be the FRC. Careful attention to the technique will minimize this error.
5. The 'nitrogen lag' effect occurs when the decreasing volume variation of the closed circuit equilibrium method is used, resulting in unequal concentration of tracer gas in the alveoli and spirometer system.

Clinical Value of the Single-Breath Test

It is implemented in routine clinical testing, determination of TLCO by the single-breath technique is simple and fast. When the above-mentioned errors are avoided and patients well instructed, results show acceptable accuracy and good reproducibility. The TLCO parameter does not only react to impairments of diffusion capacity in the sense of gas exchange over the alveolar– capillary membrane, but also to structural changes of lung tissue, independent from their cause, which might be either an increase or a reduction of alveolar space. A reduced TLCO cannot only be found in interstitial lung disease such as pulmonary brosis, sarcoidosis, alveolitis, or lung edema, but also in generalized emphysema, often characterized by loss of lung surface and increase of alveolar space. A normal or moderately reduced TLCO can also be seen in airway obstruction, while an increased TLCO may indicate obstructive hyperination, as attributed to asthma. Intrapulmonary bleeding may lead to elevated TLCO levels. TLCO is well suited for follow-up studies and therapy control and may be used as an additional parameter in the assessment of pulmonary–vascular disorders.

Due to its complexity, application of TLCO in screening may be limited to specialized studies, e.g., in workers exposed to dust. In a variation of the single-breath method using a mixture of CO, inert gas, and oxygen the diffusing capacity of the alveolar–capillary membrane, the so-called membrane component, and the capillary blood volume can be assessed, an application that might be conned to more specialized laboratories.

Additional Methods in Diffusion Assessment

In the recent years, in addition to the classical modality described above, the **IntraBreath method** was introduced, featuring a single deep inhalation but no breath-holding before exhalation, certainly advantageous in children and dyspneic patients. Using fast infrared gas analyzers for continuous reading of low dose CO, (inert) methane, and diffusible acetylene (soluble in blood), the capillary cardiac output can be determined in combination with the TLCO. The test can also be carried out under exercise. Due to its high patient exposure to CO, the previously used steady-state method has been abandoned. In addition to the TLCO test mentioned, a variety of other diffusion modalities exist, in particular those using the rebreathing technique. Nevertheless, their applicability in a regular laboratory and their international recognition might be limited.

Nitrogen dilution method

This is the other commonly used technique for measurement of the static lung volumes. In this method, the subject breathes pure oxygen in an open circuit, i.e., he or she inspires the oxygen and breathes out into room air. During the procedure, the expired nitrogen concentration (FEN2) at the mouth and the expired gas volume (VE) are measured; thus, the total amount of N2 expired is measured. The procedure is continued until the FEN2 is 0.02; this usually requires about 7 minutes in patients with lung disease. The lung volume (VL) is calculated from the formula:

$$VL = \frac{(VE+VDS)\ FE\ N2}{FAI\ N2 - FA2N2}$$

where VDS is the dead space of the apparatus, FAI N2 is the initial alveolar concentration of N2 (assumed to be equivalent to room air), and FA2 N2 is the final alveolar N concentration (assumed to be equal to the final expired N2 concentration). The measurement is mostly made at FRC.

An alternative, simpler technique is to measures the N2 concentration and the expired volume at the mouth following an inhalation of pure oxygen to total lung capacity: the area embraced by the N2 - volume plot is equivalent to the TLC. This method is subject to greater error than the open circuit techniques.

The dilution techniques will measure only those areas of the lung volume accessible to atmospheric gas; thus, a pneumothorax or emphysematous bulla not in contact with or only poorly ventilated by, atmospheric gas will not be measured by these techniques. Patients with severe obstructive lung disease, in whom a difference in static lung volumes can be demonstrated between the plethysmographic and dilutioin techniques, can be truly said to have "trapped gas" in the lungs.

Distribution of Ventilation

In many clinical situations, knowledge of distribution of ventilation in an individual patient is very useful. Two types of tests are available to the clinician: those which give an overall indication of the degree of uniformity of ventilation in the lung, and those which indicate the degree of uniformity of ventilation between specific areas of the lung.

Single-breath nitrogen test

This test is a very sensitive indicator of non-uniformity of distribution of ventilation. The subject takes in a breath of 100% oxygen to TLC: he then exhales at a submaximal rate. The exhaled volume is plotted against the N2 concentration of the exhaled gas at the mouth. The initial exhaled gas contains no N2, since it represents the previously inhaled oxygen which has stayed in the mouth and dead space; this is known as phase I. There is then an increasing N2 concentration (phase 2) as the exhaled gas changes from the dead space gas to alveolar gas. The alveolar gas consists of N2 which was diluted by the inhaled oxygen: Phase 3 indicates the alveolar gas; if the distribution of ventilation relatively uniform, the N2 concentration will be uniform, and the phase 3 tracing will inscribe a plateau. In normal subjects with no abnormalities in the distribution of ventilation, the N2 concentration in phase 2 varies by less than 2.5%L of gas exhaled. At the end of phase 3 in most, but not all, subjects there will be an upward deflection of the N2 concentration - Phase 4. This is believed to be due to the closure of the small airways (less than 2 mm in diameter) in the dependent regions of the lung due to the increased pleural pressure at RV, this results in exhalation of the gas mainly from the upper alveolar regions of the lung, which have a higher concentration of N2 since inhalation of oxygen from RV in the previous breath distributes the oxygen mainly to the lower regions of the lungs.

The single breath N2 test can be used to measure the anatomical dead space, since gas in Phase I and part of phase 2 represent this dead space. The rate of change of the N2 concentration in phase 3 gives an indication of the uniformity of the distribution of ventilation and, in this regard is a very sensitive test. The volume of phase 4 (closing volume) gives an indication of small airways function; the earlier in expiration that the small airways close, the larger the closing volume. The phase 4, or closing volume, is usually expressed as a percent of the vital capacity. Alternatively, the sum of the closing volume and the residual volume (known as the closing capacity) is expressed as a percentage of the TCL. The measurement of closing volume as an indicator of small airway function has not been proved useful, since the test is not very reproducible and there is a wide range in normal subjects.

Nitrogen-Washout Test for Determination of FRC

Widely applied for decades in the English-speaking world, this modality requires a valve and gas delivery system to allow inspiratory switching from air to pure oxygen. With each inhaled breath of oxygen, nitrogen present in the lung, not participating in the gas exchange, will be replaced. Continuous gas sampling at the mouth by either a single N2 or combined O2/CO2 analyzer allows determination of expired nitrogen volume during the N2-washout procedure. Accumulated nitrogen volume is calculated breath by breath until the N2 concentrationfallsbelow1%,marking the end of the washout sequence. Before the start of the washout, the N2 concentration (including rare inert gases) is 79.2%, which allows the functional residual capacity (FRC) to be derived as FRC= VN2 0.79 (l) .

Technical Characteristics of the N2-Washout Method is historically, this method required a fast N2 analyzer or a mass spectrometer, both expensive and demanding in operation and service. Nowadays, with the advent of fast-response combi-analyzers, the complementary gases O2 and CO2 can be determined instead of N2, involving less complex and expensive technology. However, this novel approach makes synchronization of digitized gas samples necessary. As most analyzers draw a side-stream gas sample from the mouth, causing a delay between gas sample and ow, the response characteristic of the analyzer needs adjustment and correction. In a dedicated calibration routine, the operator should be offered verication of the response compensation. The valve systems employed in N2 washout are similar to those used in diffusion testing, compromising hygiene unless a breathing lter is used.

The test duration of FRC determination by N2 washout depends on the lung distribution of the subject, taking a few minutes in a healthy and more than 20min in a severely obstructed individual. While the classical N2-washout devices use side-stream gas sampling, the novel ultrasound molar mass spirometry offers a less complex clinical approach with instantaneous gas analysis. The ultrasound sensor is able to determine both ow and molar mass, the specic weight of the gas, with a single transducer in the main stream of the respired gas. As molar masses of O2 and CO2 are distinctively different, the N2 concentration of the breathing gas can be assessed instantaneously and synchronous to ow and volume changes.

DLNO testing

The European Respiratory Society has just published the first standards for **DLNO testing**. This is a signal that DLNO is moving from a research setting into routine clinical testing. Although it is unlikely that most PFT labs will immediately jump into DLNO testing, the standard is still interesting because of an extensive discussion of DLNO, DLCO, DMCO and VC measurements and physiology. The DLNO standards (and their supplementary material) are open-access and can be downloaded from the European Respiratory Journal.

DLNO is performed in the same manner as a single-breath DLCO and it is specifically recommended that DLCO and DLNO tests be performed simultaneously. There are however, specific test system requirements based both on the properties of NO and on the two types of NO analyzers:

Nitric Oxide reacts with oxygen to form NO2 and at the levels used for DLNO testing (40-60 ppm) does so at a rate of approximately 1.2 ppm per minute. DLNO test gas is therefore usually stored as 400-1200 ppm NO in N2 and mixed into the DLCO test gas mixture (0.3% CO, 21% O2) d"2 min before the DLCO/DLNO test. This would seem to require that the DLCO/DLNO test gas mixture to be held in a reservoir of some kind and to preclude the use of a demand valve but this was not specifically discussed. Because of uncertainties that occur when mixing the DLCO/DLNO gas mixture and in how long the mixture may be held in the reservoir the inspired NO concentration must also be measured immediately before the DLCO/DLNO test is performed.

Breath-holding times of between 4 and 10 seconds have been used in DLNO research. The DLNO standard notes that breath-holding time affects the measurement of DLNO and DLCO, particularly when a ventilation inhomogeneity is present. In particular it was noted that shorter breath-hold times tended to overestimate DLCO and underestimate VA.

The standards for CO and NO analyzer linearity, accuracy and drift are essentially identical to those of the 2017 DLCO standards. The same applies for flow and volume accuracy and the need for daily volume calibrations. Recommendations that differ to one extent or another from the 2017 DLCO standards are: The gas analyzers should be zeroed before each test and the zero should be re-measured after the test. Results should be adjusted for any drift. The inspired NO concentration should be measured just before the test.

A VA measurement check by performing a DLCO/DLNO test using a calibration syringe pulled back to the 1 litre mark is recommended. VA should be between 2.7 and 3.3 litres with the syringe dead space substituted for anatomical dead space. At the same time DLCO should be <0.5 ml/min/mmHg and DLNO should be <3.0 ml/min/mmHg. Hemoglobin correction for DLNO results is not recommended but corrections in DLCO for hemoglobin and COHb remain the same.

Patient preparation and the DLNO testing manoeuvre is identical to that of the DLCO. Measuring the breath-holding period using the Jones-Meade approach is recommended. Washout and alveolar volumes are also the same as for DLCO testing. Intra-session and inter-session repeatability and reproducibility for DLCO appears to be slightly less stringent than for the 2017 DLCO standards but this may be partly due to the range of acceptable breath-holding times (5-10 seconds) for DLNO testing. Roughton and Forster's work on DLCO in the 1950's showed that diffusing capacity was a series resistance with a membrane component and a blood component:Where: DMCO = alveolar-capillary membrane conductance , Vc = pulmonary capillary blood volume, CO = rate at which CO is taken up by red blood cells

Early work showed that in normal subjects DLNO is approximately 5 times larger than DLCO. This is partly due to the fact that the difference in tissue diffusivity of NO is 1.97 times that of CO and because the reaction rate of NO with hemoglobin is approximately 1500 times faster than CO. In addition because NO does not compete for O2 binding sites on hemoglobin NO uptake is mostly independent of FiO2. In a sense DLNO is not excessively high, DLCO is low mostly because CO uptake is highly dependent on the pulmonary capillary blood volume and the alveolar oxygen concentration. NO uptake is however, more dependent than CO uptake is on alveolar surface area and lung volume.

Clinically DLNO is primarily related to membrane conductance and DLCO is primarily related to Vc. For this reason, the most common way of expressing the differences in these measurements for a given individual is the DLNO/DLCO ratio. Decreases in the DLNO/DLCO ratio tend to correlate with decreases in membrane conductance and/or increases in pulmonary capillary blood volume whereas increases in the DLNO/DLCO ratio correlate with increases in membrane conductance and/or decreases in pulmonary capillary blood volume.

In the early stages of COPD the DLNO/DLCO ratio has been shown to rise, while in established COPD the ratio appears relatively normal (although both DLNO and DLCO are reduced). In Cystic Fibrosis the DLNO/DLCO ratio is reduced. A reduced DLNO/DLCO ratio has also been shown in Sarcoidosis. Elevated DLNO/DLCO ratios have been found in hepato-pulmonary syndrome and heart failure.

In many ways the clinical use of DLNO and the DLNO/DLCO ratio is still in its early stages and comparison between different studies is made more difficult because different DLNO measurement techniques have often been used.

LCI (Lung clearance index)

What is the LCI and how is it measured?

When lung tissue and airways are normal, inhaled gas is distributed evenly throughout the lung and the mixing and turnover of alveolar gas is relatively rapid. When airway obstruction is present gas distribution tends to becomes more uneven and the mixing and turnover takes longer. The Lung Clearance Index (LCI) is a way to measure these ventilation inhomogeneities and is basically a description of how much ventilation is required to completely clear the FRC. It was first described by Margaret Becklake in 1952 but has languished for many years. It has been revived in the last decade or so, particularly because it requires only tidal breathing which allows it to be measured in infants and children.The measurement process is called **an Inert Gas Multi-Breath Washout.** It uses an open circuit and requires a tracer gas that is both inert and relatively insoluble and for these reasons has been primarily limited to helium, nitrogen and sulphur hexafluoride (SF6) although methane and argon could potentially be used as well.

At the start of the test, the tracer gas must be well distributed throughout the lung which means that for all gases except nitrogen there needs to be a wash-in period (although there of course needs to be a prolonged period of room air breathing between nitrogen washout tests).

The tracer gas mixture is breathed until 30 or 60 seconds after the inspiratory and expiratory concentrations have equalized (ERS/ATS statement says 5 minutes for adults and 4 minutes for children). The patient is then detached from the tracer gas source at end-exhalation and the washout period begins (mechanically, this process is reversed for N2 washout since wash-in occurs while breathing room air and the patient needs to breath 100% oxygen during the washout period). With each succeeding tidal breath, the tracer gas is leaves the lung. Exhaled volume is accumulated and the test continues until the exhaled gas concentration is 1/40th the initial concentration for three consecutive tidal breaths. The exhaled tracer gas volume is integrated from the flow and gas analyser signals and FRC is calculated from: where: trace = fractional concentration of tracer gas. And the Lung Clearance Index is then calculated from: The Cumulative Exhaled Volume is expressed as litres, BTPS and corrected for system dead space.

FRC tends to be lower when measured with SF6 than with N2. This is likely due to the fact that SF6 must be washed-in before it is washed-out and it may not completely equilibrate with the poorly ventilated parts of the lung. Despite this there doesn't seem to be a particularly significant difference in LCI values based on which gas is used.

LCI testing may take a prolonged period of time and this is partly because both the wash-in and the wash-out periods require at least 5 minutes each but also because the LCI test should be performed several times in order to ensure that repeatable results have been obtained. Given the length of time that patients are on a mouthpiece leaks are a potential problem and for this reason it is recommended that results with an FRC 10% greater than the mean should be discarded.

Theoretically the LCI could be measured by any test system that is able to perform N2 washout lung volumes. Despite the fact that both types of testing measure FRC the maneuvers are not the same however, and the software requirements are substantially different. At the present time there are no commercial test systems that are able to measure the LCI although this may change since the ERS/ATS released guidelines in 2013 that specifically addressed the technical and software requirements for LCI measurements (and if you read between the lines on their websites a couple of manufacturers are at least considering adding the LCI to their test systems).

The FEV1 and the FEV1/FVC ratio have been the primary focus for the detection and monitoring of airway obstruction for decades. This is in part understandable since the Forced Vital Capacity is a relatively simple and repeatable test that requires minimal equipment. Spirometry is not sensitive to all forms of airway obstruction and it has become evident in a variety of lung diseases that changes (or the lack of changes) in FEV1 does not match either disease progression or status. Ventilation inhomogeneity may be one of the missing pieces in this puzzle and as such, the LCI deserves more extensive research in a wider variety of lung diseases and age groups.

REFERENCES

1. Cotes JE, Lung Function: Assessment and application in medicine, 4 Ed. Oxford Blackwell, 1979.
2. Beclake MR A new index of intrapulmonary mixture of inspired air. Thorax 1952; 7:111-116
3. Hughs, JMB, Pulmonary gas exchange. Clin Sci 1980:58: 119
4. McHardy, GJR, Diffusing capacity and pulmonary gas exchange. Brit J.Dis. Chest 1972: 66:1'
5. Lipscombe, M. Patel, K, Hughs JMB, Interpretation of increases in the transfer coefficient for carbon monoxide (TLCO X VA of KCO) Thorax 1978:32: 728.
6. Weinberger SE, Jonson TS, Weiss ST, Use and interpretation of the single breath diffusing capacity, Chest 1980: 78; 483
7. Wanner A, Interpretation of pulmonary function test. In Sackner MA (ed): Diagnostic techniques in pulmonary disease, New York, Marcel Dekkel; 1980: p353.
8. Buist AS, Ross B, Predicted valves for closing volumes using a modified single breath nitrogen test, Am. Rev. Res. Dis. 107: 744: 1973.
9. Shankar PS, Chest Medicine, New Delhi 4th Edn. New Delhi Oxford & IBH Publications, 1994: 18.
10. Jain SK, spirometry, the need for standardization, Ind J Chest Dis & All Sci 1987: 29: 185.
11. McCarthy, Spencer R, Green R, Milic Emily, Measurements of 'closing volume' as a single and sensitive test for early detection of small airway disease. Am J. Med 1972: 52: 747-753.
12. Buist AS, vollmer WM, Johnson R, McCarrant LE, Does the single breath Nitrogen test identify the smoker who will develop chronic airflow obstruction? Am Rev Res Dis 1988: 127: 293-308.
13. Zavorsky GS, Hsia CCW, Hughes JMB, Borland CDR, Guenard H, van der Lee I, Steenbruggen I, Naeije R, Cao J, Dinh-Xuan AT. Standardisation and application of the single-breath determination of nitric oxide uptake in the lung. Eur Respir J 2017; 49: 1600-962.
14. A] Aurora P, Gustafsson P, Bush A, Lindbla A, Oliver C, Wallis CE, Stocks J. Multiple breath inert gas washout as a measure of ventilation distribution in children with cystic fibrosis. Thorax 2004; 59: 1068-1073.
15. Becklake MR. A new index of the intrapulmonary mixture of inspired air. Thorax 1952; 7: 111-116.
16. Fuchs SI, Buess C, Lum S, Kozlowska W, Stocks J, Gappa M. Multiple breath washout with a side stream ultrasonic flow sensor and mass spectrometry. A comparative study. Pediatric Pulmonology 2006; 41: 1218-1225.

17. Gustafsson PM, Aurora P, Lindblad A. Evaluation of ventilation maldistribution as an early indicator of lung disease in children with cystic fibrosis. Eur Respir J 2003; 22: 972-979.

18. Gustafsson PM, De Jong PA, Tiddens HAWN, Lindblad A. Multiple-breath inert gas washout and spirometry versus structural lung disease in cystic fibrosis. Thorax 2008; 63(2): 129-134.

19. Horsley AR, Gustafsson PM, Macleod KA, Saunders C, Greening AP, Porteous DJ, Davies JC, Cunningham S, Alton EWFW, Innes JA. Lung clearance index is a sensitive, repeatable and practical measurement of airways disease in adults with cystic fibrosis. Thorax 2008; 63(2): 135-140.

20. Jensen R, Stanojevic S, Gibney K, Slazar JG, Gustafsson P, Subbarjo P, Ratjen F. Multiple breath nitrogen washout: a feasibile alternative to mass spectrometry. PLOS One 2013; 8(2): e56868.

21. Lum S et al. Early detection of cystic fibrosis lung disease: multiple-breath washout versus raised volume tests. Thorax 2007; 62: 341-347.

22. Lum S Et al. Age and height dependence of lung clearance index and functional residual capacity. Eur Respir J 2013; 41: 1371-1377.

23. Maclead KA, Horsley AR, Bell NJ, Greening AP, Innes JA. Ventilation heterogeneity in children with well controlled asthma with normal spirometry indicates residual airways disease. Thorax 2009; 64: 33-37.

24. Robinson PD et al. ERS/ATS Consensus Statement: Consensus statement for inert gas washout measurement using multiple- and single-breath tests. Eur Respir J 2013; 41: 507-522.

25. Rowan SA et al. Lung Clearance Index is a repeatable and sensitive indicator of radiological changes in bronchiectasis. Am J Resp Crit Care Med 2014; 189: 586-592.

26. Singer F, Houltz B, Latzin P, Robinson P, Gustafsson P. A realistic validation study of a new nitrogen multiple breath washout system. Plos One 2012; 7(4): e36083.

27. Verbanck S, Paiva M, Schuermans D, Hanon S, Vincken W, Van Muylem A. Relationship between the lung clearance index and conductive and acinar ventilation heterogeneity. J Appl Physiol 2012; 112: 782-790.

9
TESTS FOR SMALL AIRWAYS FUNCTION

AJIT VIGG

Definition

Small airways refer to those airways less than 2mm in diameter. These occur from generation 8 and include a portion of both conducting airways and acinar airways. (1)

Special features

Characteristically they lack cartiliginous support and lack mucous glands. They are lined by surfactant which reduces surface tension and helps prevent their closure during expiration and at low lung volumes. The airflow is laminar and independent of gas density whereas in larger airways it is high velocity air flow which is turbulent and density dependent. The airway resistance in small airways is low in health (10-25%of total airways resistance) and is significantly increased in disease and is largely independent of lung volume; whereas the large airways resistance is altered significantly with change in lung volumes. This allows equitable ventilation of lung units at low airflow resistance and with minimal work of breathing. (2) Typically there is a disconnect between the histologic presence of small airways inflammation and the diagnosis of small airways disease (SAD).

Diseases associated with small airways obstruction

Asthma and COPD are the two major disorders studied widely. (2, 3). However several diseases which cause acute and chronic inflammation and infiltrate the airways are associated with small airways dysfunction (3) such as;

- Hypersensitivity pneumonitis
- Sarcoidosis
- Respiratory bronchiolitis interstitial lung disease
- Microcarcinoid tumourlets
- Follicular bronchiolitis
- Sjogren's syndrome

Clinical Classification of SAD

1) Bronchiolar involvement in bronchial disease (4)
   Asthma, bronchiectasis, cystic fibrosis, aspiration pneumonia and bronchial obstruction.
2) Bronchiolar involvement in parenchymal lung disease (5)
   Bronchopneumonia, eosinophilic pneumonia, cryptogenic organizing pneumonia(BOOP), extrinsic allergic alveolitis and Langerhans cell histiocytosis.
3) Disorders in which bronchiolitis is the predominant abnormality (4)
   Follicular bronchiolitis, respiratory bronchiolitis, diffuse panbronchiolitis, mineral dust bronchiolitis and constrictive obliterative bronchiolitis.

Drugs associated with SAD

1. Penicillamine
2. Gold
3. Methotrexate
4. Busulfan

Functional impact of inflammatory changes in small airways

- Mucous/fibrosis - physical obstruction
- Epithelial hyperplasia, squamous and goblet metaplasia - luminal clearance
- Cellular inflammation - oedema of airway wall
- Smooth muscle - spasm/constriction
- Scar - disrupted airflow dynamics.

Physiological assessment of small airways (6)

FEV1 mostly reflects large airways obstruction and a significant degree of small airways disease must be present before FEV1 becomes abnormal. Forced Expiratory Flow between 25 and 75 percent of FVC (FEF-25-75) is one of the most commonly used measurement of SAD. However, it is dependent on FVC and hence changes in FVC will affect the portion of flow-volume curve examined. If FEF25-75 is not adjusted for lung volume, there is poor reproducibility. Another disadvantage is the low sensitivity of this parameter, as it is frequently normal if FEV1/FVC ratio is more than 75 percent (7). The FEV3 to FVC ratio has been suggested as an alternative measure of SAD. The fraction of air not expired in the first 3 sec (1-FEV3/FVC) is also a useful measure of SAD. As FEV1/FVC falls the FEV3/ FVC also falls and the 1-FEV3/FVC rises. These measures have a better accuracy than FEF25-75 in assessment of SAD (8).

Plethysmography

Plethysmographic assessment of lung volumes provides a sensitive measure of gas trapping and lung hyperinflation. Hyperinflation is defined as an abnormal elevation of lung volumes at end expiration. It is a function of airflow limitation, lung elastic recoil and chest wall compliance. Residual volume (RV) is an important measure of SAD and may be raised before the onset of abnormal spirometry in asthma. The RV correlates with the degree of inflammatory changes in in small airways in COPD and with peripheral airway resistance in asthma. The RV/TLC ratio is a useful marker of gas trapping and is higher in patients with severe asthma compared to nonsevere asthma and correlates inversely with FVC. However, the upper limit of normal value varies with age and sex and hence predicted value may be a better measure of gas trapping than the absolute value (8).

Airways resistance (Raw) can be measured by assessing pressure and flow at mouth during body plethysmography. However, it is not specific for SAD which limits its application in diagnosing and monitoring distal airways dysfunction.

Impulse oscillometry (IOS) (9)

This involves application of oscillating pressure variations in the form of random noise to respiratory system in order to determine mechanical properties of lung. Multiple frequencies between 3 and 20 Hz are applied over normal tidal breathing from a loudspeaker. The resulting pressure and flow changes are measured at the mouth and analyzed in a Fourier transformation to determine the impedence (Z) of the respiratory system. Higher frequency signals (more than 15 HZ) are absorbed by the respiratory system before reaching the small airways and hence reflects large airway pathology. Low frequencies (5Hz) penetrate deep into the lung & therefore represent the whole lung.

The contribution of distal airways can be determined by the difference between R5 and R20 and thus give insight into SAD. IOS allows for discrimination of inspiratory and expiratory resistance and reactance. Inspiratory minus expiratory reactance at 5 Hz (delta X5) has been shown to discriminate between asthma and COPD. Additionally, it has been shown to be a sensitive noninvasive method of detecting Expiratory flow limitation (EFL) in COPD. Expiratory reactance falls when EFL is present as the pressure signals cannot pass through the obstructed small airways; this is due to enhanced collapsibility of airways in expiration and is a major factor in development of dynamic hyperinflation.

IOS is simple to use and is effort independent. It provides continuous measurement of pulmonary mechanics with high temporal resolution allowing intra-breath analysis. It does not rely on forced maneuvers and hence more suitable for children and patients with severe lung diseases.

Inert Gas Washout

Both single breath nitrogen washout and multiple breath nitrogen washout techniques can be used in assessment of SAD. However, it is not specific to small airways pathology (10).

Exhaled nitric oxide (FENO) (11)

This has been used extensively in asthma clinical research and practice. Central airways appear to be the major site of production of NO in asthma both in stable state and during exacerbations. However, results of studies assessing impact of measuring FENO have been mixed. Meta analyses of several large studies suggest no overall benefit to asthma control and quality of life. Role of FENO in COPD is less clear. An inverse correlation with FEV1, transfer factor and oxygen saturation has been reported.

Radiographic features of small airways disease

Volumetric CT scans with thin sections (0.75-1.25 mm) allow multiplanar coronal or sagittal reconstructions with maximum intensity projection(MIP) and minimum intensity projection images. The spatial resolution on a CT scan is 0.6-1.0 mm which allows direct assessment of medium sized airways (2-2.5mm) but not of smaller airways. SAD may show direct or indirect signs on a CT scan (12).

- Direct signs: thickened peripheral airways, well defined centrilobular branching nodules.
- Indirect signs: many of these are non-specific and include: - Air trapping, subsegmental atelectasis, mosaic attenuation, centrilobular nodules and tree-in-bud changes. Differentiation of air trapping from patchy areas of ground glass attenuation can be very challenging (13).

High resolution CT

High Resolution CT Scan in SAD shows most commonly gas trapping which is seen as areas of low attenuation distal to the site of obstruction. Mosaic attenuation reflects localized areas of gas trapping and suggests heterogenous distribution of airways disease. However gas trapping is best assessed on expiratory scans and may provide an indirect measure of small airways function. Comparing the mean lung density between expiratory and inspiratory CT provides a quantitative measure called MLD E/I . In asthma, MLD E/I correlate strongly with FEV1, FEV1/FVC ratio, FEF 25-75 and RV/TLC. The assessment of gas trapping in COPD is more complicated as both SAD and emphysema give rise to low attenuation areas. MLD E/I correlate with lung function measures of gas trapping. Several studies have shown that SAD contributes more strongly than emphysema to severity of COPD. MLD E/I also correlate with inflammatory changes measured by sputum neutrophils, adding further support to the inflammatory nature of SAD in COPD (14,15).

Hyperpolarised helium magnetic resonance imaging (He MRI)

It allows for the assessment of distribution of ventilation and morphometry of distal airways and lung parenchyma without exposure to ionising radiation. Quantification of regional ventilation can be achieved by both static and dynamic assessment of helium distribution. It is a useful tool for assessing airways disease with heterogenous pattern. The technique is still largely restricted to research applications and its role in clinical management of SAD is not clear yet (16).

Nuclear Medicine Techniques

- Two dimensional gamma scintigraphy (17).
- Single photon emission computed tomography (SPECT) (18).
- Positron emission tomography (PET) (19).

These are likely to be an area of exciting research in the assessment of SAD but have not become widely available because of the high cost and non-availability of radio isotopes in routine clinical practice.

Conclusions

An understanding of the role of of small airways in COPD and asthma is increasingly important as it becomes necessary to distinguish individual phenotypes of the diseases. This will lead to more tailored approach to assessment of patients with asthma and COPD specifically and various other small airways diseases generally.

REFERENCES

1) Weibel ER, Sapoval B, Filoche M et al. Design of peripheral airways for efficient gas exchange. Respir Physiol Neurobiol.2005; 148: 3-21

2) Hamid Q. Pathogenesis of small airways in asthma. Respir Int Rev Thoracic Dis. 2012; 84: 4-11

3) Hogg JC. Pathophysiology of airflow limitation in chronic obstructive airways disease. Lancet.2004; 364:709-21.

4) Verbanck S , Schuermans D, Meysman M etal. Noninvasive assessment of airway qalterations in smokers: the small airways revisited. Am J Respir Crit Care Med. 2004; 170: 414-9.

5) Burgel PR Bourdin A, Chanez P et al. Update on the role of distal airways in COPD. Eur Respir Rev. 2011; 20: 7-22.

6) Verbanck S. Physiological measurement of small airways . Respiration. 2012; 84:177-88.

7) Gelb AF, Williams AJ, Zamel N. Spirometry : FEV1 vs FEF 25-75 percent. Chest. 1983; 84: 473-4.

8) Pride NB. Tests of forced expiration and inspiration. Clin Chest Med. 2001; 22: 599-622.

9) Hira H, Munjal J, Zachariah S, etal. The site of airway obstruction in patients with emphysema: role of impulse oscillometry. Lung India. 2008; 25: 8-13.

10) Robinson PD , Goldman MD, Gustafsson PM. Inert gas washout: theoretical background and clinical utility in respiratory diseases. Respiration. 2009; 78: 399-55 . (11). Barnes P J ,Dweik RA, Gelb AF et al. Exhaled nitric oxide in pulmonary diseases: a comprehensive review. Chest 2010; 138: 682-92

12) Malani Y, Wong JC, de Jong PA et al. Prediction of small airway dimensions using computed tomography. Am J Respir Crit Care Med. 2005; 171: 142-6.

13) Hartley R, Barker B, Edwards K et al. Quantitative CT in COPD: emphysema and small airways disease independently contribute to Fev1. Eur Respr J. 2013; 42: P 2269.

14) Rossi SE, Franquet T, Volpacchio M et al. Radiographics.2005; 25:789-801.

15) Teel GS, Engeler CE, Tashijian JH et al. Imaging of small airways disease. Radiographics.1996; 16: 27-41.

10
TESTS FOR AIRFLOW

J C SURI

Introduction

Measurements of airflow provide an easy assessment of movement of air into and out of the lungs and this basic lung function test is conducted with the help of a spirometer. The yardsticks of this measurement are volume, time and flow of air during inspiration and expiration manoeuvres. Spirometry, as a measure of general respiratory health, is comparable to sphygmomanometry for assessment of cardiovascular status. It is fairly objective, non-invasive, sensitive, reproducible and can be put to use in the out-patient department, laboratory as well as workplace and field settings.

Indications for spirometry testing

The volume and flow of air movement into and out of the lungs is recorded by electronically driven computerized spirometer systems. The various indications for spirometry are enlisted in Table-1

Table 1: Indications for spirometry

Diagnostic

Evaluation of symptoms, signs or abnormal laboratory tests

Measurement of effect of disease on pulmonary function

Screening of individuals oat risk of pulmonary disease

Pre-operative evaluation

Monitoring

Assessment of any therapeutic intervention

Follow up of disease course affecting lung function

Follow up of population exposed to risk of obnoxious/ injurious substance

Follow up of drug reactions with lung texicity

Evaluation of disability / impairment

Rehabilitation programmes

Legal requirements

Insurance purposes

Public health programme

Epidemiologic survey

Clinical research

Determination of reference values

Industrial health program/ pre-employment status

Measured parameters

Measured parameters from Flow Volume graphic format (Fig 1a, b &c)

1. FVC (forced Vital capacity): The maximal volume of air exhaled with maximally forced effort from a maximal inspiration, i.e. vital capacity performed with a maximally forced expiratory effort, expressed in liters.
2. FEV_1 (forced expiratory volume in one second): the maximal volume of air exhaled in the first second of a forced expiration from a position of full inspiration

3. FEV_1/FVC ratio: the fractional percentage of FVC delivered in one second

4. $FEF_{25-75\%}$ (mean forced expiratory flow between 25% and 75% of the FVC): also known as maximum mid-expiratory flow. It is the forced expiratory flow rate during the mid-portion of the curve of FVC with effort-independent portion of the curve. It is obtained from the blow with the largest sum of FEV_1 and FVC and is dependent on the validity of the FVC measurement and the level of expiratory effort.

5. $FEF_{200-1200}$: The forced expiratory flow rate during the 1-liter volume from 200 to 1200 ml below total lung capacity (TLC) expressed in litres per minute. It correlates with the effort dependent portion of the curve and incorporates the peak flow rates.

$FIF_{200-1200}$: The forced inspiratory rate during the one litre volume portion of the inspired curve from 200 to 1200 ml above residual volume (RV)

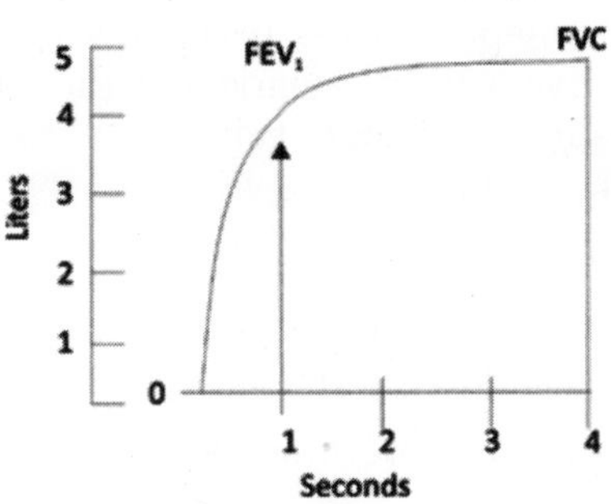

Fig 1a. Volume Time format-FEV1 and FVC in a normal subject

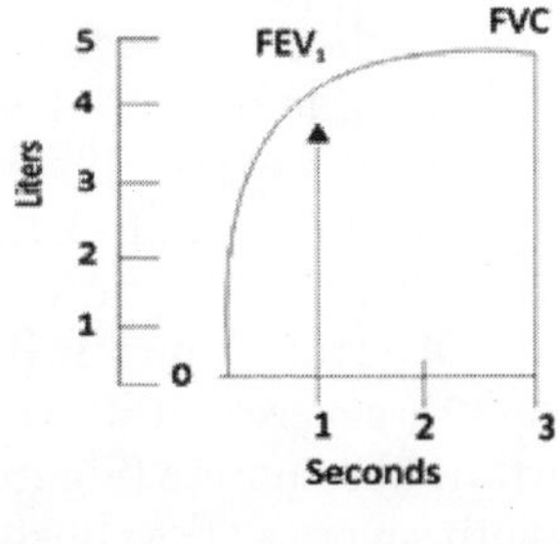

Fig 1b. Restrictive lung disease

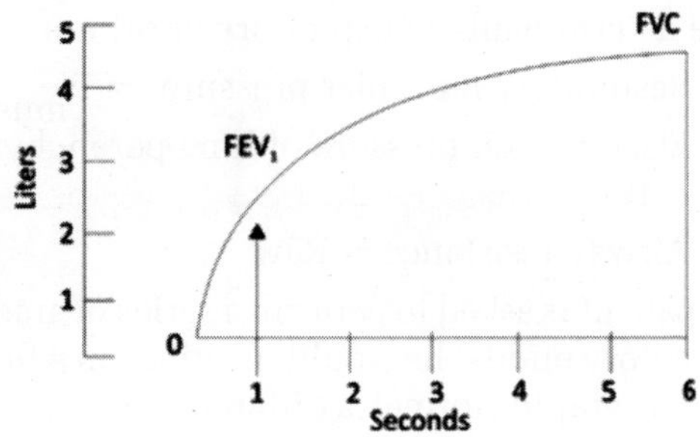

Fig. 1c. Obstructive lung disease

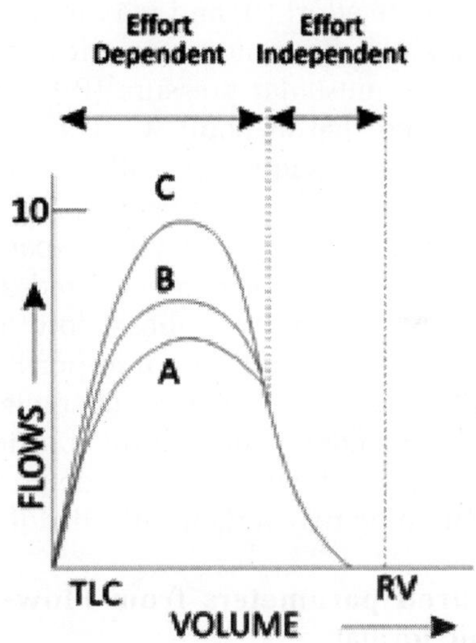

Fig 2. Flow Volume Curve

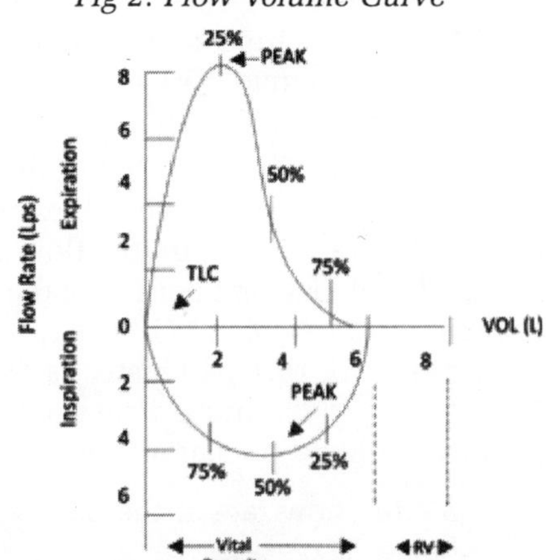

Fig 3: Expression of Expiratory and inspiratory flow

Impact of effort on flow-volume graphic format (Fig-3)

The determinants of expiratory effort are

a) Respiratory muscular pressure = P_{mus}

b) Elastic recoil pressure of lung parenchyma = Pel

c) Airway resistance = Raw

If a patient is asked to perform a series of graded expiratory efforts, he would inscribe, on a flow-volume graphic format, a different flow-volume relationship for each effort. Fig.2. shows the different curves-minimal effort (A), intermediate effort (B) and maximal effort (C). The maximal flow increases with increasing respiratory muscular pressure (P_{mus}). It may be observed that at point X, all three curves merge and subsequently follow a common pathway to residual volume (RV). At high lung volumes (the top 25% of vital capacity), the flow-volume curve is characterized as effort-dependent. During this phase flow increases with increasing effort. The mid-portion of the flow-volume curve has been characterized as effort-independent, since in this portion effort (P_{mus}) has no effect and flow is determined by the remaining two variables (V=Pel/Raw)

Measured parameters from Flow-volume graphic format

This format records every instantaneous expiratory flow rate from total lung capacity (TLC) to residual volume (RV), and inspiratory flow rate from RV back to TLC.

1. Peak expiratory flow (PEF): the maximal flow that can be exhaled when blowing out at a steady rate. Peak expiratory flow occurs in the effort-dependent portion of the curve within 20-25% of TLC; the primary determinant of this parameter is $P_{(mus)}$. This format permits immediate and reliable identification of flow parameter.
2. V_{max}25: the flow rate at the 25% volume point below TLC
3. V_{max}25: the flow rate at the 50% volume point below TLC. It occurs in the effort-independent point below TLC
4. V_{max}75: the flow rate at the 75% volume point below TLC
5. Peak inspiratory flow (PIF): the maximal flow rate that can be inhaled when breathing in at a steady state. PIF is less than PEF and occurs in the mid-portion of the inspiratory limb of flow-volume curve.
6. Inspiratory vital capacity (IVC): the maximum amount of air that can be inhaled after a full expiration.

The graphic formats namely flow-volume, loop and volume – time curve are of seminal importance in interpretation of spirometry report. Evaluation of patient's effort and other subtle features of disease is not possible without the graphic format.

Obstructive pattern

Obstructive pattern of airflow is characterized by expiratory flow limitation. A decrease in airway calibre resulting from smooth muscle contraction, inflammation, mucus plugging or airway collapse results in airflow limitation. Obstructive pattern is marked by the following changes in spirometery values

a) Reduced FEV1

b) Normal (or reduced) VC

c) Normal or reduced FVC

d) Reduced FEV1/FVC ratio

e) Concave flow-volume loop

Expiratory flow limitation

A fixed value of FEV_1 predicted is used to define normal values, with 80% predicted being the lower limit. Any value of FEV_1 less than 80% of predicted normal suggests obstructive lung disease (Fig 1-C). Any patient with post-bronchodilator FEV1/FVC ratio of < 0.7 with $\geq$80% FEV_1 predicted has mild, 50-79% moderate, 30-49% severe and <30% very severe degree of airflow obstruction (Figures 4 a, b and c). Patients with severe airflow obstruction may demonstrate the typical "dog leg" pattern of expiratory limb of flow-volume curve (Fig 4-c) with relatively high flow maintained for the first 15-25% of expired volume and abrupt fall to very low flow rates through the remaining part of the breath. Such a pattern represents the onset of marked dynamic compression of intrathoracic airways and it is less pronounced in an expiratory manoeuvre that has not been made forcibly.

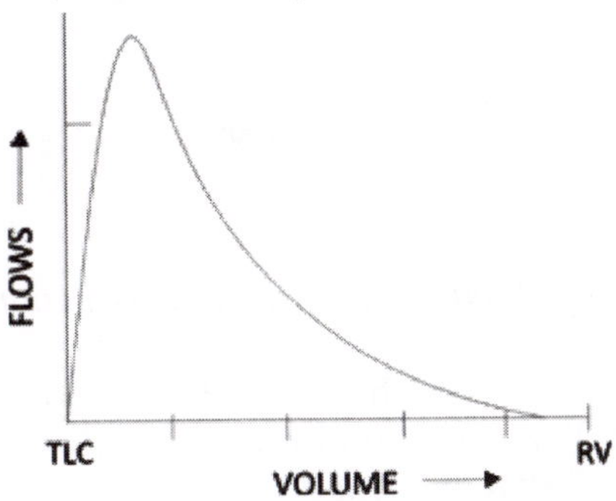

Fig 4a. Mild Obstructive disease

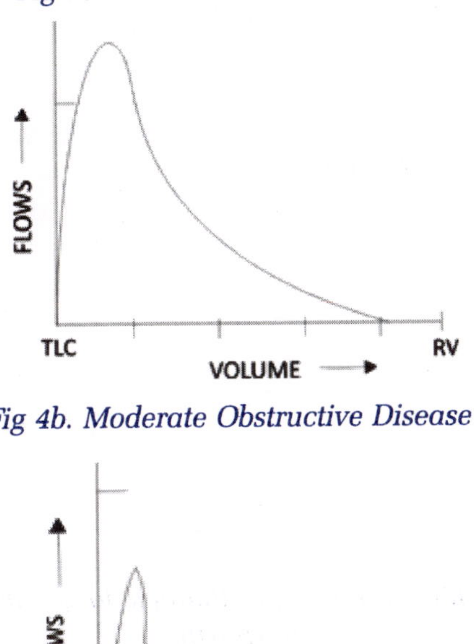

Fig 4b. Moderate Obstructive Disease

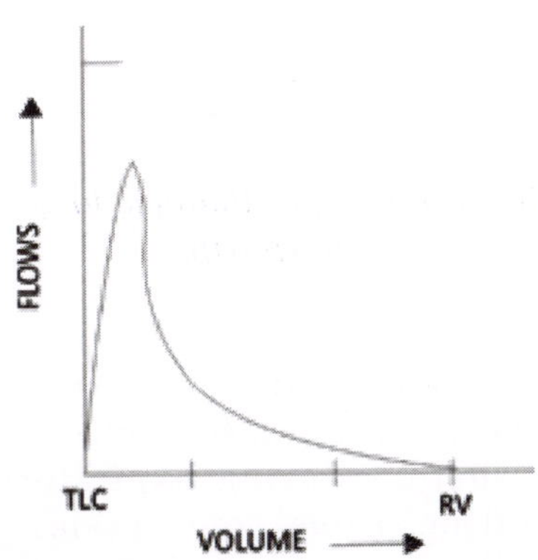

Fig 4c. Expiratory portion of Flow Volume loop showing severe obstructive disease

Table 1: obstructive Lung disease-severity staging

Severity	%FEV1
Normal	$\geq$ 80
Mild	50-79
Moderate	30-49
Severe	<30

Small airways obstruction

Small airways contribute nearly 33% of total airway resistance and are <2mm in diameter. They lack cartilaginous support and depend on elastic lung recoil for their patency. The recoil pressure decreases with decreasing lung volume, the resistance of small airways increases relative to that of the central airways during the terminal part of forced expiratory maneuver. Therefore, small airways diseases can be suspected if FEV_1 and FEF_{max} are normal, whereas measurements obtained at low lung volume are abnormally reduced. The $FEF_{25-75\%}$ has been recommended as a good way to identify small airways disease though measurement obtained entirely from the terminal part of expiration such as $FEF_{75\%}$ or $FEF_{75-85\%}$ should be more sensitive. However, the latter are difficult valves to obtain. Fig 5 shows the "slow tail" appearance of early small airway obstruction.

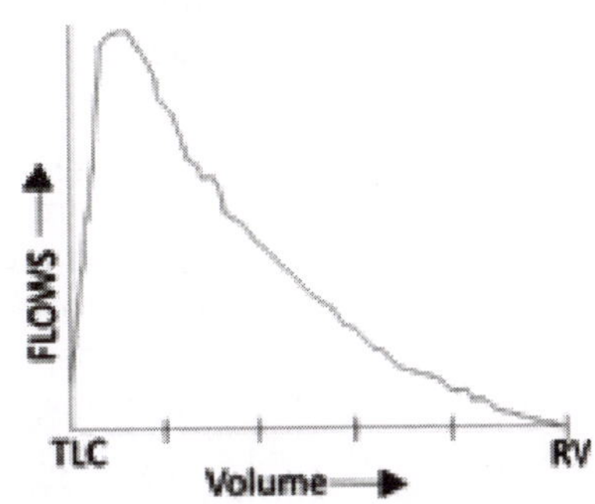

Fig 5. Early disease of small airways

Response to bronchodilators

Airflow-limitation reversibility with drug administration is commonly undertaken as part of spirometry. In case the aim is to determine whether there is any evidence of reversible airflow limitation, short-acting inhaled bronchodilator should not be used within 4 hours of testing and long acting -agonist bronchodilators stopped 12 hours prior to the test. The subject has three acceptable tests of FEV_1, FVC and PEF recorded. Four doses (100 micrograms each) of salbutamol are delivered at 30 second intervals.

Three additional acceptance tests are recorded $\geq$ 10 minutes and upto 15 minutes later. A positive response to bronchodilators is usually defined as an increase in 12% and 200 ml in the values of FEV1 or FVC and is termed as reversible airway disease.

Major airway obstruction

The portion of airway extending from oropharynx to the carina can be termed as major airways. Changes in the shape of flow-volume loop graphic can serve as pointers of major airway lesion. Determinants of the change in shape include the following factors

(a) Variability in luminal diameter during inspiration and expiration (variable vs. fixed)

(b) Location of the lesion (extrathoracic vs intrathoracic). Three distinct patterns of flow-volume loops can be identified

(c) Fixed obstruction at any site in the major airway e.g. "napkin-ring" cancer of the trachea or fixed, paralysed vocal cords. The airway lumen is not affected by changes in pressure between inspiration and expiration. A similar decrease in inspiratory and expiratory flow rates occurs irrespective of whether the narrowed airway segment is intra-thoracic or extra-thoracic. After the initial flow there is a rapid decrease in flow resulting in a uniformly decreased flow rate from TLC to RV and back, resulting in a "squared off" flow volume loop (Fig 6a)

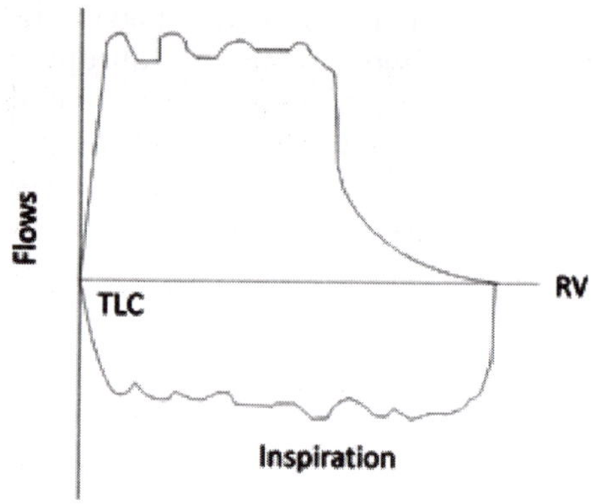

Fig 6a. Fixed upper airways obstruction

(d) Variable extrathoracic obstruction (e.g. paralysed but mobile vocal cords and subglottic stenosis) will have worse obstruction during inspiration than expiration. This results from a negative intraluminal pressure during inspiration relative to atmospheric pressure. There is a significant inspiratory reduction in flow-volume loop as compared to the expiratory limb (Fig 6-b).

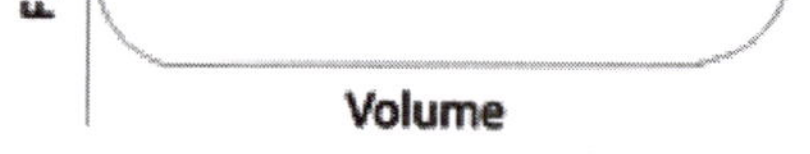

Fig 6b. Variable extra thoracic large airway narrowing

(e) Variable intrathoracic obstruction (e.g. compressible tracheal tumors and tracheomalacia) causes worsened airflow obstruction during expiratory phase resulting from compression of the intrathoracic airway during expiration. There is little impact on the inspiratory flow because pleural pressure and the lumen distend (Fig 6.c). Changes in the ratio of expiratory to inspiratory flow at 50% of the vital capacity (FEF_{50}/FIF_{50}) are observed most noticeably in cases of variable extra-thoracic lesions.

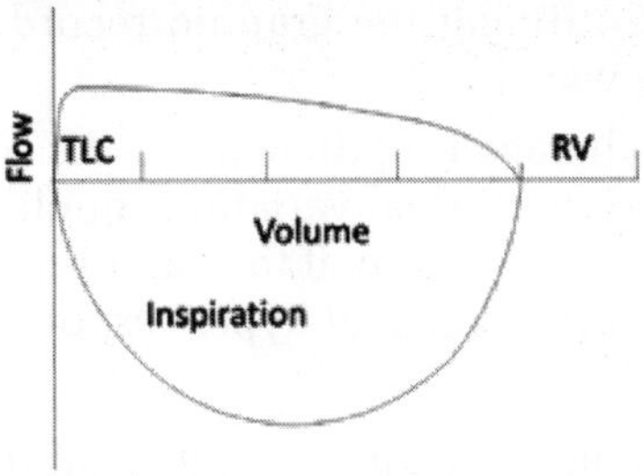

Fig 6c. Variable intrathoracic tracheal narrowing

Maximum voluntary ventilation (MVV)

During this manoeuvre one breathes as fast and as hard as possible for 10-15 seconds. The value is extrapolated to 60 seconds and measured in liters per minute. A variety of conditions can result in a fall in MVV. These include obstructive and restrictive diseases, neuromuscular disease, cardio-vascular disease as well as a poor effort on the part of the patient. MVV is often useful during pre-operative evaluation.

Air trapping

The difference between values of slow vital capacity (SVC) and forced vital capacity (FVC) is often referred to as volume of trapped air or "air trapping". Normal value of this volume of air should not exceed 250 ml. Conditions like advanced emphysema are associated with increase in airflow resistance through intrathoracic airways and loss of lung elastic recoil. Such a phenomenon leads to dynamic compression of airways due to expiratory flow limitation, which ultimately leads to increase volume of air trapping. Under such conditions the more forced the expiration, the less the volume expired and greater the degree of air trapping.

Interpretation by Gestalt approach

A predicted normal flow volume loop is superimposed over the measurement graphic. One glance at the area under the predicted curve when compared to that under the measured graphic helps in analysis. The predicted normal flow-volume curve can be taken as mechanical limit or maximal expiratory flows and volumes that can possibly be achieved by the patient under normal conditions of health. A loss of area under the maximal limits defined by this curve that may be reflected in the measured flow-volume curve is interpreted as loss of ventilatory limitation. A concave shape of the flow-volume curve and a low slope depict an obstructive pattern. The values of FVC, PEF, FEV, FEV_1/FVC ration, FEF_{25-75} and FEF_{50} are also reduced. A steep slope of the flow-volume curve and reduced FVC indicates a restrictive pattern.

Such a visual comparison of the individual flow-volume curve to a normal predicted curve is also known as Gestalt approach. Disorders in which the flow is reduced in proportion to VC i.e. FEV_1/FVC being normal or supernormal are suggestive of restrictive lung disease (Fig 7b & 8) and Table – 2

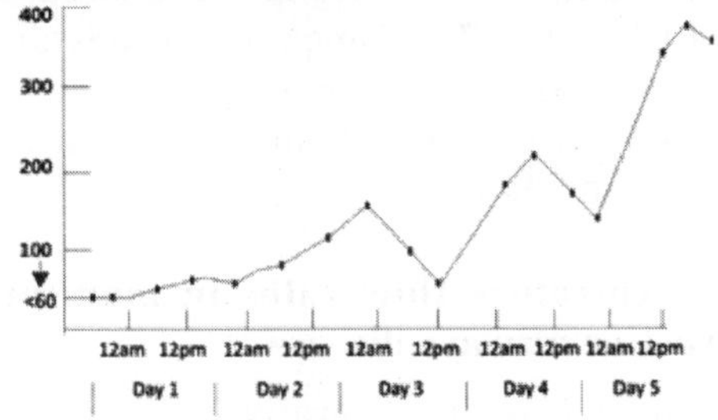

Fig 7 b. PEF chart of a patient recovering from acute severe asthma

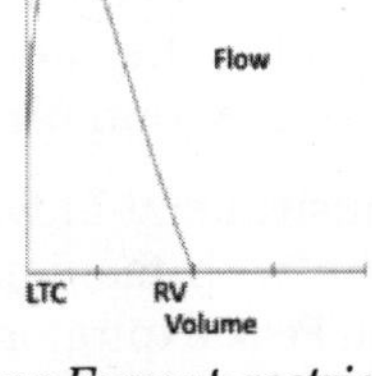

Fig 8. Flow Volume Format: restrictive lung disease

Interpretation of spirometry report

Results obtained from spirometry are compared against reference valves or predicted values that have been derived from reference equations containing data from population surveys. The surveyed population is usually very large and data gathered regarding height, weight, age, gender, ethnic origin, smoking habits, environment, working conditions and physical fitness are also factored into its estimation.

1. Look at the FVC and FEV_1/FVC ratio
2. Look for obstruction (scooped out pattern), restriction (witch's hat pattern) disorders
3. If FEV_1/FVC <70%: obstructive pattern (mild, moderate or severe based on FEV_1)
4. If FEV_1/FVC is normal: restrictive pattern (mild, moderate, or server based on FVC)
5. Bronchodilator response is positive (FEV_1 increases by 12% and 200 ml) is helpful in obstructive pattern.
6. Shape of flow-volume curve indicates obstructive or restrictive pattern, major (upper) airway obstruction
7. Methacholine challenge: a decrease in FEV1>20% after 25 mg/ml indicates airway hyper-responsiveness and variable obstruction over time due to airway inflammation.

Peak expiratory flow rates in monitoring obstructive airways disease

For optimizing the therapy, following the progress of a patient and titrating the dose of bronchodilators and steroids, three times daily measurements of peak expiratory flow rates by a hand held peak flow meter serves the ideal way of managing a patient of obstructive airway disease. This is also the method by which patient can themselves optimize the therapy.

This is a small instrument in which one needs to blow or expire with maximal force after a deep inspiration. Peak expiratory flow rates are expressed in litre/minute. By obtaining three daily readings in the morning, evening and at night one can plot a graphic record. This record on a daily basis reflects the diurnal variation of peak expiratory flow and indirectly the degree of bronchial hyper reactivity.

Obstructive airway disease therapy can be followed utilizing the graphic record in the following way:

1. If the therapy is optimal or the disease is in remission, diurnal variation should not be more than 501/min. if the variation is more it suggests bronchial hyper-responsiveness (Fig. 7.a).
2. If patient is seen in an acute condition and treatment is started, improvement in PEFR suggests a successful therapeutic response and this treatment should be continued till the graph reaches a maximum and the daily record becomes plateaued (Fig. 7.b).
3. The drug therapy should be slowly tapered, while the graphic record remains stable till the minimal daily requirements of inhaled bronchodilators and steroids is reached.
4. If during the follow-up one finds the PEFR fluctuating more than 50L/min then one should increase the dosage of therapy and see that it reduces the increased diurnal fluctuation. If this does not happen so and patient continues to have a fall in PEFR with worsening symptoms, patient should seek expert medical attention.

Using this modality both patients and treating physician can get an objective assessment of the severity of underlying obstructive lung disease and match the minimal therapy with maximal benefit.

Restrictive pattern

A restrictive defect pattern indicates a reduction in lung volume as depicted by an FVC value of <80%. The severity of restrictive defect is staged on the basis of FVC valve (Table-2). Various examples of restrictive defect are enlisted in Table-3.

Restrictive pattern is characterized by

- Reduced FVC
- Normal to high FEV1/FVC ratio
- Normal looking shape on spirometry trace
- Possibly a relatively high PEF

Table 2: Staging of restrictive lung disease

Category	VC (% of predicted normal)
Normal	>80
Mild	60-79
Moderate	40-59
Severe	<40

Table 3: Examples of restrictive defect pattern

A.	Lung	Lobectomy, pneumonectomy, atelectasis, pulmonary fibrosis, congestive heart failure, lung mass/ tumor
B.	Pleural	Effusion, thickened pleura
C.	Chest wall	Kyphoscoliosis, obesity, ascites, scleroderma, pregnancy
D.	Muscular	Neuromuscular disease, post-poliomyelitis, residual paralysis, diaphragmatic paralysis

Acceptable spirometry maneuver

A reliable spirometry maneuver is the one that represents a true maximal effort. The single best out of the three efforts is accepted. A satisfactory effort is associated with a rapid climb to peak flow, continuous decrease in flow and subsequent termination at 0 to 0.1 L/S of zero flow. It should be free of coughs, false starts and interruptions of expiration by artificial teeth, tongue in mouthpiece and closure of glottis. Hesitating start, sub-maximal effort at start of expiration and early quit of maneuver are unacceptable.

A submaximal effort is suspected if FEF_{max} is much lower fraction of the predicted valve than the FEV_1; if flow-volume curve shows an ill-defined peak resembling the non-forced curves, and an abrupt fall to zero at the end of expiration. The maneuver should meet the end-of-test criteria (exhaling for >6s with <50 ml being exhaled in the last 2 sec).

Recommendations

It is very important for those using this very convenient device to recognize its limitations since even with very elaborate approach, the error in this system cannot be completely corrected. The following measures will keep the error to a minimum:

1. Flow meters should be calibrated in the system in which they will be used over the entire range of flows that will be measured.
2. Changes in the system may necessitate recalibration and re-evaluation of the linearity of the flowmeter.
3. If flow is to be measured in two directions, the upstream and downstream geometries of the system should be similar.
4. If possible, the calibrating gas should reproduce the temperature, humidity, and composition of the gas whose flow will be measured.
5. If the pneumotocahograph is used to monitor expired volume and is calibrated with room air at ambient temperature, the heater should be on and the pneumotachograph warm. A conversion factor for ATPS to BTPS should be applied if the pneumotachograph is used to measure inspiratory flow or inspired volume.
6. If only inspiratory flow is to be measured in a non-rebreathing system, the device should be calibrated and used with the heater off, and a correction factor for ATPS to BTPS should be applied if appropriate.

Inspite of its limitations the reader should not take the impression that the pneumotachograph is inherently less accurate than the conventional spirometer.

Summary

Spirometry is of immense help for detection of early airflow abnormalities. Progression of disease and response to therapy can be accurately estimated. It is easy to perform and has options for portability. It is of seminal importance that besides accuracy, technical requirements of the equipment, optimal effort of the patient and availability of a persuasive technologist are also ensured.

REFERENCES

1. Miller MR, Hankinson J, Brusasco V, et al ATS/ERS Task Force. Standardisation of spirometry. Eur Respir J. 2005;26(2):319-38.
2. Mead J, Turner JM, Macklem PT, Little JB. Significance of the relationship between lung recoil and maximum expiratory flow. J Appl Physiol. 1967 ;22(1):95-108.
3. Moore VC. Spirometry: step by step. Breathe 2012 8: 232-240
4. Buist AS. Evaluation of lung function: concept of normality in Simmons DH (ed): Current Pumonolgy IV, Boston, Hoghton Mifflin, 1982
5. Dawson A. Pneumotachography, Pulmonary Function testing – Guidelines and controversies. Academic Press, 1982; 91-97
6. Mead J. Problems in interpreting common tests of pulmonary function, in: Macklem PT, Permutt S (eds): The lung in the transition between health and disease. New York, Marcel Dekker; 1978; 43-51.
7. Mead J, Turner JM, Macklem PT, Little JB: Significance of the relationship between lung recoil and maximum expiratory flow. J appl Physiol. 1967;22:95.
8. Miller RW, Hyatt RE. Evaluation of obstructive lesion of the trachea and larynx by flow volume loops. Am Rev Respir Dis. 1973;108:475.
9. Miller RW, Hyatt RE. Obstructing lesions of the larynx and trachea: Clinical and Physiological Characteristics. Mayo Clin Proc. 1969;44:145-161.
10. Tifeneau R, Pinelli A. Air Circulant et air Captif dans L'xploration de la function ventilatrice pumonaire. Paris Med, 1947;37:624.
11. Tisi GM: Pulmonary physiology in Clinical Medicine, Ch 3, 1980;3-73
12. Wilson AF. Pulmonary Function Testing-Indications and Interpretations, Orlando, Grune and Stratton, Ch2, 1985;9-32
13. Pellegrino R, Viegi G, Brusasco V, et al Interpretative strategies for lung function tests. Eur Respir Jour 2005 26: 948-968;
14. Guidelines for the measurement of respiratory function. Recommendations of the British Thoracic Society and the Association of Respiratory Technicians and Physiologists. Respir Med March 1994;88(3): 165–194
15. Quanjer PH. Standardized lung function testing. Report working party. Bull Eur Physiopathol Respir. 1983;19 Suppl 5:1-95.

16. Tweeddale PM, Alexander F, McHardy GJ. Short term variability in FEV1 and bronchodilator responsiveness in patients with obstructive ventilatory defects. Thorax. 1987; 42(7): 487–490.

17. Chhabra SK, Kumar R, Mittal V. Prediction Equations for Spirometry for Children from Northern India. Indian Pediatr. 2016 Sep 8;53(9):781-785.

18. Desai U, Joshi JM, Chhabra SK, Rahman MU. Prediction equations for spirometry in adults in western India. Indian J Tuberc. 2016;63(3):176-182.

19. Heffler E, Crimi C, Campisi R, et al Bronchodilator response as a marker of poor asthma control. Respir Med. 2016 Mar;112:45-50.

20. Maree DM. Five tips for good office spirometry. South Afr Med Jour 2015;105 (9), 791-792

21. Chhabra SK. Interpretation of Spirometry: Selection of Predicted Values and Defining Abnormality. Indian J Chest Dis Allied Sci. 2015;57(2):91-105.

22. Czajkowska-Malinowska M, Tomalak W, Radliñski J Quality of spirometry in the elderly. Pneumonol Alergol Pol 2013;81(6):511-517.

11

ASSESSMENT OF PULMONARY FUNCTION IN CHILDREN

NIKHIL SARANGDHAR

Introduction

Lung function tests are increasingly gaining importance as tools for the diagnosis, assessment and management of pulmonary diseases in children. The assessment of pulmonary function in young children with early onset of respiratory disease greatly assists in:

1. Diagnosis
2. Monitoring
3. Evaluation of therapeutic interventions early in the course of disease
4. Treatment modification and Efficacy of therapy
5. Documentation of lung function with age and anthropometric variables for population based studies/surveys or derivation of reference equations

Tests for assesement of Pulmonary function in Children

1. Spirometry

Spirometry, though extremely useful for the diagnosis, assessment and monitoring of respiratory disease is often difficult to perform on very young children aged between 2-6 years. Important practical and technical difficulties which arise while performing spirometry in children include:

1. Apprehension of the young child in unfamiliar surroundings.
2. Inadequate understanding of verbal communication while explaining instructions for the forced expiratory maneuver.
3. Physical discomfort and agitation produced when the transducer is inserted in the mouth or nose clip on the nose .
4. Short attention and performance span and poor effort or cooperation while performing the maneuver.
5. In contrast to adults and older children , younger children have relatively smaller lungs and larger airways in proportion to lung volume, as a result of which forced expiration is completed faster in a shorter time, often well before the recommended 6 seconds .
6. Paucity of population data for spirometric variables in children leading to difficulty while computing standard predicted (reference) values or developing reference equations .
7. Inspite of all these issues , there is growing evidence that young children might be able to perform spirometry satisfactorily, however it may not be possible to for them to fulfil all quality criteria enumerated in spirometry guidelines[1,2]. Due to smaller lung volumes and larger airways, children tend to complete the forced expiratory maneuver in a short time , hence the reliability of FEV_1 as a parameter of airway obstruction in them is questionable. Recent studies have also explored the utility of

forced expiratory volume in 0.5 seconds ($FEV_{0.5}$) and 0.75 seconds ($FEV_{0.75}$) as substitutes for FEV_1 for young children, with varying results.[1]

The operator or technician should express patience with the child while explaining and performing the test as often repeated instructions are necessary to make the child comprehend the performance and implications of a forced expiratory maneuver. The child should be explained that the test is being performed to find out how their breathing can be made better. If possible, the test should be scheduled at a time of the day when the child is usually attentive and not hungry or tired[3,4].

Children can be encouraged to perform acceptable spirometry by a variety of methods. The child may be encouraged to blow a "whistle" or "toy horn" to practice forced expiration with maximal effort before the test. Attractive "incentive" spirometry programs in the form of real-time interactive cartoons, videos or games can be used to stimulate the child's interest, attention and effort while performing the forced expiratory maneuver. The incentive in this case is often the objective of the cartoon or game which is achieved if the child successfully performs a complete forced expiration with maximal effort (e.g. blowing out all candles on a cake [Fig.1]

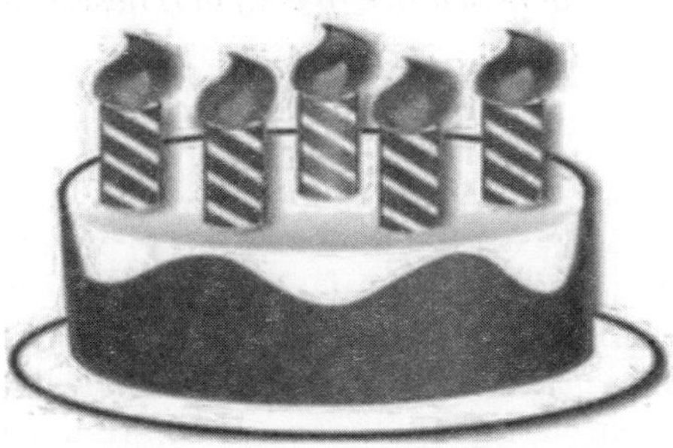

Fig. 1: Computerized incentive spirometry program (Object - All candles on the cake will be extinguished if the child performs a complete forced expiration with maximal effort)

2. **Forced Oscillation technique (FOT)**

Forced oscillation technique (FOT) is a non-invasive test of pulmonary function which requires minimal cooperation as it is performed during normal tidal breathing and has been used to measure airway function in preschool children. FOT estimates airway impedance by forcing the imposition of external pressure signals (positive and negative pressure oscillations and flow impulses) on airways during tidal breathing[5].

The imposed oscillations may be mono-sinusoidal (mono-frequency FOT), multi-sinusoidal (multi-frequency pseudo-random noise FOT) or time discrete pressure signals (impulses) as in Impulse Oscillometry (IOS) and they cause minor alterations in airflow leading to changes in airway pressure. The resultant peaks in pressure and flow signals are measured and used to calculate Resistance (Rrs) , Impedance (Zrs) and Reactance (Xrs) which are expressed in values of Kpa/L/s or $cmH_2O/L/s$. At higher frequencies (20 Hz), the oscillation influences flow in the large (upper & central) airways whereas at lower frequencies (5 Hz) it influences flow in the entire lung. Hence, R20 (resistance at 20 Hz) denotes resistance in the large airways , whereas R5 (resistance at 5Hz) denotes the sum total of resistance in all airways. The difference (R5 - R20) is an accurate measure of peripheral (small airway) resistance.

For clinical application of FOT, it is standard practice to apply medium frequency oscillatory signals within the range of 4–20 Hz to the airway opening via a mouthpiece and measure the resultant pressure and flow changes. In Impulse Oscillometry a short recording of 30 seconds during tidal breathing, with impulses delivered at intervals of 0.02 seconds is taken.

An ATS/ERS statement on lung function testing in preschool children attempted to standardize FOT measurements by recommending that the optimal measurement frequencies be between 4 and 8 Hz[2,9]. Many studies in healthy young children have formulated reference equations for FOT Rrs, unfortunately these tend to be of limited utility as there is significant variability between such studies in equipment, frequency and measurement protocols[6-9].

Estimation of respiratory impedance shows promising utility for the measurement of changes in lung mechanics in young children. FOT overcomes the drawbacks of spirometry induced bronchoconstriction , is able to differentiate between the resistive and elastic components of tidal breathing , is sensitive for small airway disease and is able to identify airway obstruction and bronchodilator response reliably.

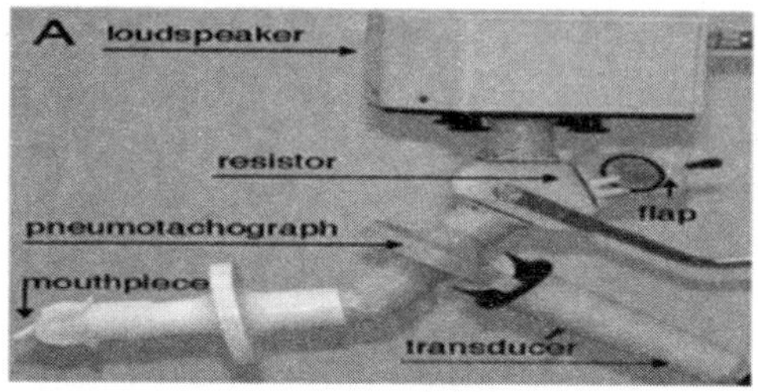

Fig. 2. Equipment for Impulse Oscillometry

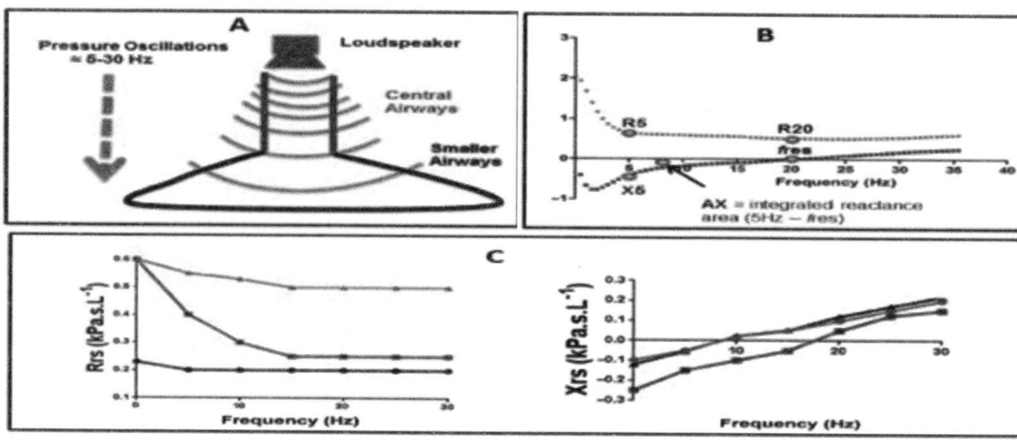

Fig. 3. Principle of Impulse Oscillometry (A) and Measurement of Reactance (B & C) and Resistance (C)

3. *Whole body Plethysmography*

Whole body plethysmography is the gold standard for the estimation of specific airway resistance (*sR*aw) and lung volumes like functional residual capacity (FRC), residual volume (RV) and total lung capacity (TLC) . Plethysmographic measurement of specific airway resistance (*sR*aw) is a useful test for assessment of pulmonary function in children above 2 years of age. In the original DuBois' method, airway resistance (*R*aw) was calculated by Boyle's law, which required measurement of FRC during shutter occlusion which children find difficult[5]. Hence for young children , *sR*aw is measured by the method introduced by Dab and Alexander[10].

Smaller plethysmograph chambers have been developed for the examination of infants and young children. In infants, the procedure can be performed in the supine position using a face mask taking care to avoid air leaks. The child sits upright in the sealed plethysmography box and breathes quietly until resting FRC level is achieved. Changing thoracic dimensions with inspiration and expiration also result in pressure changes within the chamber which are measured simultaneously. The flow at the mouth is then plotted versus the change in volume. At first, *s*Raw is determined during uniform tidal breathing without any active effort by the child . The slope of the curve obtained during quiet tidal breathing equals *s*Raw, which is calculated as the median value of three technically acceptable specific resistance loops[3,10].

For the measurement of lung volumes at end expiration [intrathoracic gas volume (ITGV) or FRC_{pleth}] the airway is transiently occluded by closing a shutter located close to the mouth at this phase of the respiratory cycle. Thereafter the child continues to breathe against the closed shutter with lips closed tightly over the mouthpiece for about 3 seconds , after which the shutter is reopened. During these efforts, the intrathoracic gas volume is compressed and decompressed and airway and plethysmograph pressures are recorded simultaneously. After the determination of FRC, the child is instructed to fully exhale and then to fully inhale which allows the measurement of RV and TLC[3,10,11].

Studies from some centres show that *s*Raw is increased in preschool children with recurrent wheezing or asthma as compared to healthy children . Limited data also exists to suggest that in older subjects *s*Raw may be more sensitive to assess bronchodilator responsiveness than spirometry. *s*Raw has also been demonstrated to improve following treatment with inhaled corticosteroids[12], bronchodilators[13] and leukotriene receptor antagonists[14]. Reference equations for derivation of *s*Raw in children have also been developed [15]. Still, certain factors like the lack of consensus regarding standardization of measurement, equipment and interpretation limit the clinical application of s*R*aw in the diagnosis or monitoring of asthma or recurrent wheeze in young children .

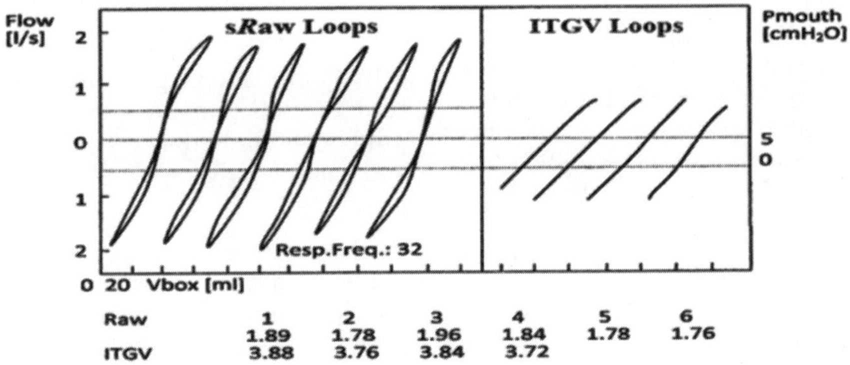

Fig. 4 . Specific airway resistance (sRaw) and Thoracic gas volume recordings

4. Interrupter technique

The measurement of airway resistance using the interrupter technique (*R*int) is useful in children as young as 3 years of age as it is a noninvasive and effort independent test which requires minimal cooperation.

*R*int measurements may be obtained by a plethysmograph or more portable equipment (Micro*R*int device with flowmeter), a pressure measurement device and a flow interruption (occlusion) system. The interrupter technique is based on the principle that during a sudden and brief interruption of airflow at the mouth, the mouth pressure equilibrates with the alveolar pressure. *R*int is defined as this pressure (mouth pressure) divided by the airflow measured immediately before interruption[16,17]. The availability of reference values for preschool children has made clinical interpretation of the interrupter technique convenient[18].

Some studies have demonstrated significantly higher *R*int values in young children with recurrent wheeze or asthma as compared to healthy controls, whereas others have noted significant overlap in distribution of *R*int values between healthy infants and asthmatics[19,20]. Current understanding is that *R*int is of limited value to diagnose or predict asthma or assess bronchodilator responsiveness in preschool children, but may be used to evaluate therapeutic interventions in them .

5. Multiple breath inert gas washout

The multiple breath inert gas washout (MBW) technique assesses the distribution of ventilation as well as FRC during washout of an inhaled inert tracer gas (or gas mixture). Inert gases are harmless, tend to have low blood and tissue solubility and are not absorbed into the body in significant amounts. The most well known of all inert gases is nitrogen (N_2), which can be washed out from the lungs by letting the patient breathe pure oxygen. The advantage of multiple breath washout lies in the fact that it is effort independent and can be applied from infancy to adulthood using tidal breathing techniques. The equipment consists of a flowmeter, a gas analyser (mass spectrometer or ultrasonic sensors which estimate tracer gas concentrations by measuring molecular mass derived from absolute transit times of the ultrasonic pulses) and a computer with the necessary application software.

Initially, the child is instructed to breathe through a mask or mouthpiece for 2–3 minutes. The child is asked to breathe the tracer gas or gas mixture through a face mask until the lungs are equilibrated with this gas (the wash-in phase) (Fig. 5a) . The gas supply is then removed (the wash-out phase), and the child breathes air (if nitrogen is used, the wash-out is performed by breathing pure oxygen) . After the gas supply is removed, the inert gas is cleared from the child's lungs over a number of breaths. During wash-out, airflow and the respective tracer gas concentration are continuously measured at the airway opening(Fig. 5b). The change in concentration of inert gas through this wash-out period is monitored until the concentration of expired inert gas has fallen to $1/40^{th}$ (2.5%) of the original value . Since the initial and final tracer concentrations are known and the total volume of the expired tracer is calculated from the flow and tracer concentration signals, the FRC can be determined.

A number of parameters can be derived from this technique. The most widely used is the Lung clearance index (LCI), which is defined as the cumulative expired volume required to clear (lower) the inert gas concentration to $1/40^{th}$ (2.5%) of its initial (end tidal) value, divided by the FRC.

MBW appears to be particularly attractive as a tool to evaluate lung function in young preschool children as it is effort independent and requires only passive cooperation and tidal breathing[2,3,21].

LCI can detect inhomogeneity of global ventilation early during the onset of lung disease and also functional changes resulting from structural alterations of the lung tissue which are not possible with spirometry[22,23]. However, further work needs to be done to understand the relevance of abnormalities in LCI and their clinical correlation . Furthermore, the technique is currently available commercially using different devices and as yet standardization in test methodology, protocol and reporting is lacking .

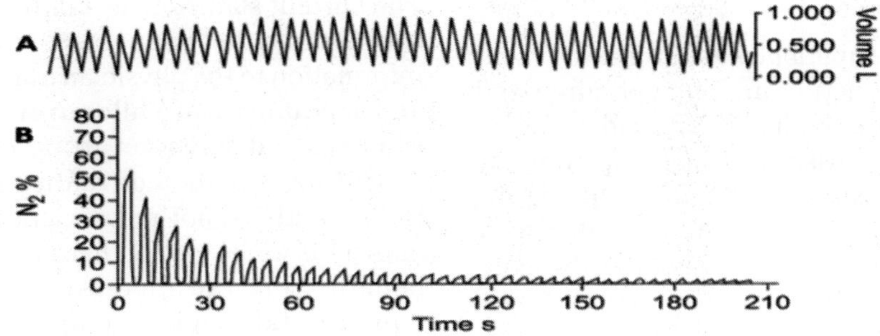

Fig. 5. Tracing of Multiple breath inert gas washout technique with nitrogen showing Equilibration (A) and Wash-out (B) phases

6. Fractional concentration of Exhaled Nitric Oxide (FE_{NO})

The fractional concentration of exhaled nitric oxide (FE_{NO}) is a marker of airway inflammation in asthmatics which has been demonstrated to be elevated in children as well as adults with allergic rhinitis and asthma[24]. Nitric Oxide (NO) is an inflammatory mediator synthesized from L-arginine by the enzyme Nitric Oxide synthase(NOS). 3 isoforms of NOS are known to exist, of which the cytokine inducible NOS (iNOS) present in airway epithelium and inflammatory cells is responsible for NO production in the airways.

Before measurement of FE_{NO}, the child is instructed to sit comfortably and breathe quietly for 5 minutes. A nose clip is not used. The child is asked to take the mouthpiece into his/her mouth and to inhale ambient (NO free) air quickly and deeply to TLC. Following this, the child is instructed to continuously exhale without breath holding at a constant expiratory flow of 50 ml/second maintained within 10% for at least 4-6 seconds with a mouth pressure of 5 to 20 cm H_2O (adequate to close the velum to prevent contamination with nasal nitric oxide) until a NO concentration plateau of at least 2 seconds duration (which corresponds to NO concentration in the lower airways) is identified . Measurement is expressed as NO concentration in parts per billion (ppb) based on the mean of 2 or 3 values within 10% of each other [25]. For children, FE_{NO} levels are classified as low (< 20 ppb), intermediate (20-35 ppb) or high (> 35 ppb).

FE_{NO} levels correlate well with sputum and BAL eosinophilia in school children with atopic asthma, peak flow variability and airway hyperresponsiveness and also decrease following corticosteroid therapy (inhaled as well as oral) in a dose dependent manner[26,27].

Despite its promise as a surrogate marker of airway inflammation in asthma in infants and young children, FE_{NO} has not yet been approved as a tool for diagnosis of asthma in this age group due to several limitations, which include the lack of a standardized measurement protocol, variable expiratory airflow in children (FE_{NO} measurement is flow dependent), contamination of tidal breath with nitric oxide from the upper airways, inability of children less than 5 years of age to generate a stable concentration of NO, inability of elevated FE_{NO} levels to distinguish between asthma and non-eosinophilic bronchitis, a variable upper limit of normal (12.7 to 22.8 ppb) for FE_{NO} in children and significant differences in absolute values of FE_{NO} measured between different analysers, including some of the newer inexpensive portable models[28,29]. Currently, FE_{NO} is recommended only as an additional diagnostic investigation for children in whom the diagnosis of asthma remains unclear despite standard evaluation .

Summary

No single test is superior by itself for assessment of pulmonary function in young children and each test has its individual merits and demerits. Despite evident disadvantages, spirometry provides useful objective data which aids the physician during assessment of the wheezy or asthmatic child and still remains the gold standard for diagnosis and assessment of airway obstruction. Other methods like the forced oscillation technique, whole body plethysmography for measurement of specific airway resistance and lung volumes, the interrupter technique, multiple breath inert gas washout and fractional concentration of exhaled nitric oxide are being increasingly studied throughout the world as surrogate methods for estimation of lung function in children with varying results.

The current status of most of these tests is that they provide valuable supplementary information to the physician during assessment and monitoring of children with respiratory illnesses but have yet to be established as substitutes for the conventional methods of testing and are not recommended for routine clinical use. Several of these tests are likely to benefit from the increasing availability of commercial devices and their technical modifications and research. Standardization of test procedures, protocols, equipment, analysis and interpretation and the availability of valid accurate reference values for children are necessary before their efficacy or clinical utility can be established.

REFERENCES

1. Gaffin JM, Shotola NL, Martin TR, Phipatanakul W. Clinically useful spirometry in preschool-aged children: evaluation of the 2007 American Thoracic Society Guidelines. J Asthma 2010; 47 : 762-67.
2. Beydon N, Davis SD, Lombardi E, Allen JL, Arets HG, Aurora P, et al. An official American Thoracic Society/European Respiratory Society statement: pulmonary function testing in preschool children. Am J Respir Crit Care Med 2007; 175 : 1304-45.
3. Vogt B, Falkenberg C, Weiler N, Frerichs I. Pulmonary function testing in children and infants. Physiol. Meas. 2014; 35(3) : R59-90
4. Eigen H, Bieler H, Grant D, Christoph K, Terrill D, Heilman DK et al. Spirometric pulmonary function in healthy preschool children. Am. J. Respir. Crit. Care Med. 2001; 163 (3) : 619-23.
5. Aggarwal AN. Pulmonary function testing . Textbook of Pulmonary and critical care medicine 1st Ed. 2009; 26A : 331-45
6. Lebecque P, Desmond K, Swartebroeckx Y, Dubois P, Lulling J, Coates A. Measurement of respiratory system resistance by forced oscillation in normal children: a comparison with spirometric values. Pediatr Pulmonol 1991; 10 : 117-22.
7. Klug B, Bisgaard H. Specific airway resistance, interrupter resistance and respiratory impedance in healthy children aged 2–7 years. Pediatr Pulmonol 1998; 25 : 322-31.
8. Ducharme FM, Davis GM, Ducharme GR. Pediatric reference values for respiratory resistance measured by forced oscillation. Chest 1998; 113 : 1322-28.
9. Solymar L, Aronsson PH, Bake B, Bjure J. Respiratory resistance and impedance magnitude in healthy children aged 2–18 years. Pediatr Pulmonol 1985; 1 : 134-140.
10. Dab I, Alexander F. A simplified approach to the measurement of specific airway resistance. Pediatr Res 1976; 10 : 998-9.

11. Stocks J, Godfrey S, Beardsmore C, Bar-Yishay E, Castile R. Plethysmographic measurements of lung volume and airway resistance. ERS/ATS Task Force on Standards for Infant Respiratory Function Testing. European Respiratory Society/ American Thoracic Society. Eur Respir J 2001; 17 : 302-312.

12. Nielsen KG, Bisgaard H. The effect of inhaled budesonide on symptoms, lung function, and cold air and methacholine responsiveness in 2- to 5-year-old asthmatic children. Am J Respir Crit Care Med. 2000; 162(4.1) : 1500-6.

13. Nielsen KG, Bisgaard H. Discriminative capacity of bronchodilator response measured with three different lung function techniques in asthmatic and healthy children aged 2 to 5 years. Am J Respir Crit Care Med. 2001; 164 : 554-59.

14. Bisgaard H, Nielsen KG. Bronchoprotection with a leukotriene receptor antagonist in asthmatic preschool children. Am.J. Respir. Crit. Care Med. 2000; 162 : 187-90

15. Kirkby J, Stanojevic S, Welsh L, Lum S, Badier M, Beardsmore C, et al. Reference equations for specific airway resistance in children: the Asthma UK initiative. Eur Respir J. 2010; 36 : 622-29.

16. Child F. The measurement of airways resistance using the interrupter technique (*R*int). *Paediatr Respir Rev.* 2005; 6 : 273-7.

17. Beydon N. Interrupter resistance: what's feasible? Paediatr Respir Rev 2006; 7 (1) : S5-S7.

18. Merkus PJ, Stocks J, Beydon N, Lombardi E, Jones M, McKenzie SA, et al. Reference ranges for interrupter resistance technique: the Asthma UK Initiative. Eur Respir J 2010; 36 : 157-63.

19. Brussee JE, Smit HA, Koopman LP, Wijga AH, Kerkhof M, Corver K, et al. Interrupter resistance and wheezing phenotypes at 4 years of age. Am J Respir Crit Care Med 2004; 169 : 209-13

20. Black J, Baxter-Jones AD, Gordon J, Findlay AL, Helms PJ. Assessment of airway function in young children with asthma: comparison of spirometry, interrupter technique, and tidal flow by inductance plethsmography. Pediatr Pulmonol 2004; 37 : 548-53.

21. Robinson PD, Goldman MD, Gustafsson PM. Inert gas washout : theoretical background and clinical utility in respiratory disease. Respiration 2009; 78 : 339-55.

22. Macleod KA, Horsley AR, Bell NJ, Greening AP, Innes JA, Cunningham S. Ventilation heterogeneity in children with well controlled asthma with normal spirometry indicates residual airways disease. Thorax 2009; 64 : 33-37

23. Downie SR, Salome CM, Verbanck S, Thompson B, Berend N, King GG. Ventilation heterogeneity is a major determinant of airway hyperresponsiveness in asthma, independent of airway inflammation. Thorax 2007; 62 : 684-89.

24. Taylor DR, Pijnenburg MW, Smith AD, de Jongste JC. Exhaled nitric oxide measurements: clinical application and interpretation. Thorax 2006; 61 : 817-87.

25. D'Silva L, Nair P. Asthma diagnosis. Textbook of Pulmonary and critical care medicine 1st Ed. 2009; 66 : 847-65

26. Shaw DE, Berry MA, Thomas M, et al. The use of exhaled nitric oxide to guide asthma management: a randomized controlled trial . Am. J. Respir. Crit. Care Med. 2007; 176(3) : 231-7

27. Sivan Y, Gadish T, Fireman E, Soferman R. The use of exhaled nitric oxide in the diagnosis of asthma in school children. J Pediatr 2009; 155 : 211-6.

28. Muller KC , Jorres RA, Magnussen H, et al. Comparison of exhaled nitric oxide analysers. Respir. Med. 2005; ; 99(5) : 631-7.

29. Borill Z, Clough D, Truman N, et al. A comparison of exhaled nitric oxide measurements performed using three different analysers. Respir. Med. 2006; 100(8) : 1392-6.

12

EVALUATION OF PULMONARY FUNCTION BY RADIOLOGY

AMITA NENE, VIKAS AGRAWAL

Introduction

Advances in thoracic imaging, such as high-resolution computed tomography (HRCT) scanning of the lungs, multi-detector helical scanners, together with newer volumetric image analysis tools, has greatly advanced anatomic imaging of the airways and the lung parenchyma. However, static structural images do not reflect the highly physiologic nature of the lungs.

Functional imaging of the lungs has largely been indirect, correlating the structural changes depicted on these scans with conventional pulmonary function tests (PFTs). The introduction of static inspiratory-expiratory CT scanning and dynamic imaging with electron beam CT, as well as multi-row detectors for helical CT, has enabled evaluation of abnormal tracheo-bronchial collapse and/or gas trapping.

Several new approaches to direct imaging of pulmonary ventilation have emerged, using magnetic resonance (MR) and CT techniques. The introduction of new MR contrast agents, including the hyperpolarized noble gases ^{3}helium (^{3}HE) and ^{129}Xenon (^{129}XE) among others, along with more rapid pulse sequences, have enabled direct imaging of gas wash-in, distribution in the lungs, and wash-out with unprecedented spatial and temporal resolution. Likewise, dynamic, high-resolution, contrast-enhanced CT ventilation scanning using stable nonradioactive xenon gas has been shown to be feasible. These new techniques offer substantial advantages over traditional methods of assessing pulmonary function.

Although conventional PFTs have become an indispensable tool in pulmonary medicine, and have revealed a wealth of information about lung physiology in normal and diseased states, they are limited to global measurements of total lung function. The image-based methods, on the other hand, can provide quantitative displays of regional lung function, not only of individual lungs but also of lobes, segments, and even smaller regions. This represents a major step forward, since the physiology of both the normal lung and virtually all lung disorders are heterogeneous to some degree. Common examples include:

- Centrilobular emphysema, which is predominant in the upper zones;
- Usual interstitial pneumonia, a typically basilar disease with temporal and spatial heterogeneity in its pathologic evolution;
- Asthma and small airway disease, in which the airway abnormalities are heterogeneously distributed both spatially and temporally;
- Pulmonary embolism, which involves select pulmonary vascular distributions; and
- Adult respiratory distress syndrome (ARDS), in which the lung involvement and resulting mechanical impairment are typically heterogeneously distributed.

These evolving functional imaging techniques also hold promise, as a means, to monitor new therapies, such as surgical and mechanical approaches to advanced emphysema, new medical treatments for asthma and chronic interstitial disease, or tailoring of mechanical ventilatory parameters in ARDS.

This chapter describes the new applications of CT and MRI in relation to obtaining functional and quantifiable tools for the study of pulmonary diseases.

The upper airway

Upper airway is the portal of entry for ventilation. The upper airway must be rigid enough to withstand collapse by the negative intra-luminal pressures generated during inspiration. The upper airway is a finely controlled apparatus in which the calibre of the airway lumen is maintained by active dilator muscle activity counterbalancing the inspiratory negative intra-luminal pressure. Upper airway imaging studies using both ultrafast MR, in conjunction with physiologic monitoring of respiration, are providing new insights into the biomechanical functioning of the normal upper airway, as well as clues to the patho-physiology of obstructive sleep apnoea (OSA). Furthermore, these upper airway imaging techniques are helping to elucidate the mechanisms underlying the efficacy of various therapeutic interventions for this disorder.

MRl evaluation is helpful in determining the level of obstruction i.e. whether the collapse of airway is retropalatal or retroglossal or at multiple levels. A retropalatal level of narrowing can be rectified by Uvulopalatopharyngoplasty while retroglossal narrowing due to retrognathism may require mandibular advancement. Macroglossia may require genioplasty. Multiple levels of obstruction may require more than one surgery[1].

The trachea

Using dynamic CT in normal subjects, Stern et al[2] found that the tracheal airway surface decreased 35% from full inspiration to expiration (280 mm^2 to 178 mm^2). Normal bowing of the posterior membranous trachea is thus observed in expiration. In tracheobronchomalacia, damage to the tracheal cartilage with resultant loss of the normal structural integrity of the airway wall leads to an increase in tracheal compliance and increased flaccidity. The latter is most evident during coughing or forced expiration. The coronal diameter of the trachea substantially exceeds the sagittal diameter, resulting in a so-called lunate configuration. The acquisition of paired inspiratory and dynamic expiratory images with multi-section helical CT is a promising method for diagnosing tracheobronchomalacia. The low-dose technique performs as well, as the standard-dose technique for the dynamic expiratory phase, with a similar degree of confidence for measuring the tracheal lumen[3].

The Bronchi and the Peripheral airways

Despite dramatic developments in HRCT and helical CT for anatomic imaging of the lungs, radiologic techniques including CT cannot directly resolve the individual distal airways and airspaces at the gas exchange level in the lung parenchyma. However, functional imaging techniques are available to visualize ventilation and gas exchange in the lung parenchyma. This has traditionally been performed with nuclear medicine techniques. More recently, however, MR and CT based methods have been developed that have greatly expanded our ability to image a variety of functional parameters related to ventilation. These exciting methods, many of which are still under development, provide quantitative imaging of regional lung function with high temporal and spatial resolution

The introduction of multi-detector row CT (MDCT) has enabled coronal, sagittal, and oblique reformatting at greater spatial resolution than before. The techniques using spirometric controlled MDCT allow for quantification of presence and distribution of parenchymal and airway pathology. Xenon gas can be employed to assess regional ventilation of the lungs. Magnetic resonance imaging (MRI) of the lung is developing its own arsenal for lung assessment, both in terms of morphology, pulmonary circulation, ventilation, and right heart assessment. It is clear that the inherent advantage of MRI over CT – its lack of ionizing radiation – makes it of primary interest in the field of lung diseases which tend to be chronic with acute exacerbations, thus requiring multiple investigations during the life-span of the patient.

COMPUTED TOMOGRAPHY

1. Development of the scanners:

Volumetric physiological imaging via x-ray CT had its beginning in the mid 1970's with the Dynamic Spatial Reconstructor (DSR), the prototype of dynamic volumetric X-ray CT designed and installed at the Mayo Clinic[4]. Much of the work establishing the accuracy and precision of volumetric lung imaging was performed on the DSR[4,5]. The primary lesson learned from the DSR was that lungs must be studied dynamically and volumetrically. Commercial imaging technology lagged significantly behind this early work. The electron beam CT[6], used parallel X-ray targets to get improved scan speeds up to 50 msec per slice pair, acquiring eight stacked slices in approximately 224 milliseconds. There have been rapid advances in speed and resolution with the advent of MDCT[7]. Its cone-beam spiral CT uses a 2D detector array, allowing larger scanning range in shorter time with higher image resolution[8,9].

From the initial beginnings of computed transverse axial scanning tomography[10], *via* electron beam CT[6] to the current 16-cm coverage electrocardiography-gated imaging within a single heart beat[11], CT has been at the heart of changes in medical diagnosis and management. It is difficult to imagine that even Hounsfield in his visionary acceptance speech of the Nobel Prize could have quite foreseen the impact CT has made[12]. Apart from the high temporal resolution now available on CT systems, the spatial resolution has also improved and 0.4-mm isotropic resolution is now achievable using the latest scanner technology[13]. Furthermore, the application of novel reconstruction methods has resulted in significant reductions in radiation dose, and all vendors now routinely include iterative reconstruction as part of their standard protocols with the latest techniques resulting in very low-dose CT with exposure for lung parenchymal disease in the order of 0.15 mSv[14] and for lung nodule detection with exposures less than traditional chest radiographs at 0.06 mSv[15].

The advanced technologies now enable structural imaging of the chest in great detail and with 0.4 to 0.6 mm isotropic resolution. This is all achieved with a z-axis coverage of 4 to 16 cm in a rotation time of 0.3 seconds or less. This speed makes the examination more robust and full coverage of the chest in a single breath-hold is easier to achieve. At the same time, it is crucial to coach patients to full inspiration as well as forced residual volume expiration where air trapping or airway collapse is being investigated.

With the introduction of dual source CT, there is a growing interest in the use of dual energy[16-19] as a means of characterizing tissues regionally as well as quantitating local amounts of a contrast agent. Dual energy imaging permits mathematical separation of the contrast signal from the background tissue signal on a single scan acquisition.

The application of contrast has yielded anatomic images of the vasculature in the chest, including the coronary arteries, aorta, and pulmonary vessels. However, with dual-energy application, where 2 scans are performed using different keV settings, it is feasible to separate out particular high-density compounds such as iodine or xenon. Thus, it is now feasible to obtain the distribution of vascular contrast (resulting in a measure of pulmonary blood volume)[20,21], as well as to evaluate the distribution of inhaled contrast like xenon gas[22,23]. Similarly, dynamic contrast-enhanced methods can track a tight contrast bolus of 5 to

9 mL/s during a 20-second period to yield true perfusion, mean transit times and even assess pulmonary and systemic supply of the pulmonary vascular bed.

2. Image Analysis:

With the advent of MDCT and isotropic voxels, it is now possible to reliably segment the airway tree to approximately the 5th generation (trachea being generation 0) and many of the 6th and 7th generation branches are captured in the segmentation. Airway wall thickness is commonly expressed as wall area percent (percent of the area defined by the outer wall of the airway segment occupied by the airway wall)[24].

Clinical Applications: These measures are being used to assess airway remodelling in both asthma and chronic obstructive pulmonary disease (COPD). **Fig. 1** shows a depiction of the airway tree and lobe segmentation from both a normal non-smoker and a patient with COPD. These images can be used to not only quantify the airway and parenchyma characteristics but also to provide a roadmap linking airway paths to sub-lobar segment[25].

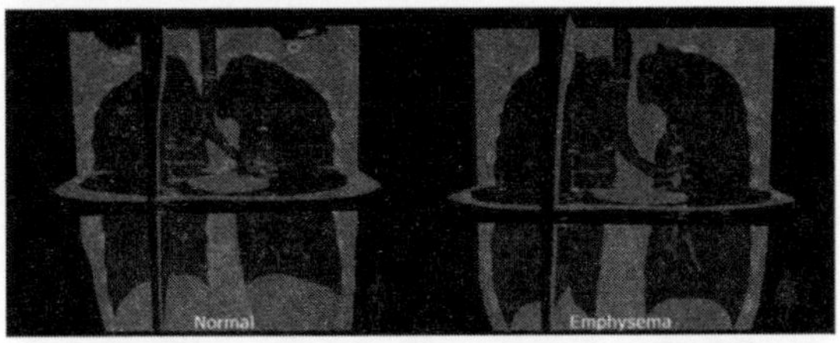

Fig. 1: *Images derived from MDCT-based imaging of a normal non-smoker (left) and a smoker with emphysema (right). These images demonstrate the automatic segmentation of the lungs, lobes and bronchial tree with automatic bronchial tree labelling.*

3. Ventilation Assessment:

The measurement of lung ventilation, lung volume, and tidal volume has traditionally been made for the entire lung, despite the fact that lung function in both health and disease is inhomogeneous. Xenon-enhanced MDCT (Xe-MDCT) is a method for the non-invasive measurement of regional pulmonary ventilation, determined from the wash-in and/ or wash-out rates of the radiodense, non-radioactive gas xenon as measured in serially acquired, axial MDCT scans[25].

Clinical Application: The technique is used for evaluation of ventilation in various conditions, such as COPD[26], asthma[27], bronchiolitis obliterans[28].

4. Perfusion Imaging:

There have been a growing number of studies, demonstrating the use of MDCT with infusion of iodinated contrast agent to assess the presence of pulmonary emboli via visualization of flow voids in peripheral lung segments, and the improved ability to detect pulmonary emboli, aortic dissection and coronary atherosclerosis have resulted in the "triple rule out" method for use in patients with chest pain[29].

Many studies have reported the application of perfusion CT in assessment of pulmonary thromboembolism. A small observational study comparing dual energy CT (DECT) perfusion with CT pulmonary angiogram (CTPA) demonstrated a sensitivity and specificity of 100% on a per-patient basis, and 60% to 66.7%, and 99.5% to 99.8% on a per-segment basis, the sensitivity and specificity ranged between 60% and 66.7%, and 99.5% and 99.8%[30]. Compared with scintigraphy, the reported sensitivity and specificity of DECT perfusion on a per-patient basis was 75% and 80%, and 83% and 99% on a per-segment basis[31]. **Fig. 2** shows the advantage of CT perfusion over CTPA in the detection of peripheral pulmonary arterial vascular obstruction that is often missed on CTPA, especially in the subacute cases of pulmonary embolism.

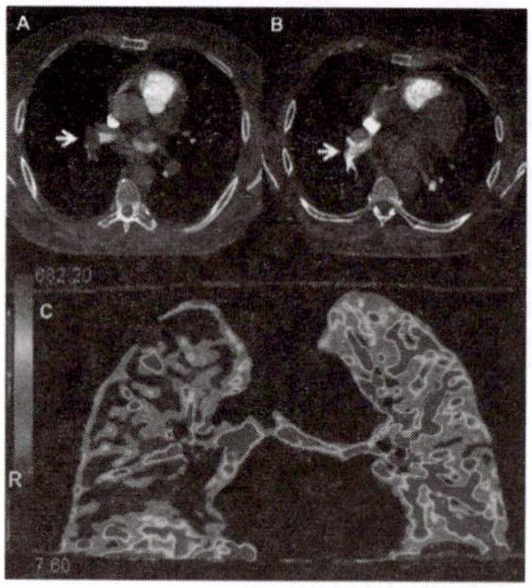

Fig. 2: Pulmonary perfusion changes in a 52-year-old female smoker with a recent episode of pulmonary embolism(PE). This patient presented with large volume bilateral PE (arrow; A). The patient remained symptomatic at 6 months despite treatment. (B) Resolution of PE in the lobar and segmental branches (arrow). (C) Dynamic CT perfusion, however, demonstrated significant residual perfusion reduction in the right lung accounting for patient's symptoms. Pixels are colour coded in the parametric maps according to the degree of perfusion (from high to low perfusion values: red, yellow, green, blue/black).

A study of dynamic CT perfusion in patients with minor emphysema versus control (healthy volunteers and smokers without emphysema) reported globally increased heterogeneity in the early emphysema group, but not in the control group. The authors suggested that the CT perfusion might be able to differentiate smokers at risk of emphysema[32]. When emphysema is established, alveolar surface reduction is associated with reduction in capillary volume[33,34]. As a result, the reduction in perfusion on CT correlated with severity of emphysema[35]. **Fig. 3** shows diffuse perfusion changes in a patient with emphysema.

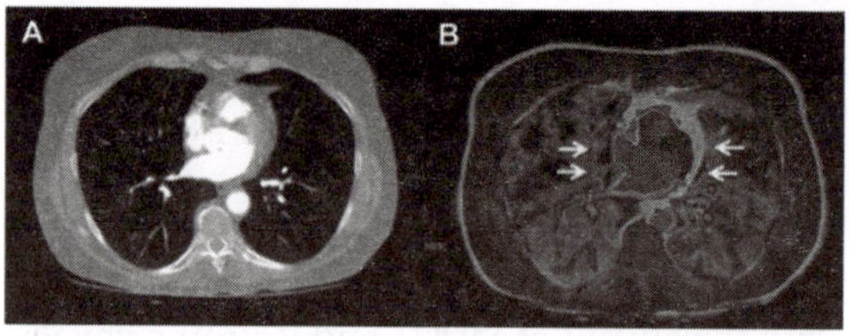

Fig. 3: Pulmonary perfusion changes in a 63-year-old female smoker with diffuse emphysema (A, lung window CT; B, parametric perfusion map). Perfusion map from dynamic contrast-enhanced CT shows diffusely abnormal perfusion throughout both lungs. Pixels are colour coded in the parametric maps according to the degree of perfusion (from high to low perfusion values: red, yellow, green, blue/black). The perfusion is much better in the right lower lobe, compared with the other lobes (note homogenous higher perfusion as coded in green/yellow in the right posterior zone, compared with patchy darker pixels in the other regions indicating lower perfusion). Note artifactual increased perfusion around the heart (arrows) secondary to cardiac motion.

Clinical Applications: i) Perfusion CT is superior to CTPA and scintigraphy in detection of pulmonary embolism, ii) CT perfusion might be able to differentiate smokers at risk of emphysema, and iii) Dynamic perfusion CT is reported to be more specific and accurate than static positron emission tomography/CT for differentiating malignant from benign pulmonary nodules of less than 3 cm[36].

MAGNETIC RESONANCE IMAGING

1. Development of the scanners:

During the past several years there has been accelerated development of pulmonary MRI. This has been driven in part by concerns regarding ionizing radiation using MDCT. However, MRI also offers capabilities for fast multi-spectral and functional imaging using gas agents that are not technically feasible with CT. Recent improvements in gradient performance and radial acquisition methods using ultra-short echo time have contributed to advances in these functional pulmonary MRI techniques. Functional lung MRI methods using the gas agents are improving our understanding of a wide range of chronic lung diseases, including COPD, asthma, and cystic fibrosis in both adults and children.

Pulmonary MRI has conventionally been limited by low signal to noise in the lung parenchyma. This limitation stems from the combined effects of low proton density and high local susceptibility induced by the numerous air tissue interfaces intrinsic to the lung parenchyma that facilitate gas exchange. Because of these challenges, significant research focus has been dedicated to developing methods to enhance contrast in the lungs, particularly in the lung parenchyma[37-40].

Multiple methods of functional lung imaging using MRI exist with trade-offs and imaging strategies that are dependent on the properties of the gas used. The most mature of these are the hyperpolarized gases, ^{3}He and ^{129}Xe, but the new implementations of oxygen enhanced and fluorinated gas methods are re-emerging as competitive alternatives thanks to technical advances in scanner hardware and software that enable dynamic imaging of gas wash-in and wash-out.

These advances have further improved the traditional advantages of MRI over nuclear medicine such as higher 3D spatial and temporal resolution and non-ionizing radiation[41]. Improved 3D temporal-spatial resolution of pulmonary ultra-short echo time MRI is now approaching that of CT[42] while the myriad of tools for assessing lung function exceed those available with CT[43]. These factors coupled with concerns over X-ray radiation dose for longitudinal studies using CT have made MRI especially attractive for paediatric and young adult populations[44-46].

2. Proton imaging:

As with any MRI technique, proton imaging uses the large magnetic field and the free moving protons to derive signal from changes in proton orientation due to radiofrequency pulses. The lungs are different from the rest of the body, as there is a relative low number of protons and most of the lung parenchyma consists of air. Although this is a problem, it can be used to advantage as pathological processes tend to increase the number of protons (haemorrhage, oedema, inflammation, or tumour) or alternatively lead to relative voids of proton density (as with calcification or fibrosis).

Clinical Applications:

i) Several pathological processes can be evaluated using proton imaging, including pleural effusions, pneumonia, lung tumours (particularly useful in Pancoast tumours and for determination of tumour invasion in mesothelioma) and the assessment of the mediastinum[47-49] **(Fig. 4)**. The technique is complementary to CT, although tissue plane definition and characterization is better using MRI.

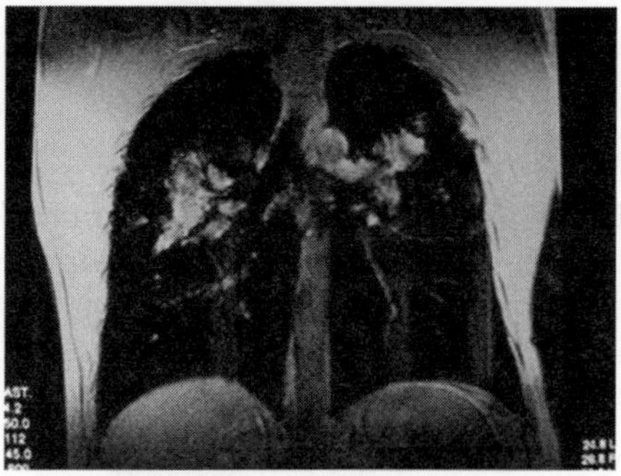

***Fig. 4:** Patient with sarcoidosis. Coronal proton single shot fast spin echo sequence, demonstrating black lungs with some interstitial markings and extensive mediastinal and bilateral hilar lymphadenopathy.*

ii) Assessment of respiratory dynamics has become feasible with the advent of ultrafast proton imaging capabilities. This has resulted in novel approaches for assessment of diaphragm and chest wall motion assessment and breathing mechanics[50,51].

3. Gadolinium-enhanced imaging:

The use of Gadolinium contrast has enabled a rapid expansion of chest MR imaging, as it became feasible to assess enhancement of pathological processes as well as visualization of the pulmonary vascular tree (both as static component and dynamics of perfusion) and the other large arteries[52].

Clinical Applications:

i) This has allowed MRI to become competitive with more traditional CT techniques in several aspects of chest imaging, particularly imaging of the large vessels, including congenital anomalies such as patent ductus arteriosus **(Fig. 5)** and the assessment of pulmonary hypertension[53,54] **(Fig. 6)**.

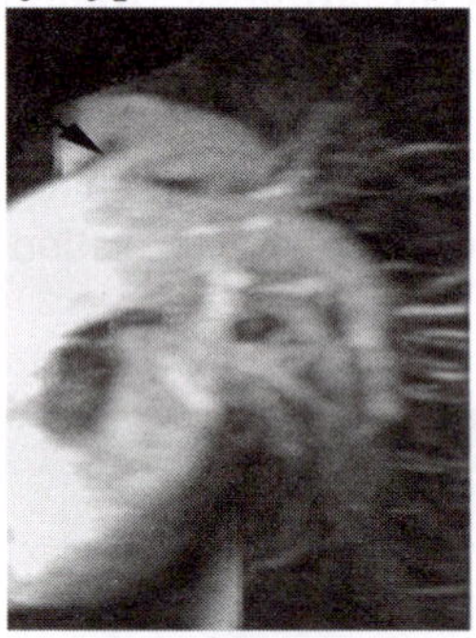

Fig. 5: *Sagittal 3D-Gadolinium enhanced MR angiogram, demonstrating direct connection between aorta and pulmonary artery (arrow), consistent with patent ductus arteriosus in a patient with pulmonary hypertension*

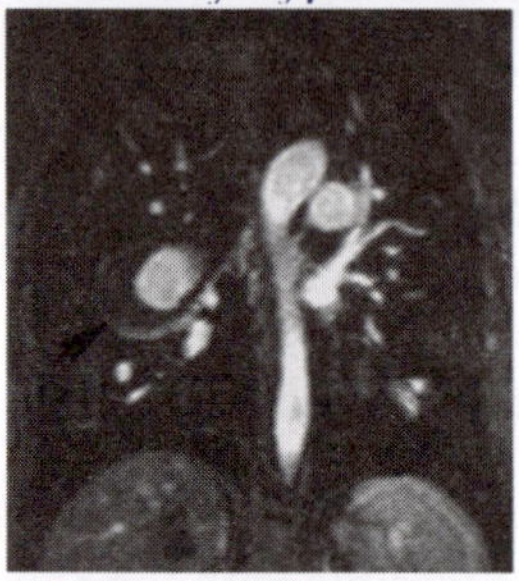

Fig. 6: *Coronal 3D-Gadolinium-enhanced MR angiogram, demonstrating enhancement of an aneurysm of the right pulmonary artery with a black rim of mural organized thrombus (arrow) in a patient with pulmonary hypertension.*

ii) Although CT has maintained a primary role in the diagnosis of pulmonary embolism, the application of MRI for subsets of patients like pregnant women or those that will require follow-up imaging to assess response to therapy is now feasible with very high-resolution MR angiographic imaging[55-57].

iii) Dynamic contrast-enhanced MRI offers the capability to study the contrast bolus traveling through the entire cardiac cycle, giving rise to perfusion, blood volume, and transit time measurements. The technique is increasingly finding use in routine clinical practice, particularly in centres of excellence where patients are investigated for pulmonary hypertension[58,59].

4. Hyperpolarized gas imaging:

MRI is based on tuning radio frequency (RF) amplifiers to a particular transmission/ receiving frequency, which is 64 MHz at 1.5 T for proton. By changing this frequency, it is possible to tune into other nuclear signals (referred to as multinuclear spectroscopy), and this has been successfully applied for lung imaging of inert noble gases, like ^{3}He, and ^{129}X, whereas other gases are also undergoing tests (^{19}Flourine, for instance)[60,61]. These gases have no signal in their normal resting state, but they can be excited by laser light, resulting in a hyperpolarized state. This state can then be used to visualize these nuclei during MRI, where the loss of polarization results in an RF signal that can be detected by appropriately tuned RF coils.

Three types of imaging are available with hyperpolarized gas image MRI. These are i) Images of Ventilation, ii) Diffusion Weighted Imaging, iii) pO_2 Mapping.

All hyperpolarized gas imaging techniques rely on the delivery of a single breath of gas mixture into the airways, with the hyperpolarization either performed on site or by a central distribution network[62].

i) Images of Ventilation:

Spin density images during breath-hold represent a snapshot of gas distribution. The resulting "ventilation defects" **(Fig. 7)** are influenced by regional airway obstruction and air trapping[63,64]. The ventilation defect volume[63,65,66], ventilated volume[65,67], and coefficient of variation[68,69] derived from these images **have all proven useful for demonstrating regional heterogeneity of ventilation in a wide range of obstructive lung diseases.**

Measures of ventilation defects are also sensitive to subclinical decline in function due to aging in healthy never-smokers[64,69] as well as smokers[70-72]. One semi-automated measure that is emerging as a biomarker is the ventilation defect percentage (VDP), defined as the defected lung volume normalized by the total lung volume[73-76]. Multiple groups have demonstrated repeatability and validity of this measure compared to pulmonary function testing and severity of disease[60,66,69,77-80]. In mild to moderate COPD, the VDP in particular is associated with severe outcomes such as hospitalizations for exacerbations – an association that is not observed using conventional measures, including CT[80].

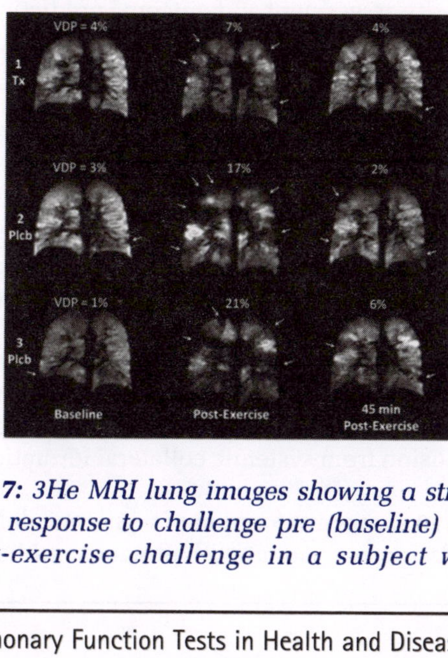

***Fig. 7:** 3He MRI lung images showing a strong VDP response to challenge pre (baseline) and post-exercise challenge in a subject with exercise-induced bronchoconstriction and treatment with Montelukast (visit 1 vs. visits 2 and 3). Defects (arrows) occur most prominently after exercise challenge and post-challenge decreases in FEV1 for this subject coincide with decreases in VDP as indicated. Recovery 45 minutes post-exercise shows residual VDP for visit 3. Overall, residual VDP after recovery was significantly higher on 3He MRI but not on FEV1. Plcb = "placebo visit"; Tx = "treatment visit."*

ii) Diffusion Weighted Imaging (DWI):

DWI exploits the high free diffusion of ^{3}He and ^{129}Xe gases. In the context of restriction by the lung micro-structure, this allows indirect measurement of the average dimensions of the lung airspaces. When ^{3}He or ^{129}Xe gas is restricted by tissue boundaries, the diffusivity is referred to as the apparent diffusion coefficient (ADC). A semi-quantitative ADC map – a surrogate for airspace size – is easily derived. Regional ADC changes have been observed in response to increases in lung volume, gravity dependence **(Fig. 8)**, age, and aetiology of emphysema, i.e. COPD or alph1-antitrypsin[67,81-87]. **The ^{129}Xe ADC in human subjects is strongly associated with increased COPD severity** and correlates well with ^{3}He ADC reported in previous studies[85,88,89].

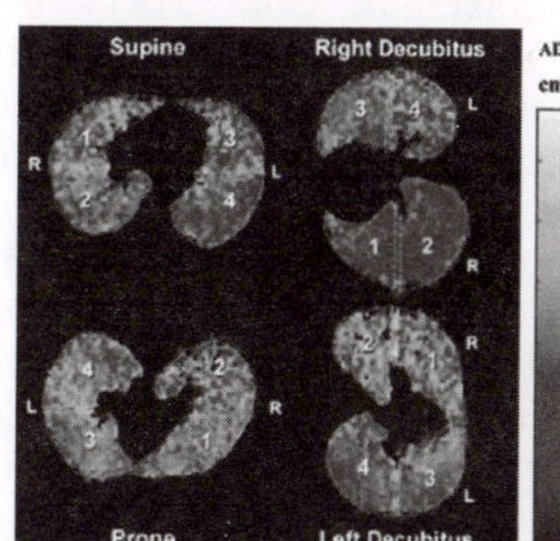

***Fig. 8:** Apparent diffusion coefficient (ADC) imaging in a normal volunteer in different positions, demonstrating gravity dependent changes with decreased ADC values in dependent lung portions.*

iii) pO_2 Mapping:

The paramagnetic effects of oxygen reduce the T1 and T2 of hyperpolarized gases (as well as proton signals)[39] and can therefore be exploited to provide a quantitative estimate of regional pO_2[90-92]. Regional pO_2 measures can potentially be used to calculate the ratio of ventilation to perfusion (V/Q)[93]. In fact, pO_2 measurements have recently been used as a marker of disease severity in a study of V/Q heterogeneity in smokers[94,95].

Clinical Applications:

i) The vast majority of clinical research studies using hyperpolarized gas MRI have been performed in asthma[63,68,75,78,79,96,97] and COPD[69,87,98], with a growing number of recent studies focusing on cystic fibrosis in children and adults[77,99,100]. It has been shown that the extent of non-ventilated lung regions seen in patients with airflow obstruction correlated with pulmonary function tests.

ii) This technique offers a direct spatial delineation, which may be important for therapy planning. This method has been used to study asthma , COPD, measuring response to treatment in cystic fibrosis and COPD, and also in predicting risk of COPD exacerbations.

iii) Perhaps the greatest advantage of hyperpolarized gas MRI is for characterizing, or "phenotyping," disease progression and severity. The ADC has found particular utility in studies of COPD that have shown that ADC correlates with pulmonary function[87,101,102], is highly reproducible[82], and is sensitive to subclinical disease[70-72,103] and disease progression[84,98]. Thus there is potential use of hyperpolarized gas MRI to identify patients most likely to have severe outcomes at an earlier stage of disease progression. This, in turn, could allow more aggressive treatment to be targeted at these higher-risk individuals – an example of hyperpolarized gas MRI providing the means to personalized medicine[104].

iv) Other important emerging applications using hyperpolarized gas MRI include image-guided therapy, characterization of gas exchange, and combined structure-function MRI.

v) Image guided interventions using hyperpolarized ^{3}He MRI show promise for evaluating the effects of stent placement in COPD[105-107], smooth muscle ablation treatments in asthma[108,109] and radiation treatment planning in lung cancer[110-115].

vi) Moreover, gas exchange imaging with ^{129}Xe MRI shows promise for detection of gas diffusion block in idiopathic pulmonary fibrosis (IPF), a disease that is presently untreatable and for which conventional diagnostic imaging methods such as CT are insensitive[116]. However, with promising drug trials currently in progress early detection and prognosis may be sensitively detected with hyperpolarized ^{129}Xe MRI.

Perfusion Imaging:

Pulmonary perfusion imaging has been used in many benign and malignant lung diseases. A study reported application of dynamic MR perfusion imaging to be superior to MR and CT angiography in extent assessment of disease severity assessment and outcome prediction for acute pulmonary embolism[117]. Both CT and MR pulmonary perfusion imaging are being used in the assessment of pulmonary arteries and right ventricular function in patients with chronic thromboembolic disorders.

Fig. 9 shows an example of ventilation and perfusion assessment in a patient with chronic thromboembolic pulmonary hypertension. Various studies reported delayed regional perfusion in chronic thromboembolic disease when compared with acute pulmonary embolism[118]. This phenomenon is explained by perfusion from systemic collateral formation[118].

Fig. 10 shows an example of segmental delayed perfusion in a patient with previous pulmonary embolism and apparent perfusion defect in the pulmonary artery phase.

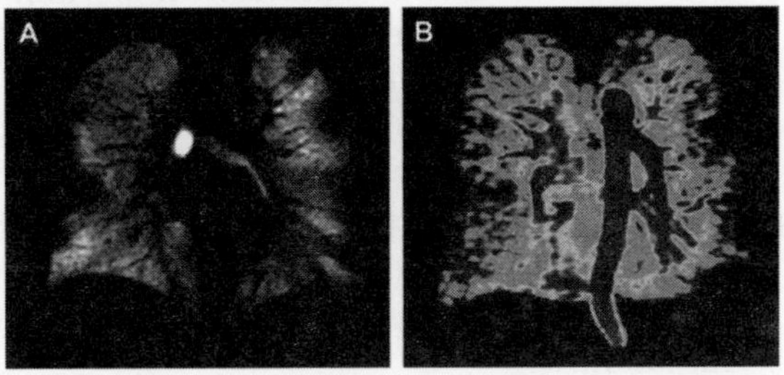

Fig. 9: MR ventilation and perfusion imaging in a patient with chronic thromboembolic pulmonary hypertension. Hyperpolarized ^{3}He MRI (A) demonstrated multiple peripheral ventilation defects. The dynamic gadolinium enhanced ^{1}H perfusion study (B) showed more extensive bilateral segmental perfusion abnormalities in segments with abnormal and normal ventilation (matched and mismatched VQ). (B) Pixels are colour coded in the parametric maps according to the degree of perfusion (from high to low perfusion values: red, yellow, green, blue/black).

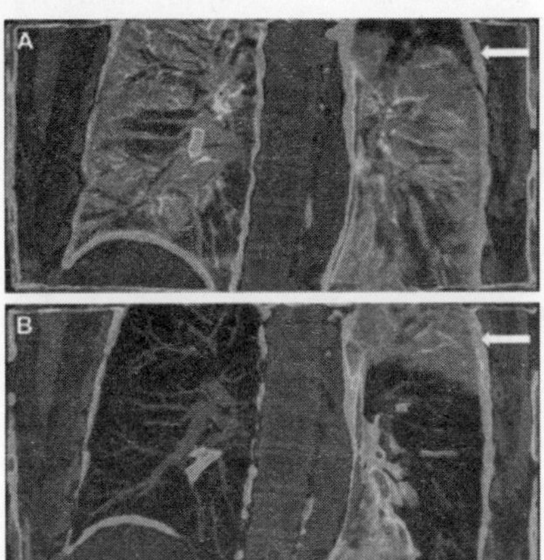

Fig. 10: Delayed perfusion after an episode of recent pulmonary embolism. Pixels are colour coded in the parametric maps according to the degree of perfusion (from high to low perfusion values: red, yellow, green, blue/black). Dual phase perfusion analysis shows lack of perfusion from pulmonary artery in the left upper lobe (arrow; A), but perfusion from other sources (arrow; B). The time delay was approximately 4 seconds.

Clinical Applications: These measures are being used to assess airway remodelling in both asthma and chronic obstructive pulmonary disease (COPD). **Figure 1** shows a depiction of the airway tree and lobe segmentation from both a normal non-smoker and a patient with COPD. These images can be used to not only quantify the airway and parenchyma characteristics but also to provide a roadmap linking airway paths to sub-lobar segment[25].

Ventilation Assessment:

The measurement of lung ventilation, lung volume, and tidal volume has traditionally been made for the entire lung, despite the fact that lung function in both health and disease is inhomogeneous. Xenon-enhanced MDCT (Xe-MDCT) is a method for the non-invasive measurement of regional pulmonary ventilation, determined from the wash-in and/or wash-out rates of the radiodense, non-radioactive gas xenon as measured in serially acquired, axial MDCT scans[25].

Clinical Application: The technique is used for evaluation of ventilation in various conditions, such as COPD[26], asthma[27], bronchiolitis obliterans[28].

Perfusion Imaging:

There have been a growing number of studies, demonstrating the use of MDCT with infusion of iodinated contrast agent to assess the presence of pulmonary emboli via visualization of flow voids in peripheral lung segments, and the improved ability to detect pulmonary emboli, aortic dissection and coronary atherosclerosis have resulted in the "triple rule out" method for use in patients with chest pain[29].

Many studies have reported the application of perfusion CT in assessment of pulmonary thromboembolism. A small observational study comparing dual energy CT (DECT) perfusion with CT pulmonary angiogram (CTPA) demonstrated a sensitivity and specificity of 100% on a per-patient basis, and 60% to 66.7%, and 99.5% to 99.8% on a per-segment basis, the sensitivity and specificity ranged between 60% and 66.7%, and 99.5% and 99.8%[30]. Compared with scintigraphy, the reported sensitivity and specificity of DECT perfusion on a per-patient basis was 75% and 80%, and 83% and 99% on a per-segment basis[31]. **Figure 2** shows the advantage of CT perfusion over CTPA in the detection of peripheral pulmonary arterial vascular obstruction that is often missed on CTPA, especially in the subacute cases of pulmonary embolism.

A study of dynamic CT perfusion in patients with minor emphysema versus control (healthy volunteers and smokers without emphysema) reported globally increased heterogeneity in the early emphysema group, but not in the control group. The authors suggested that the CT perfusion might be able to differentiate smokers at risk of emphysema[32]. When emphysema is established, alveolar surface reduction is associated with reduction in capillary volume[33,34]. As a result, the reduction in perfusion on CT correlated with severity of emphysema[35]. **Figure 3** shows diffuse perfusion changes in a patient with emphysema.

Clinical Applications: i) Perfusion CT is superior to CTPA and scintigraphy in detection of pulmonary embolism, ii) CT perfusion might be able to differentiate smokers at risk of emphysema, and iii) Dynamic perfusion CT is reported to be more specific and accurate than static positron emission tomography/CT for differentiating malignant from benign pulmonary nodules of less than 3 cm[36].

Advantages of pulmonary MRI over pulmonary function testing and scintigraphy:

Pulmonary MRI approaches have important advantages over established clinical methods such as pulmonary function testing and scintigraphy that could change the current cost-benefit calculus.

1) Pulmonary function testing cannot easily characterize different phenotypes of disease.
2) Furthermore, pulmonary function testing is a global assessment of the lungs and is generally insensitive to clinically important changes in disease severity that might impact patient management, especially as more therapy options become available and more mild disease is targeted.
3) The spatial resolution of scintigraphy is generally poorer than that achievable with MRI and scintigraphy requires ionizing radiation.
4) The use of X-ray based methods, including CT, diminish the numbers and types of imaging sessions that are practical for longitudinal assessment of lung disease due to the potentially harmful effects of accumulated ionizing radiation exposure in patients with chronic lung disease.

   The continued development of ultra-low dose CT[126] may impact this assessment, but it should also be noted that newer functional lung imaging methods using x-ray CT – for example, perfusion and dual energy xenon CT[127] – require more radiation than standard chest CT.
5) Furthermore, recent advances in gradient performance and image reconstruction have significantly improved image quality for structural MRI of the lungs.

Summary

This chapter shows the breadth of functional lung assessment that can now be achieved with excellent image quality in the chest. A combination of perfusion and ventilation assessment is feasible with great detail, and this may help study the effects of treatments. Assessment of regional lung ventilation and gas exchange can be done by oxygen enhanced MRI, hyperpolarized gas MRI and Xenon CT whereas pulmonary perfusion can be assessed by CT and MRI after administration of contrast material. The technologies have clearly made significant strides over the past 5 to 10 years, and there is an increasing role for functional imaging for study of pathophysiologic processes in the lungs.

Glossary

ADC	Apparent Diffusion Coefficient
COPD	Chronic Obstructive Pulmonary Disease
DLCO	Diffusing Capacity of the Lungs for Carbon Monoxide
FEV1	Forced Expiratory Volume in 1 Second
VDP	Ventilation Defect Percentage

REFERENCES

1. Roy BS, Sujai A, et al. Role of dynamic MR imaging in obstructive sleep apnoea. Indian J. Otolaryngol. Head Neck Surg. 2008;60:25–29.
2. Stern EJ, Graham CM, Webb WR, et al. Normal trachea during forced expiration: dynamic CT measurements. Department of Radiology, University of California San Francisco. 1993;187.1
3. Jingbo Z, Ichiro S, David F, et al. Dynamic Expiratory Volumetric CT Imaging of the Central Airways: Comparison of Standard-Dose and Low-Dose Techniques. 2003;10(7):719-724.
4. Ritman, EL. Robb, RA, Harris, LD. Imaging Physiological Functions: Experience with the DSR. Philadelphia: Praeger; 1985.
5. Hoffman EA, Larsen RL. Regional Pulmonary Blood Flow via X-ray CT and Biodegradable Radiopaque Microspheres. Circulation 1990;4:111–124.
6. Boyd, DP. Lipton, MJ. Cardiac computed tomography; Proceedings of the IEEE; 1983. p. 298-307.
7. Saito T, Misaki M, Shirato K, Takishima T. Three-dimensional quantitative coronary angiography. IEEE Trans Biomed Eng 1990;37:768–777
8. Saito Y. Multislice X-ray CT scanner. Med Rev 1998;98:1–8.
9. Wang G, Lin TH, Cheng PC, Shinozaki DM. A general cone-beam reconstruction algorithm. IEEE Trans Medical Imaging 1993;12:486–496.
10. Hounsfield GN. Computerized transverse axial scanning (tomography). Description of system. Br J Radiol 1973;46:1016–22.
11. Kasai J, Sugiura T, Tanabe N, et al. Electrocardiogram-gated 320-slice multidetector computed tomography for the measurement of pulmonary arterial distensibility in chronic thromboembolic pulmonary hypertension. PLoS One 2014;9:e111563.
12. Hounsfield GN. Computed medical imaging. Nobel lecture, December 8, 1973. J Comput Assist Tomogr 1980;4:665–74.
13. Meyer M, Haubenreisser H, Raupach R, et al. Initial results of a new generation dual source CT system using only an in-plane comb filter for ultra-high resolution temporal bone imaging. Eur Radiol 2015; 25(1):178–85.
14. Newell JD Jr, Fuld MK, Allmendinger T, et al. Very low-dose (0.15 mGy) chest CT protocols using the COPDGene 2 test object and a third-generation dual source CT scanner with corresponding thirdgeneration iterative reconstruction software. Invest Radiol 2015;50(1):40–5.
15. Gordic S, Morsbach F, Schmidt B, et al. Ultra low dose chest computed tomography for pulmonary nodule detection: first performance evaluation of single energy scanning with

spectral shaping. Invest Radiol 2014;49:465–73.

16. Johnson TR, Nikolaou K, Fink C, et al. Dual-source CT in chest pain diagnosis. Radiol 2007;47:301–309.
17. Johnson TR, Krauss B, Sedlmair M, et al. Material differentiation by dual energy CT: initial experience. Eur Radiol 2007;17:1510–1517.
18. Saba, OI.; Fuld, MK.; Krauss, B.; Van Beek, EJ.; McLennan, G.; Hoffman, EA. Dual Energy MDCT for Volumetric Assessment of V/Q: Initial Experiences; American Thoracic Society Annual Meeting; San Francisco, CA. 2007. p. A938
19. Fuld, M.; Saba, O.; Krauss, B.; Van Beek, EJ.; McClennan, G.; Hoffman, EA. Dual Energy Xe-MDCT for Automated Assessment of the Central airway Tree: initial Experiences; American Thoracic Society Annual Meeting; San Francisco, CA. 2007. p. A250
20. Ameli-Renani S, Rahman F, Nair A, et al. Dual-energy CT for imaging of pulmonary hypertension: challenges and opportunities. Radiographics 2014; 34:1769–90.
21. Sakamoto A, Sakamoto I, Nagayama H, et al. Quantification of lung perfusion blood volume with dualenergy CT: assessment of the severity of acute pulmonary thromboembolism. Am J Roentgenol 2014;203:287–91.
22. Zhang LJ, Zhou CS, Schoepf UJ, et al. Dual-energy CT lung ventilation/perfusion imaging for diagnosing pulmonary embolism. Eur Radiol 2013;23:2666–75.
23. Fuld MK, Halaweish AF, Newell JD Jr, et al. Optimization of dual-energy xenon-computed tomography for quantitative assessment of regional pulmonary ventilation. Invest Radiol 2013;48:629–37.
24. Nakano Y, Wong JC, de Jong PA, et al. The prediction of small airway dimensions using computed tomography. Am J Respir Crit Care Med 2005;171:142–146.
25. van Beek EJ, Hoffman EA. Functional imaging: CT and MRI. Clin Chest Med 2008;29:195–216.
26. Park EA, Goo JM, Park SJ, et al. Chronic obstructive pulmonary disease: quantitative and visual ventilation pattern analysis at xenon ventilation CT performed by using a dual-energy technique. Radiol 2010;256:985–97.
27. Chae EJ, Seo JB, Lee J, et al. Xenon ventilation imaging using dual-energy computed tomography in asthmatics: initial experience. Invest Radiol 2010; 45:354–61.
28. Goo HW, Yang DH, Hong SJ, et al. Xenon ventilation CT using dual-source and dual-energy technique in children with bronchiolitis obliterans: correlation of xenon and CT density values with pulmonary function test results. Pediatr Radiol 2010;40:1490–7.
29. Johnson TR, Nikolaou K, Wintersperger BJ, et al. ECG-gated 64-MDCT angiography in the differential diagnosis of acute chest pain. AJR Am J Roentgenol 2007;188:76–82.
30. Fink C, Johnson TR, Michaely HJ, et al. Dual-energy CT angiography of the lung in patients with suspected pulmonary embolism: initial results. Rofo 2008;180(10):879–83.
31. Thieme SF, Becker CR, Hacker M, et al. Dual energy CT for the assessment of lung perfusion: correlation to scintigraphy. Eur J Radiol 2008;68(3):369–74.
32. Alford SK, van Beek EJ, McLennan G, et al. Heterogeneity of pulmonary perfusion as a mechanistic image-based phenotype in emphysema susceptible smokers. Proc Natl Acad Sci U S A 2010;107(16): 7485–90.
33. Morrison NJ, Abboud RT, Muller NL, et al. Pulmonary capillary blood volume in emphysema. Am Rev Respir Dis 1990;141(1):53–61.

34. Barbera' JA, Riverola A, Roca J, et al. Pulmonary vascular abnormalities and ventilation-perfusion relationships in mild chronic obstructive pulmonary disease. Am J Respir Crit Care Med 1994;149(2 Pt 1):423–9.
35. Pansini V, Remy-Jardin M, Faivre JB, et al. Assessment of lobar perfusion in smokers according to the presence and severity of emphysema: preliminary experience with dual-energy CT angiography. Eur Radiol 2009;19(12):2834–43.
36. Ohno Y, Koyama H, Matsumoto K, et al. Differentiation of malignant and benign pulmonary nodules with quantitative first-pass 320-detector row perfusion CT versus FDG PET/CT. Radiol 2011; 258(2):599–609.
37. Edelman RR, Hatabu H, Tadamura E, Li W, Prasad PV. Noninvasive assessment of regional ventilation in the human lung using oxygen-enhanced magnetic resonance imaging. Nat Med. 1996; 2(11):1236–1239.
38. Kuethe DO, Caprihan A, Fukushima E, Waggoner RA. Imaging lungs using inert fluorinated gases. Jour Mag Reson Med. 1998; 39(1):85–88.
39. Fain S, Schiebler ML, McCormack DG, Parraga G. Imaging of lung function using hyperpolarized helium-3 magnetic resonance imaging: Review of current and emerging translational methods and applications. Jour Mag Res Imag JMRI. 2010; 32(6):1398–1408.
40. Mugler JP 3rd, Altes TA. Hyperpolarized 129Xe MRI of the human lung. Jour Magnetic Reson Imag : JMRI. 2013; 37(2):313–331.
41. Melo V. Quantification of Regional Ventilation-Perfusion Ratios with PET. Jour Nucl Med 2003; 44:1982–1991.
42. Johnson KM, Fain SB, Schiebler ML, Nagle S. Optimized 3D ultrashort echo time pulmonary MRI. Jour Mag Reson Med 2012
43. Bauman G, Eichinger M. Ventilation and perfusion magnetic resonance imaging of the lung. Polish Jour Radiol 2012; 77(1):37–46.
44. Kuo W, Ciet P, Tiddens H, Zhang W, Guillerman RP, van Straten M. Reply: Cumulative radiation exposure to abdominal organs in patients with cystic fibrosis should not be forgotten. Amer J Respir Crit Care Med 2014; 190(8):962.
45. Kuo W, Ciet P, Tiddens HA, Zhang W, Guillerman RP, van Straten M. Monitoring cystic fibrosis lung disease by computed tomography. Radiation risk in perspective. Amer J Respir Crit Care Med 2014; 189(11):1328–1336.
46. de Jong PA, Tiddens HA, Lequin MH, Robinson TE, Brody AS. Estimation of the radiation dose from CT in cystic fibrosis. Chest. 2008; 133(5):1289–1291. author reply 1290–1281.
47. Benamore RE, O'Doherty MJ, Entwisle JJ. Use of imaging in the management of malignant pleural mesothelioma. Clin Radiol 2005;60:1237–1247.
48. Erasmus JJ, Truong MT, Munden RF. CT, MR, and PET imaging in staging of non-small-cell lung cancer. Semin Roentgenol 2005;40:126–142.
49. Puderbach M, Hintze C, Ley S, Eichinger M, Kauczor HU, Biederer J. MR imaging of the chest: A practical approach at 1.5T. Eur J Radiol. 2007
50. Swift AJ, Woodhouse N, Fichele S, et al. Rapid lung volumetry using ultrafast dynamic magnetic resonance imaging during forced vital capacity maneuver: correlation with spirometry. Invest Radiol 2007;42:37–41.

51. Eichinger M, Tetzlaff R, Puderbach M, Woodhouse N, Kauczor HU. Proton magnetic resonance imaging for assessment of lung function and respiratory dynamics. Eur J Radiol. 2007
52. Pedersen MR, Fisher MT, van Beek EJ. MR imaging of the pulmonary vasculature—an update. Eur Radiol 2006;16:1374–1386.
53. Kreitner KF, Kunz RP, Ley S, et al. Chronic thromboembolic pulmonary hypertension – assessment by magnetic resonance imaging. Eur Radiol 2007;17:11–21.
54. Ley S, Zaporozhan J, Arnold R, et al. Preoperative assessment and follow-up of congenital abnormalities of the pulmonary arteries using CT and MRI. Eur Radiol 2007;17:151–162.
55. Meaney JF, Weg JG, Chenevert TL, Stafford-Johnson D, Hamilton BH, Prince MR. Diagnosis of pulmonary embolism with magnetic resonance angiography. N Engl J Med 1997;336:1422–1427.
56. Oudkerk M, van Beek EJ, Wielopolski P, et al. Comparison of contrast-enhanced magnetic resonance angiography and conventional pulmonary angiography for the diagnosis of pulmonary embolism: a prospective study. Lancet 2002;359:1643–1647.
57. Ohno Y, Higashino T, Takenaka D, et al. MR angiography with sensitivity encoding (SENSE) for suspected pulmonary embolism: comparison with MDCT and ventilation-perfusion scintigraphy. AJR Am J Roentgenol 2004;183:91–98.
58. Rajaram S, Swift AJ, Telfer A, et al. 3D contrast enhanced lung perfusion MRI is an effective screening tool for thromboembolic pulmonary hypertension: results from the ASPIRE registry. Thorax 2013;68:677–8.
59. Swift AJ, Wild J, Nagle S, et al. Quantitative MR imaging of pulmonary hypertension: a practical approach to the current state of the art. J Thorac Imaging 2014;29:68–79.
60. De Lange EE, Altes TA, Patrie JT, et al. Changes in regional airflow obstruction over time in the lungs of patients with asthma: evaluation with 3He MR imaging. Radiol 2009;250:567–75.
61. Mugler JP 3rd, Altes TA, Ruset IC, et al. Simultaneous magnetic resonance imaging of ventilation distribution and gas uptake in the human lung using hyperpolarized xenon-129. Proc Natl Acad Sci U S A 2010;107:21707–12.
62. Wild JM, Schmiedeskamp J, Paley MN, et al. MR imaging of the lungs with hyperpolarized helium-3 gas transported by air. Phys Med Biol 2002;47:N185–N190.
63. Fain SB, Gonzalez-Fernandez G, Peterson ET, et al. Evaluation of structure-function relationships in asthma using multidetector CT and hyperpolarized He-3 MRI. Acad Radiol 2008; 15(6):753–762.
64. Sheikh K, Paulin GA, Svenningsen S, et al. Pulmonary ventilation defects in older never-smokers. Jour Appl Physiol 2014; 117(3):297–306.
65. Woodhouse N, Wild JM, Paley MN, et al. Combined helium-3/proton magnetic resonance imaging measurement of ventilated lung volumes in smokers compared to never-smokers. Jour Mag Res Imag JMRI. 2005; 21(4):365–369.
66. Mathew L, Evans A, Ouriadov A, et al. Hyperpolarized 3He magnetic resonance imaging of chronic obstructive pulmonary disease: reproducibility at 3.0 tesla. Acad Radiol 2008; 15(10):1298–1311.
67. van Beek EJ, Dahmen AM, Stavngaard T, et al. Hyperpolarised 3He MRI versus HRCT in COPD and normal volunteers: PHIL trial. Eur Respir Jour. 2009; 34(6):1311–1321.
68. Tzeng YS, Lutchen K, Albert M. The difference in ventilation heterogeneity between asthmatic and healthy subjects quantified using hyperpolarized 3He MRI. Jour Appl Physiol 2009; 106(3):813–822.

69. Virgincar RS, Cleveland ZI, Kaushik SS, et al. Quantitative analysis of hyperpolarized 129Xe ventilation imaging in healthy volunteers and subjects with chronic obstructive pulmonary disease. NMR in biomedicine. 2013; 26(4):424–435.

70. Fain SB, Panth SR, Evans MD, et al. Early emphysematous changes in asymptomatic smokers: detection with 3He MR imaging. Radiol 2006; 239(3):875–883.

71. Quirk JD, Lutey BA, Gierada DS, et al. In vivo detection of acinar microstructural changes in early emphysema with (3)He lung morphometry. Radiol 2011; 260(3):866–874.

72. Kirby M, Owrangi A, Svenningsen S, et al. On the role of abnormal DL(CO) in ex-smokers without airflow limitation: symptoms, exercise capacity and hyperpolarised helium-3 MRI. Thorax. 2013; 68(8):752–759.

73. Tustison NJ, Avants BB, Flors L, et al. Ventilation-based segmentation of the lungs using hyperpolarized (3)He MRI. Jour Mag Res Imag JMRI. 2011; 34(4):831–841.

74. Kirby M, Heydarian M, Svenningsen S, et al. Hyperpolarized 3He magnetic resonance functional imaging semiautomated segmentation. Acad Radiol 2012; 19(2):141–152.

75. Niles DJ, Kruger SJ, Dardzinski BJ, et al. Exercise-induced bronchoconstriction: reproducibility of hyperpolarized 3He MR imaging. Radiol 2013; 266(2):618–625.

76. He M, Kaushik SS, Robertson SH, et al. Extending semiautomatic ventilation defect analysis for hyperpolarized (129)xe ventilation MRI. Acad Radiol. 2014; 21(12):1530–1541.

77. Kirby M, Svenningsen S, Ahmed H, et al. Quantitative evaluation of hyperpolarized helium-3 magnetic resonance imaging of lung function variability in cystic fibrosis. Acad Radiol 2011; 18(8):1006–1013.

78. de Lange EE, Altes TA, Patrie JT, et al. Evaluation of asthma with hyperpolarized helium-3 MRI: correlation with clinical severity and spirometry. Chest. 2006; 130(4):1055–1062.

79. Kruger SJ, Niles DJ, Dardzinski BJ. Exercise-Induced Bronchoconstriction: Hyperpolarized Helium-3 MRI During Challenge and Therapy Jour Mag Reson Med 2013

80. Kirby M, Pike D, Coxson HO, McCormack DG, Parraga G. Hyperpolarized (3)he ventilation defects used to predict pulmonary exacerbations in mild to moderate chronic obstructive pulmonary disease. Radiol. 2014; 273(3):887–896.

81. Kauczor HU, Ebert M, Kreitner KF, et al. Imaging of the lungs using 3He MRI: preliminary clinical experience in 18 patients with and without lung disease. Jour Mag Res Imag: JMRI. 1997; 7(3):538–543.

82. Diaz S, Casselbrant I, Piitulainen E, et al. Hyperpolarized 3He apparent diffusion coefficient MRI of the lung: reproducibility and volume dependency in healthy volunteers and patients with emphysema. Jour Mag Reson Imag: JMRI. 2008; 27(4):763–770.

83. Halaweish AF, Hoffman EA, Thedens DR, Fuld MK, Sieren JP, van Beek EJ. Effect of lung inflation level on hyperpolarized 3He apparent diffusion coefficient measurements in never-smokers. Radiol 2013; 268(2):572–580.

84. Diaz S, Casselbrant I, Piitulainen E, et al. Progression of emphysema in a 12-month hyperpolarized 3He-MRI study: lacunarity analysis provided a more sensitive measure than standard ADC analysis. Acad Radiol 2009; 16(6):700–707.

85. Kaushik SS, Cleveland ZI, Cofer GP, et al. Diffusion-weighted hyperpolarized 129Xe MRI in healthy volunteers and subjects with chronic obstructive pulmonary disease Jour Mag Reson Med 2011; 65(4):1154–1165.

86. Fain SB, Altes TA, Panth SR, et al. Detection of age-dependent changes in healthy adult lungs with diffusion-weighted 3He MRI. Acad Radiol 2005; 12(11):1385–1393. [PubMed: 16253850]

87. Salerno M, de Lange EE, Altes TA, Truwit JD, Brookeman JR, Mugler JP 3rd. Emphysema: hyperpolarized helium 3 diffusion MR imaging of the lungs compared with spirometric indexes—initial experience. Radiol 2002; 222(1):252–260.

88. Kirby M, Svenningsen S, Kanhere N, et al. Pulmonary ventilation visualized using hyperpolarized helium-3 and xenon-129 magnetic resonance imaging: differences in COPD and relationship to emphysema. Jour Appl Physiol 2013; 114(6):707–715.

89. Kirby M, Parraga G. Pulmonary functional imaging using hyperpolarized noble gas MRI: six years of start-up experience at a single site. Acad Radiol 2013; 20(11):1344–1356.

90. Fischer MC, Spector ZZ, Ishii M, et al. Single-acquisition sequence for the measurement of oxygen partial pressure by hyperpolarized gas MRI. Jour Mag Reson Med 2004; 52(4):766–773.

91. Deninger AJ, Eberle B, Ebert M, et al. Quantification of regional intrapulmonary oxygen partial pressure evolution during apnea by (3)He MRI. Jour Mag Reson 1999; 141(2):207–216.

92. Deninger AJ, Eberle B, Bermuth J, et al. Assessment of a single-acquisition imaging sequence for oxygen-sensitive (3)He-MRI. Jour Mag Reson Med 2002; 47(1):105–114.

93. Rizi RR, Baumgardner JE, Ishii M, et al. Determination of regional VA/Q by hyperpolarized 3He MRI. Mag Reson Med 2004; 52(1):65–72.

94. Hamedani H, Kadlecek SJ, Ishii M, et al. A variability study of regional alveolar oxygen tension measurement in humans using hyperpolarized (3) He MRI. Jour Mag Reson Med 2013; 70(6):1557–1566.

95. Hamedani H, Kadlecek SJ, Ishii M, et al. Alterations of Regional Alveolar Oxygen Tension in Asymptomatic Current Smokers: Assessment with Hyperpolarized He MR Imaging. Radiol. 2014:132809.

96. Altes TA, Powers PL, Knight-Scott J, et al. Hyperpolarized 3He MR lung ventilation imaging in asthmatics: preliminary findings. Jour Mag Res Imag : JMRI. 2001; 13(3):378–384.

97. Samee S, Altes T, Powers P, et al. Imaging the lungs in asthmatic patients by using hyperpolarized helium-3 magnetic resonance: assessment of response to methacholine and exercise challenge. Jour Allerg Clin Immunol . 2003; 111(6):1205–1211.

98. Kirby M, Mathew L, Wheatley A, Santyr GE, McCormack DG, Parraga G. Chronic obstructive pulmonary disease: longitudinal hyperpolarized (3)He MR imaging. Radiol. 2010; 256(1):280–289.

99. Mentore K, Froh DK, de Lange EE, Brookeman JR, Paget-Brown AO, Altes TA. Hyperpolarized HHe 3 MRI of the lung in cystic fibrosis: assessment at baseline and after bronchodilator and airway clearance treatment. Acad Radiol . 2005; 12(11):1423–1429.

100. Paulin GA, Svenningsen S, Jobse BN, et al. Differences in hyperpolarized He ventilation imaging after 4 years in adults with cystic fibrosis. Jour Mag Reson Imag JMRI. 2014

101. Morbach AE, Gast KK, Schmiedeskamp J, et al. Diffusion-weighted MRI of the lung with hyperpolarized helium-3: a study of reproducibility. Jour Mag Res Imag : JMRI. 2005; 21(6):765–774.

102. Diaz S, Casselbrant I, Piitulainen E, et al. Validity of apparent diffusion coefficient hyperpolarized 3He-MRI using MSCT and pulmonary function tests as references. Europ J Radiol 2009; 71(2):257–263.

103. Wang C, Mugler JP 3rd, de Lange EE, Patrie JT, Mata JF, Altes TA. Lung injury induced by secondhand smoke exposure detected with hyperpolarized helium-3 diffusion MR. Jour Mag Res Imag: JMRI. 2014; 39(1):77–84.

104. Kirby M, Kanhere N, Etemad-Rezai R, McCormack DG, Parraga G. Hyperpolarized helium-3 magnetic resonance imaging of chronic obstructive pulmonary disease exacerbation. Jour Mag Res Imag : JMRI. 2013; 37(5):1223–1227.

105. Mata J, Altes T, Truwit J, et al. Characterization and detection of physiologic lung changes before and after placement of bronchial valves using hyperpolarized helium-3 MR imaging: preliminary study. Acad Radiol 2011; 18(9):1195–1199.

106. Snell GI, Holsworth L, Borrill ZL, et al. The potential for bronchoscopic lung volume reduction using bronchial prostheses: a pilot study. Chest. 2003; 124(3):1073–1080.

107. Mathew L, Kirby M, Farquhar D, et al. Hyperpolarized 3He functional magnetic resonance imaging of bronchoscopic airway bypass in chronic obstructive pulmonary disease. Canadian Respir Jour 2012; 19(1):41–43.

108. Thomen RP, Sheshadri A, Quirk JD, et al. Regional Ventilation Changes in Severe Asthma after Bronchial Thermoplasty with (3)He MR Imaging and CT. Radiol. 2015; 274(1):250–259.

109. Cox G, Thomson NC, Rubin AS, et al. Asthma control during the year after bronchial thermoplasty. New Engl J Med. 2007; 356(13):1327–1337.

110. Ireland RH, Bragg CM, McJury M, et al. Feasibility of image registration and intensity-modulated radiotherapy planning with hyperpolarized helium-3 magnetic resonance imaging for non-small-cell lung cancer. Internat Jour Radiat Oncol Biol Physic. 2007; 68(1):273–281.

111. Ireland RH, Woodhouse N, Hoggard N, et al. An image acquisition and registration strategy for the fusion of hyperpolarized helium-3 MRI and x-ray CT images of the lung. Physic Med Biol 2008; 53(21):6055–6063.

112. Bates EL, Bragg CM, Wild JM, Hatton MQ, Ireland RH. Functional image-based radiotherapy planning for non-small cell lung cancer: A simulation study. Radiotherapy and oncology Jour Eur Sic Therapeut Radiol Oncol. 2009; 93(1); 32-36

113. Hodge CW, Tome WA, Fain SB, Bentzen SM, Mehta MP. On the use of hyperpolarized helium MRI for conformal avoidance lung radiotherapy. Medical dosimetry : Jour Amer Assoc Med Dosimetrists. 2010; 35(4):297–303.

114. Tahir BA, Swift AJ, Marshall H, et al. A method for quantitative analysis of regional lung ventilation using deformable image registration of CT and hybrid hyperpolarized gas/(1)H MRI. Physic Med Biology. 2014; 59(23):7267–7277.

115. Cai J, McLawhorn R, Altes TA, et al. Helical tomotherapy planning for lung cancer based on ventilation magnetic resonance imaging. Medical dosimetry : Jour Amer Assoc Med Dosimetrists. 2011; 36(4):389–396.

116. Kaushik SS, Freeman MS, Yoon SW, et al. Measuring diffusion limitation with a perfusion-limited gas—hyperpolarized 129Xe gas-transfer spectroscopy in patients with idiopathic pulmonary fibrosis. Jour Appl Physiol 2014; 117(6):577–585.

117. Ohno Y, Koyama H, Matsumoto K, et al. Dynamic MR perfusion imaging: capability for quantitative assessment of disease extent and prediction of outcome for patients with acute pulmonary thromboembolism. J Magn Reson Imag 2010;31(5): 1081–90.

118. Hong YJ, Kim JY, Choe KO, et al. Different perfusion pattern between acute and chronic pulmonary thromboembolism: evaluation with two-phase dualenergy perfusion CT. AJR Am J Roentgenol 2013; 200(4):812–7.

119. Schaefer JF, Vollmar J, Schick F, et al. Solitary pulmonary nodules: dynamic contrast-enhanced MR imaging– differences in malignant and benign lesions. Radiology 2004;232:544–53.

120. Dean PB, Niemi P, Kivisaari L, et al. Comparative pharmacokinetics of gadolinium DTPA and gadolinium chloride. Invest Radiol 1988;23(Suppl 1): S258–60.

121. Milne EN, Noonan CD, Margulis AR, et al. Vascular supply of pulmonary metastases: experimental study in rats. Invest Radiol 1969;4:215–29.

122. Milne EN, Zerhouni EA. Blood supply of pulmonary metastases. J Thorac Imaging 1987;2:15–23.

123. Ohno Y, Iwasawa T, Seo JB, et al. Oxygen-enhanced magnetic resonance imaging versus computed tomography: multicentre study for clinical stage classification of smoking-related chronic obstructive pulmonary disease. Am J Respir Crit Care Med 2008;177:1095–102.

124. Ohno Y, Nishio M, Koyama H, et al. Asthma: comparison of dynamic oxygen-enhanced MR imaging and quantitative thin-section CT for evaluation of clinical treatment. Radiol 2014;273:907–16.

125. Wild JM, Woodhouse N, Fichele S, et al. 3D volume-localized pO2 measurement in the human lung with 3He MRI. Magn Reson Med 2005;20:1055–64.

126. Yu H, Zhao S, Hoffman EA, Wang G. Ultra-low dose lung CT perfusion regularized by a previous scan. Academic Radiol 2009; 16(3):363–373.

127. Kim WW, Lee CH, Goo JM, et al. Xenon-enhanced dual-energy CT of patients with asthma: dynamic ventilation changes after methacholine and salbutamol inhalation. AJR Amer J Roentgenol 2012; 199(5):975–981.

13

RADIONUCLEIDES IN REGIONAL LUNG FUNCTION SCINTILLATION AND PERFUSION STUDIES

AMITA NENE, SWAPNIL KULKARNI

Introduction

Lung function has to be evaluated not only globally but also regionally because some of the abnormalities may occur focally. Ventilation-Perfusion scans (V/Q Scans) are specialized radiological techniques to examine lungs in which tiny amount of a radioactive substance is used.[1]

There are two types of scans:

- Ventilation scan- It evaluates ventilation or air in and out of airways.
- Perfusion scan- It evaluates blood flow within the lungs.

Radionuclide or radioactive substance will get collected at abnormal blood flow in perfusion scan, while in ventilation scan radionuclide will fill all over lungs except in parts in which air cannot move. The emitted radionuclide is then detected by scanner. Areas are then divided into 'hot spots' where radionuclide collects and 'cold spots' where it does not.[1]

The information gained from these studies may be used to diagnose and determine treatment of lung diseases. While radionuclide lung studies are essentially qualitative, they have an advantage over most quantitative tests of global lung function in distinguishing between diffuse and regional lung disease with the option of loco-regional semi quantitation.

The use of radioactive tracers to study lung functions dates back to 1955 when Knipping et al[2] and his team used $Xenon^{133}$ (Xe^{133}) to examine regional ventilation. Later Dyson and Sinclair used $Oxygen^{15}$ to study pulmonary blood flow in 1960. Contribution of many such scientists has led to the development of far sophisticated and noninvasive techniques available at present.

Definitions

Lung scintigraphy is a diagnostic imaging procedure that uses ventilation scintigraphy, perfusion scintigraphy, or both to evaluate cardiovascular and pulmonary disorders. [3]

Aerosol ventilation scintigraphy is a diagnostic imaging test that records the bronchopulmonary distribution of an inhaled radioactive aerosol within the lungs. [3]

Gas ventilation scintigraphy is a diagnostic imaging test that records the pulmonary distribution of a radioactive gas during breathing. [3]

Pulmonary perfusion scintigraphy is a diagnostic imaging test that records the distribution of pulmonary arterial blood flow. [3]

Common clinical indications for lung scintigraphy

Indications for lung scintigraphy include, but are not limited to, the following:

A. Most common clinical indication

The most common clinical indication for lung scintigraphy is to determine the likelihood of pulmonary embolism.[4]

B. Less common clinical indications

- Document the degree of resolution of pulmonary embolism.[5]
- Quantify differential pulmonary function before pulmonary surgery for lung cancer.[6]
- Evaluate lung transplants. [7]
- Evaluate congenital heart or lung disease such as (cardiac shunts, pulmonary arterial stenoses, and arteriovenous fistulae and their treatment. [8]
- Confirm the presence of bronchopleural fistula. [9]
- Evaluate chronic pulmonary parenchymal disorders such as cystic fibrosis. [10]
- Evaluate the cause of pulmonary hypertension.[11]

Procedure / Specification of the examination

A. Gathering clinical history and other important information:

1) Important clinical history includes - right-to-left shunt, severe pulmonary hypertension, chest pain, dyspnea, hemoptysis, syncope, symptoms of deep venous thrombosis, oral contraceptive use, recent surgery, prior pulmonary embolism, cancer, congestive heart failure, antecedent illness, smoking and intravenous drug abuse.[1]
2) In women of childbearing age, pregnancy and lactation status should be noted and the procedure is performed in a manner to minimize radiation exposure.[12]
3) Important clinical findings on physical examination include, a) vital signs, particularly respiratory rate; b) chest examination; c) cardiac examination; and d) leg findings.
4) Results of D-dimer test, if obtained, should be noted.
5) Review of prior lung scintigraphy should be reviewed. Defects from prior pulmonary emboli do not always resolve completely.[13]
6) Pertinent chest radiographic findings include, consolidation, atelectasis, effusions, masses, cardiomegaly and decreased pulmonary vasculature. Chest radiograph may be normal in patients with pulmonary embolism.
7) Treatment with anti-coagulant or thrombolytic therapy should be noted.

B. Patient Preparation:

1) A routine chest radiograph obtained in both the posterior-anterior and lateral projections is preferred. In patients who have no changes in signs or symptoms, a chest radiograph within 1 day of scintigraphy is adequate. A more recent chest radiograph (preferably within 1 hour) is necessary in patients whose signs and symptoms are changing.
2) A CT scan can substitute for the chest radiography.
3) Before administration of the radiopharmaceutical, the patient should be instructed to cough and to take several deep breaths.

C) Radionuclides:

1) Ventilation Imaging –

i) Aerosols:

Tc^{99m} diethylenetriamine - pentaacetic acid (DTPA) is the preferred radionuclide. Aerosol inhalation scans have been used as an indication of regional ventilation. Tc^{99m} labeled DTPA is the most widely used aerosol which clears from the lungs with a half-life of 60 minutes. The usual administered activity of Tc^{99m} DTPA is 900-1300 MBq (0.5-1.0 mCi) to the lungs. Aerosol imaging is usually performed before perfusion imaging because it is more difficult to deliver a larger dose of Tc^{99m} MAA (macroaggregated albumin) as both are labeled with Tc^{99m} , it's important that the count rate of the second study is at least 3-4 times the first study.

ii) Krypton^{81m}:

Krypton^{81m} is a noble gas that can be used to evaluate regional ventilation. This radioactive gas has a very short physical half-life (13 sec), and images acquired with this agent reveal ventilation to major airway systems only. However, the short physical half-life of Krypton^{81m} allows generation of images of the lungs in multiple projections. Krypton^{81m} is produced from a rubidium 81 generator. The parent radionuclide has a physical half-life of 4.7 hours, which limits the useful lifetime of the generator to only 1 day. Imaging with Krypton^{81m} is generally performed following the perfusion scan. The usual administered activity of Krypton^{81m} 40-400 MBq (1-10mCi).

iii) Xenon (Xe ^{133}) :

Xe ^{133} has been widely used to determine regional ventilation in the lungs. For technical reasons (lower energy of gamma radiation of Xe^{133} compared to Tc^{99m}), ventilation images with Xe^{133} are obtained before perfusion imaging [11]. With Xe^{133}, images can be obtained only in a limited number of views in contrast to perfusion images, which are obtained in multiple projections. The usual administered activity is 200-750 MBq (5-20mCi).

2) Perfusion Imaging –

Tc^{99m} macroaggregated albumin (Tc^{99m}MAA):[13,14]

Currently, the agent of choice for pulmonary perfusion imaging is technetium 99m–labeled macroaggregated albumin (Tc^{99m}MAA). These particles range in size from 10 to 150 m. Tc^{99m}MAA is considered the agent of choice for routine perfusion lung scanning because of its availability, short residence time in the lungs, and relatively low cost. The usual administered dose of radioactivity is between 74 and 148 MBq (2 to 4 mCi).

D. Precautions:

Reduced numbers of macroaggregated albumin (MAA) particles should be considered for patients with pulmonary hypertension or right-to-left shunting, and in infants and children. In adults, the number may be reduced to 100,000–200,000 particles without altering the quality of the images for detection of perfusion defects.

E. Image Acquisition

1. Sequence of Imaging

a. A chest radiograph should be obtained and reviewed before lung scintigraphy.

b. Ventilation scintigraphy using 133Xe is usually performed before perfusion scintigraphy using 99mTc. Alternately, perfusion scintigraphy can be performed first and ventilation scintigraphy omitted if not needed.

c. The **disadvantages** of performing perfusion imaging first are:

   i. With 133 Xe gas or 99mTc aerosol imaging, the perfusion image contributes background activity to the ventilation image.

   ii. A decision to perform or not to perform the ventilation study must be made in a timely manner.

d. The **advantages** of performing perfusion imaging first are:

   i. If the perfusion study is normal or matches the chest radiographic findings, the ventilation study can be omitted.

   ii. For single-projection ventilation studies, the projection that best shows the defect can be obtained.

2. Technique of ventilation imaging:

In a ventilation scan, the patient inhales a mixture of air and radioactive gas (xenon-133, krypton-85, krypton-81m, or 99m Tc-DTPA) through the mouthpiece of a face mask. The radioactive gas follows the same pathway as the air in normal breathing. A nuclear scan is performed at three phases: during the buildup of gas, after the patient rebreathes from a bag and the radioactivity reaches a steady level, and after removal of the radioactive gas from the lungs. Ventilation imaging lasts about 30 minutes. A typical xenon ventilation study consists of 3 phases.

a) A wash in phase: It is obtained after a single breath inhalation of the tracer.
b) An equilibrium phase which is obtained after 3-5 minutes of rebreathing of radioactive gas.
c) Washout phase which consists of successive images while Xenon is being washed out of the lungs by atmospheric air.

Both single breath and intravenous injections of Xenon can be combined with a rebreathing method. Inhalation of boluses of Xe^{133} during particular phases can be used to study the distribution of air under special circumstances and to measure closing volume. A wash in period of 3-5 minutes followed by a washout of upto 10 minutes, with serial images taken at 30 second interval provides sufficient information. [Fig. 1].

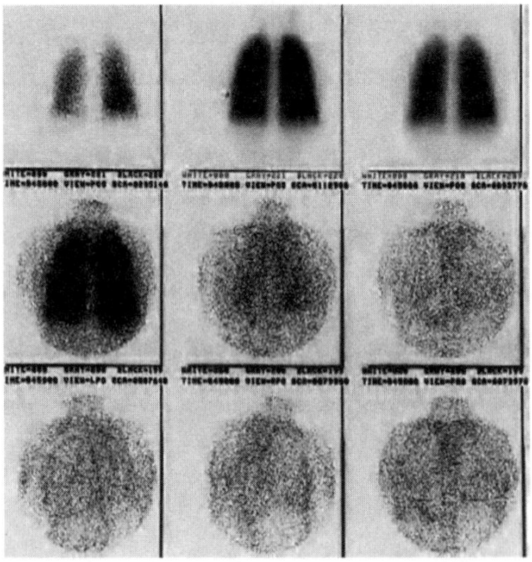

Fig 1: Normal Ventilation Scan

***Image courtesy:** Dr Shwetal Pawar, Assistant Professor, Department of Nuclear Medicine, Seth G S Medical College and KEM hospital, Mumbai, India.

At the end of wash in, there is an even distribution of activity which corresponds to lung volume. The clearance is rapid and lung outlines are no longer visible in 2-3 minutes after washout starts.

Ventilation studies should be performed in upright position when it is most efficient. Posterior projection is the preferred view as it encompasses larger lung volume.

The distribution of a single breath of Xe^{133} is compared to its distribution at equilibrium to give an index of ventilation per unit lung volume.

3. Technique of perfusion imaging:

Regional perfusion is most commonly studied following intravenous injection of Tc^{99m}MAA.[1] It is preferred because of its favourable physical properties.

In a perfusion scan, a radionuclide-tagged MAA is injected slowly intravenously over several respiratory cycles. Half is injected while the patient is sitting up, and the other half while lying down. The patient is placed in the supine, prone, and various lateral positions on the nuclear medicine table under the camera. Scanning with a gamma-ray detector is begun immediately. The scintillation camera takes several single stationary images of the anterior, posterior, and lateral areas of the chest. A routine perfusion scan should include at least six views of the lungs; anterior, posterior, right and left lateral, and right and left posterior oblique views.

Perfusion imaging lasts about 45 minutes. After intravenous injection, radioactive particles are trapped in the pulmonary microcirculation. The distribution of particles in the lungs is proportional to regional pulmonary blood flow at the time of injection. Approximately 200,000 to 500,000 particles are injected during a routine clinical perfusion lung scan. The normal adult human lung contains approximately 300 million precapillary arterioles and 300 billion capillaries. Therefore, only about 0.1 percent of precapillary arterioles are blocked following the procedure. In addition, the blockage of pulmonary precapillary arterioles by 99mTc MAA is transient; it's biologic half-life in the lung ranges between 2 and 6 h.

In pediatric patients and patients with suspected or known right-to-left shunts, pulmonary hypertension, prior pneumonectomy, or a single lung transplant, the number of particles injected should be reduced. A minimum of 60,000 particles is required to obtain an even distribution of activity within the pulmonary arterial circulation and avoid potential false-positive interpretations.

Perfusion lung scans are routinely utilized to examine patients with suspected pulmonary embolism. Unfortunately, perfusion imaging is sensitive, but not specific, for diagnosing pulmonary embolism. Virtually all lung diseases (including tumors, infections, asthma, and chronic obstructive pulmonary disease) may cause decreased pulmonary arterial blood flow in the affected lung zones. Therefore, combined use of perfusion and ventilation studies can improve the diagnostic specificity of lung scanning for pulmonary embolism. Pulmonary embolism almost always causes abnormal perfusion, while ventilation is preserved **(mismatched defects).** In contrast, in parenchymal pulmonary disorders, decreased ventilation and perfusion are noted in the same lung region **(matched defects).** Conditions in which the ventilation abnormality may appear larger than the perfusion abnormality **(reverse mismatch)** include airway obstruction, mucus plug, atelectasis, and pneumonia.

4. Interventions:

i) In patients with acute obstructive lung disease, the use of bronchodilator therapy before lung scintigraphy may decrease ventilatory defects and improve the accuracy of the study. Because perfusion defects often change as acute obstruction resolves, patients are best imaged when bronchospasm has resolved.

ii) In patients with congestive heart failure, improved specificity will be obtained if imaging can be delayed until therapy for heart failure has been instituted.

F. Interpretive considerations:

Ventilation–perfusion mismatch can result from any cause of pulmonary arterial blood flow obstruction. We need to know these causes for correct interpretation of our results.

Common causes of V/Q mismatch:

- Pulmonary embolism: Impaired perfusion with normal ventilation. [14,15] Fat emboli typically produce a mottled appearance due to the presence of many small fat emboli.
- Pneumonia/pleural effusion/atelectasis: Usually, there is more ventilation abnormality with normal or minimally reduced perfusion.
- Obstruction of pulmonary artery by a tumor or hilar lymphadenopathy: Bronchi are more resistant to extrinsic compression than are the pulmonary arteries because of their rigid cartilaginous rings and perfusion will be affected more than the ventilation.
- Radiation treatment/vasculitis: Can reduce regional lung perfusion. Radiation treatment results in the obliteration of the microvasculature. Perfusion defects from radiation are usually geometric and follow the treatment port. They are typically nonsegmental. Ventilation may also be reduced in the irradiated area, but it is usually less affected than perfusion.
- Pulmonary artery atresia or hypoplasia.
- Segmental or branch pulmonary artery stenosis.
- Fibrosing mediastinitis: Can lead to central vascular obstruction.

G. Sources of error on V/Q images:

- Perfusion images can show hot spots in the lungs, if clotting of blood occurs in the syringe during the injection or if the injection is made through an indwelling catheter that is not well flushed. Therefore the syringe containing Tc99m MAA should be vigorously shaken before injection. Moreover, at the time of injection, blood should not be withdrawn in the syringe.

Injection of 99mTc-MAA through a central line can result in inadequate mixing of activity in the pulmonary artery. This inadequate distribution of activity is especially true if the activity is injected through a pulmonary artery line. [1]

- Attenuation defects due to effusions: When the patient is scanned in the supine position, effusions may collect posteriorly/ superiorly and mimic a defect.

  Ventilation scintigraphy may be obtained with the patient upright, while the radiopharmaceutical for perfusion scintigraphy typically is injected with the patient supine. These changes in position may also affect the comparability of the 2 scintigrams.

- Liver uptake: Xenon is fat soluble and may get deposited in the liver, especially in case of fatty liver.

Clinical applications of V/Q scan:

1) Pulmonary embolism:

Ventilation-perfusion lung imaging has been shown to be a safe, noninvasive technique in evaluating pulmonary embolism (PE). A normal V/Q scan essentially excludes the possibility of recent significant pulmonary embolus. Ventilation perfusion mismatch (an area of normal ventilation corresponding to a segmental wedge-shaped area of decreased or absent perfusion) is the hallmark of a pulmonary embolism on V/Q scanning.

Interpretation criteria: [15-17]

Traditionally, the V/Q scans are interpreted using the PIOPED criteria, though original interpretation was based on Biello's criteria.[18] In PIOPED criteria, planar perfusion scan is compared with planar ventilation scan and interpreted along with a recent chest X-ray (<12 hours old). The perfusion defects are classified as small (<25% of a segment), medium (25% to 75% of a segment) and large (>75% of a segment) defects. Two or more large mismatched perfusion defects with a normal chest X-ray indicate the high probability of PE. One to three moderate-sized mismatched perfusion defects are considered as intermediate probability. Less than three small-sized mismatched perfusion defects are considered to be low probability. Modifications to PIOPED criteria were suggested on the bases of retrospective PIOPED data review. Gottschalk suggested that a high probability study should be interpreted as PE present and that normal and very low probability exams be interpreted as PE absent for a more conclusive interpretation.

2009 European Association of Nuclear Medicine Guidelines for Ventilation-Perfusion Interpretation [19]

1. No PE

   Normal perfusion conforming to anatomical lung boundaries.

   - Matched or reverse mismatch V/Q defects of any size in absence of mismatched defects.
   - Mismatch without lobar, segmental or subsegmental pattern.

2. PE present

   - V/Q mismatch at least one segment or two subsegments conforming to pulmonary vascular anatomy

3. Non diagnostic for PE

   - Multiple V/Q abnormalities not specific of particular disease.

The 2009 European Association of Nuclear Medicine Guidelines has a reported sensitivity of 96% to 99%, specificity of 97% to 99%, and negative predictive value of 97% to 99%. Rates of non-diag-nostic examinations were low, at 1% to 3%.

2) Fat Embolism:

Classically, a heterogeneous perfusion pattern (multiple small to moderate perfusion defects scattered through out both lungs) is observed. Segmental perfusion defects are rarely present. However, in the majority of cases due to small-sized emboli, V/Q scan may be normal. Unfortunately, the lung scan is not very useful in diagnosing fat emboli, but can be used to exclude thromboembolism as the cause of the patient's hypoxia in these patients. [1]

3) Pulmonary Infarction:

Pulmonary infarction may occur as a complication of PE. The perfusion defect is usually larger than the chest X-ray consolidation. [1]

4) Pre-operative lung assessment [Fig. 2]

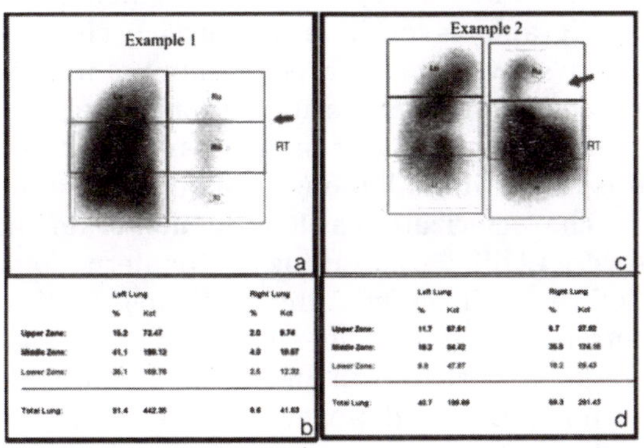

***Fig. 2: Sample case** - A case of post tuberculosis sequelae with atelectatic collapse of right lung planned for right pneumonectomy. a) Tc^{99m} MAA lung perfusion image shows minimal perfusion in entire right lung (green arrow), b) quantification shows right lung contributing 8.6% to the total lung perfusion. Predicted FEV_1 post right pneumonectomy using given formula was 1.15L.*

Example 2: a case of emphysematous bulla in the upper lobe of right lung planned for bullectomy.

a) Tc^{99m} Lung Perfusion image shows no perfusion corresponding to the bulla in right upper lobe involving majority of upper and part of middle segment (red arrow),

b) The upper segment of right lung was contributing 5.7% to the total lung perfusion Predicted approximate FEV_1 post bullectomy was 970ml.

Quantitative measures of relative lung perfusion (comparing lungs or dividing each lung into thirds and calculating the percentage of total counts in each region) may be useful in preoperative lung assessment of high risk patients before planned lung resection for malignancy, dead-space lung volume reduction and lung transplantation.[20] This information is used in conjunction with spirometry to determine how much function each lung or lung region contributes.

Preoperative lung imaging is often performed to assess the regional lung function to predict expected residual function after surgery. A forced expiratory volume in 1 second (FEV1) > 2L or greater than 60% of the predicted value and FEV1 > 1.5 or over 40% of predicted values are essential for pneumonectomy and lobectomy, respectively in order to prevent unexpected postoperative respiratory failure (assessment of functional inoperability). Quantitation of perfusion (right to left, upper to lower lung fields) is indicated when spirometric measurements are borderline and serves as the basis for calculation of postoperative ventilation. These studies are particularly important in patients with lung cancer since coexistence of COPD is frequent in these patients.[21]

a) Pneumonectomy/Sleeve resection/ lobectomy for lung carcinoma

Lung scintigraphy provides a fairly accurate determination of the patient's ability to undergo surgery. The American College of Chest Physicians recommends that quantitative perfusion scintigraphy should be used in patients with borderline lung function to predict postoperative lung function. The postoperative FEV1 can be calculated by multiplying the global preoperative FEV1 by the split function of the remaining lung. Ventilation scintigraphy may be a better predictor of postoperative function, but central airway tracer deposition can potentially limit the results.[22-27]

b) Preoperative evaluation of bullectomy / pneumonectomy for patients with obstructive airway disease- e.g surgery for emphysematous bullae:

V/Q studies are of value in studying how well the lung functions be preserved after surgery. When the tissue surrounding the bullous area is well perfused and there is little evidence of obstructive disease elsewhere, some improvement in lung functions can be expected postoperatively. When surrounding lung is poorly perfused, operation is best avoided as the disability is more related to the parenchymal disease rather than bulla.[23]

c) Preoperative evaluation for lung transplant:

There is increasing interest in V/Q imaging in cryptogenic fibrosing alveolitis because of the data these scans provide in the dynamic V/Q relationships in such patients undergoing single lung transplantation. V/Q imaging complements the data obtained from the lung function tests and is particularly useful in defining the differential function of each lung which is particularly important in the assessment of patients for single lung transplantation. This can also be used in children. [24]

5) Pulmonary Hypertension:

In secondary pulmonary hypertension, perfusion is typically heterogeneous, with small peripheral defects on V/Q scintigraphy. However, the scan may also be normal. In primary pulmonary hypertension, the presence of reverse mismatch (diminished ventilation, normal perfusion) representing failure of hypoxic vasoconstriction has been described.

6) Hemoptysis:

Labeled RBCs can also be used in cases of hemoptysis to localize the site of pulmonary hemorrhage. About 50% of patients may show positive scan and bleeding rates as low as 50 ml/day may be detected.[26]

7) Chronic obstructive pulmonary disease (COPD):

Patients with a chronic bronchitic phenotype may temporarily show ventilation defects due to mucous plugging of bronchi [28]. During an acute exacerbation, ventilation and accompanying perfusion abnormalities in ventilation/perfusion scintigraphy are common. These abnormalities usually affect both lungs. In patients with a phenotype defined by predominant emphysema with loss of respiratory bronchioles, **ventilation scintigraphy is sensitive to even early changes,** when 'slow paces' delayed washout of inhaled xenon or 'hot spots' (accumulation of the tracer at the branching site of airways) is encountered. **It is an additional, though not official tool for the characterization as to mild, moderate and severe COPD** [29], according to the international GOLD-classification. Although there is no strict correlation between hot spots with the clinical stage, a correlation between ventilation abnormality and pulmonary function, in particular using aerosol ventilation, has been claimed. In earlier stages, usually the aerosol exhibits enhanced central deposition with normal peripheral ventilation, while in more severe stages areas of little or even absent aerosol transportation to the periphery of the lung are seen.

In patients with early or mild COPD, the perfusion scan may be normal or near normal. However, as the destruction of lung parenchyma progresses, it characteristically produces multiple nonsegmental perfusion defects, which may be relatively focal and discrete or diffusely scattered throughout the lungs. Perfusion defects may also be caused by regional hypoxia producing reflex vasoconstriction and by bullae themselves or their compression of adjacent lung. Large apical bullae may render reduced or absent perfusion to the upper lung zones. COPD is thus characterized by matched ventilation and perfusion defects. A phenomenon named 'reverse mismatch' is encountered when perfusion exceeds in the same area ventilation (low ventilation/perfusion-ratio). In acute bronchial constriction (asthma, acute exacerbation of COPD), bronchodilator therapy before lung scintigraphy may decrease ventilatory defects and thereby improve the accuracy of the study.

In Emphysema, ventilation imaging is most helpful in characterizing the regional distribution of abnormalities and to a lesser extent in delineating the clinical severity.

Emphysema is likely if in the perfusion scan all the defects are small, subsegmental, and have matched ventilation defects. However, widely differing patterns of regional ventilation are seen, ranging from predominantly upper lobe involvement (smokers) and predominantly lower lobe disease (emphysema in alpha-1-antitrypsin deficiency) [30] to diffuse involvement.

Besides CT scan, perfusion scans also help in the assessment of the type of regional involvement, which is crucial for the indication of procedures for reducing lung volume by surgery or bronchial interventions causing atelectasis.

133Xenon has been found useful for the assessment of interaction between intra-bullous and surrounding lung ventilation which is difficult to judge by CT.

8) Bronchiectasis and cystic fibrosis: [31]

Patients with bronchiectasis show perfusion defects that are constant in location and generally restricted to the lung bases; they are mainly related to reflex vasoconstriction secondary to local hypoxia.

Cystic fibrosis, with its onset in early childhood is characterized by regionally irregular ventilation and perfusion, with patchy nonsegmental defects in perfusion and markedly disturbed ventilation. In general, both lungs are affected to a similar, though rarely identical, degree. Usually, the upper parts of the lung are more severely involved, the involvement mostly being not symmetrical. The prominent delineation of the interlobar fissures, often called the 'fissure sign', is seen frequently in this disease. **The extent of scintigraphic abormalities is related to the severity of the disease.** As differentiation from other clinical problems such as asthma is not possible, lung scintigraphy plays no role in either diagnosis or monitoring. [31,32]

9) Sarcoidosis:

Gallium scintigraphy has been used since long for diagnosis and staging of sarcoidosis [33,34]. Diffuse as well as focal radionuclide uptake has been reported in this entity. However, FDG PET scan is useful in assessing inflammatory activity in sarcoidosis, seems to be more suitable for evaluating the mediastinum and mediastinal lymph nodes as well as posterior regions of the lung and non-thoracic lesions.

10) Radiation therapy:

Pneumonitis and pulmonary fibrosis secondary to irradiation may present as non-segmental process. These effects depend on the radiation dosage, fractionation schedule, lung volume irradiated, and biological factors. Optimization of the radiation therapy plan for lung carcinoma can be supported by a lung perfusion scintigraphy. [35]

A quantitative ventilation/perfusion scintigraphy giving regional and functional information that morphological methods cannot provide, **allows for a better prediction of the effects of radiation upon the pulmonary tissue.** Furthermore, information based on perfusion can help to prevent radiation damage to the remaining functioning lung parenchyma, especially in patients with major perfusion deficiencies. The best predictors of pulmonary function following radiation therapy are variables obtained from lung perfusion scintigraphy such as the "predicted perfusion reduction" and the "mean perfusion weighed lung dosage"

11) Congenital heart disease [36]:

Lung perfusion scintigraphy is a simple and cheap procedure with **high specificity for detection and quantification of a right-to-left shunt and for estimating the consecutive right ventricular strain.** The presence of a right-to-left shunt is identified by the deposition of injected particles in systemic, extra pulmonary vascular beds, mainly in the brain, the liver and the kidneys. The absence of tracer accumulation in the brain virtually excludes a significant right to left shunt.

The fraction of right-to-left shunting can be approximated by comparing the activity in the lungs to the activity in the rest of the body.

12) Post-transplantation lung scintigraphy:

In the immediate post-transplantation setting, perfusion imaging documents the patency of the vascular anastomoses. In single-lung transplantation, the ratio of right-to-left lung perfusion and the change in ratio correlate with rejection. Analysis of regional changes in ventilation and perfusion may also be useful. Development of matched ventilation perfusion abnormalities consistent with obstructive lung disease often reflects rejection (bronchiolitis obliterans).

13) Bronchopleural Fistula:

Ventilation studies may be used in the diagnosis of bronchopleural fistulas. They can also be used in follow up to check whether the fistula is closed or not. Xenon or Crypton gas can be used as a radioactive inhalational agent. In presence of bronchopleural fistula, these gases accumulate in pleural space within and remain in the pleural space in washout study. But the limitation is that this procedure can give us a clue regarding presence of the fistula but if present, its size cannot be determined.

There have been few reports in the literature advocating the use of ventilation scintigraphy for the diagnosis of post pneumonectomy bronchopleural fistula. Neilsen and associates [37] have suggested this method to localize the site of persistent air leak in post thoracotomy patients. Moote and colleagues [38] used ventilation lung scanning to image a post pneumonectomy bronchopleural fistula.

14) Quantitative V/Q scanning is useful for **estimating regional pulmonary functions in infants and children.**

Summary

Ventilation perfusion scan or lung scintigraphy is a very good tool which can be used in various conditions apart from the pulmonary embolism. It has role in not only diagnosis but also in monitoring the treatment as well as predicting the outcome of treatment especially in lung resection surgeries. As it is noninvasive, less time consuming, and relatively free from adverse effects, patient acceptability is very high. As it does not involve injection of contrast agent, it can be safely used in patients with history of allergy to contrast agents and those with renal impairment. It has excellent sensitivity and specificity. The radiation exposure is low. With efficient technique and effective organization, V/Q acquisition time is only 20-30 minutes. Though it has many advantages, availability and high cost are the issues leading to its limited use.

REFERENCES

1. Parker JA, Coleman RE, Grady E et al. SNM practice guideline for lung scintigraphy 4.0. J Nucl Med Technol 2012; 40: 57-65
2. Knipping HW, Bolt W, Ventrath H et al. Eine neue Methode zur Prüfung der Herz-und Lungenfunktion die regionale Funktionsanalyse in der Lungen und Herzklinik mit Hilfe des Radioaktiven Edelgases Xenon 133 (isotopen-thorakographie). Dtsch Med Wochenschr 1955; 80:1146–1147
3. Bajc M, Neilly JB, Miniati M et al. EANM guidelines for ventilation/perfusion scintigraphy. Eur J Nucl Med Mol Imaging 2009; 36: 1356-70
4. PIOPED Investigators. Value of the ventilation/perfusion scan in acute pulmonary embolism: results of the prospective investigation of pulmonary embolism diagnosis (PIOPED). JAMA. 1990;263:2753–2759
5. Freeman LM, Krynyckyi B, Zuckier LS. Enhanced lung scan diagnosis of pulmonary embolism with the use of ancillary scintigraphic findings and clinical correlation. Semin Nucl Med. 2001;31:143–157
6. Beckles MA, Spiro S, Colis G, Rudd R. The physiologic evaluation of patients with lung cancer being considered for resectional surgery. Chest. 2003;123(suppl): 105S–114S.
7. Starobin D, Shitrit D, Steinmetz A, Fink G, Hardoff R, Kramer MR. Quantitative lung perfusion following single lung transplantation. Thorac Cardiovasc Surg. 2007;55:48–52
8. Gates GF, Orme HW, Dore EK. Measurement of cardiac shunting with technetium-labeled albumin aggregates. J Nucl Med. 1971;12:746–749
9. Hollett P, Wright E, Wesolowski C, Harris R. Aerosol ventilation scintigraphy in the evaluation of bronchopleural fistula: a case report and literature review. Can J Surg. 1991;34:465–467
10. Stanchina ML, Tantisira KG, Aquino SL, Wain JC, Ginns LC. Association of lung perfusion disparity and mortality in patients with cystic fibrosis awaiting lung transplantation. J Heart Lung Transplant. 2002;21:217–228
11. Fukuchi K, Hayashida K, Nakanishi N, et al. Quantitative analysis of lung perfusion in patients with primary pulmonary hypertension. J Nucl Med. 2002; 43(6):757-61.
12. Freeman LM. Don't bury the V/Q scan: it's as good as multidetector CT angiograms with a lot less radiation exposure. J Nucl Med. 2008; 49(1):5-8.
13. Ell PJ, Gambhir SS, Ed. Nuclear medicine in clinical diagnosis and treatment. 3rd ed. Edinburgh, Scotland: Churchill Livingstone 2004.
14. Stein PD, Gottschalk A. Critical review of ventilation/perfusion lung scans in acute pulmonary embolism. Prog Cardiovasc Dis. 1994; 37(1):13-24.
15. Stein PD, Woodard PK, Weg JG, et al. Diagnostic pathways in acute pulmonary embolism: recommendations of the PIOPED II Investigators. Radiol 2007; 242(1):15-21.
16. Freeman LM, Stein EG, Sprayregen S, et al. The current and continuing important role of ventilation-perfusion scintigraphy in evaluating patients with suspected pulmonary embolism. Semin Nucl Med. 2008; 38(6):432-40.
17. Sostman HD, Stein PD, Gottschalk A, et al. Acute pulmonary embolism: sensitivity and specificity of ventilation-perfusion scintigraphy in PIOPED II study. Radiol 2008;246:941–946.
18. Lee ME, Biello DR, Kumar B, et al. "Low-probability" ventilation perfusion scintigrams: clinical outcomes in 99 patients. Radiol 1985;156:497–500

19. Bajc M, Neilly JB, Miniati M, Schuemichen C, Meignan M, Jonson B. EANM guidelines for ventilation/perfusion scintigraphy: part 2. Algorithms and clinical considerations for diagnosis of pulmonary emboli with V/P_{SPECT} and MDCT. *Eur Jour Nuc Med Mol Imag* 2009;36(9):1528–1538
20. Humplik BI, Sandrock D, Aurisch R, Richter WS, Ewert R, Munz DL. Scintigraphic results in patients with lung transplants: a prospective comparative study. Nuklearmedizin. 2005;44:62–68
21. Win T, Tasker AD, Groves AM, et al. Ventilation-perfusion scintigraphy to predict postoperative pulmonary function in lung cancer patients undergoing pneumonectomy. AJR Am J Roentgenol.. 2006; 187(5):1260-5.
22. Yuan ST, Frey KA, Gross MD et al. Semi-quantification and classification of local pulmonary function by V/Q SPECT in patients with non-small cell lung cancer: potential indication for radiotherapy planning. J Thorac Oncol 2011; 6: 71-8.
23. Fessler HE, Feller-Kopman D. Helping the homogeneous. Eur Respir J 2010; 36: 8-9
24. Mettler FA GM, Ed. Essentials of nuclear medicine imaging, 6th ed. Philadelphia, PA:Saunders Elsevier 2012.
25. Sarlin RF, Schillaci RF, Georges TN, Wilcox JR. Focal increased lung perfusion and intrapulmonary venoarterial shunting in broncho-alveolar cell carcinoma. Am J Med 1980; 68: 618-23
26. Zeissman HA, Thrall J. Nuclear medicine: the requisites. 3rd ed. St. Louis, MO: Mosby 2007
27. Taube K, Konietzko N. Prediction of postoperative cardiopulmonary function in patients undergoing pneumonectomy. Thor Cardiovasc Surg 1980; 23: 348-51
28. National Emphysema Treatment Trial (NETT) Research Group. A randomized trial comparing lung volume reduction surgery with medical therapy for severe emphysema. New Engl J Med 2003; 348: 2059-73
29. Travaline JM, Maurer AH, Charkes ND et al. Quantitation of regional ventilation during the washout phase of lung scintigraphy: measurement in patients with severe COPD before and after bilateral lung volume reduction surgery. Chest 2000; 118: 721-7
30. Welch MH, Richardson RH, Whitcomb WH et al. The lung scan in alpha-1-antitrypsin deficiency. J Nucl Med 1969; 10: 687-90
31. Piepsz A, Wetzburger C, Spehl M et al. Critical evaluation of lung scintigraphy in cystic fibrosis: study of 113 patients. JNM 1980; 21: 909-13
32. Itti E, Fauroux B, Pigeot J, et al. Quantitative lung perfusion scan as a predictor of aerosol distribution heterogeneity and disease severity in children with cystic fibrosis. Nucl Med Commun. 2004;25:563–569
33. Braun JJ, Kessler R, Constantinesco A, Imperiale A. 18F-FDG PET/ CT in sarcoidosis management: review and report of 20 cases. Eur J Nucl Med Mol Imaging 2008; 35: 1537-43
34. Prager E, Wehrschuetz M, Bisail B et al. Comparison of 18F-FDG and 67Ga-citrate in sarcoidosis imaging. Nuklearmedizin 2008; 47: 18-23
35. De Jaeger K, Seppenwoolde Y, Boersma LJ et al. Pulmonary function following high-dose radiotherapy of non-small-cell lung cancer. Int J Radiat Oncol Biol Phys 2003; 55: 1331-40
36. Tamir A, Melloul M, Berant M, Horev G, Lubin E, Blieden LC, et al. Lung perfusion scans in patients with congenital heart defects. J Am Coll Cardiol. 1992;19:383–8.
37. Neilsen K, Blake LM, Mark J. Localization of bronchopleural fistula using ventilation scintigraphy. J Nucl Med 1994;35: 867-9
38. Moote D, Ehrlich L, Martin RH. Postpneumonectomv bronchopleural fistula imaged by ventilation lung scanning. Clin Nucl Med 1987;12:337-8.

14

NORMAL VALUE OF PULMONARY FUNCTIONS TESTS

KT PRASAD, D. BEHERA

Introduction

Spirometry is one of the most important tests for assessing pulmonary function. It is imperative that one should have a thorough knowledge of the various technical and biological factors which may influence the measured variables to ensure accurate test results. Besides, interpretation of the results of pulmonary function tests requires knowledge of the 'normal' values for a given population. These normal values are calculated using prediction equations developed by studying pulmonary function of a large number of \healthy\ individuals. Selection and application of appropriate prediction equations is of paramount importance as it can profoundly influence the interpretation of the test results.

Sources of variation in spirometry

Most factors may affect the parameters measured during lung function testing. These include technical factors related to the equipment and the procedure, and biological factors related to the subject performing spirometry.

Technical factors

A number of technical factors related to the device and the performance of the procedure can affect the test results. To avoid errors related to these technical factors, recommended spirometry standard need to be strictly followed (1). Adequate quality control of the spirometer device should be ensured by performing validation and calibration of recommended intervals. The spiromery measurements should meet the standard criteria for acceptability and reproducibility (1).

Utmost care must be taken while collecting information from the subjects performing spirometry. As discussed below, age and height are an integral part of any spirometry prediction equation, and hence they should be measured as accurately as possible. Truncating the age to the last decimal may introduce a 1-year bias which may result in bias of up to 8.5% in predicted FEV1 or FVC values, especially in children and adolescents less than 18 years of age (3). Similarly, an error of only +1% in the height may result in variations in FEV1 and/or FVC ranging from 1% to 40% (2).

Biological factors

Age: In general, pulmonary function continues to improve with age as long as physical growth occurs. In males, the increase in VC may continue even after maximal height is attained, usually be the age of 18 years. This increase may continue may continue up to about 25 years of age and is attributable to the increase in chest dimensions. However, in females, maximal VC is reached at about 16 years of age (3). Thereafter, pulmonary function usually remains constant up to an age of about 40 years. Beyond this age, pulmonary function starts to decline. This decline is attributed to the progressive loss of elastic recoil of the lung with age (4).

Height: Height is the most important factor among the parameters used in the prediction of lung function. Addition of other factors like chest circumference has been shown to only slightly improve the prediction.

Weight: Lung function declines at both extremes of weight. Obese subjects have lower ERV and FRC; however RV, TLC, FEV1 and FVC are not affected significantly unless the patient is massively obese (5, 6). Airway resistance is usually increased in obese subjects.

Gender: FVC and FRV1 values of adult males tend to be 10-15% higher than that of adult females. However, in studies of younger individuals, girls have been to show have greater expiratory flow rates compared to boys. This may be because girls have a smaller VC and lesser airway resistance as compared to boys (3).

Ethnicity: Caucasians have been shown to have FVC and FEV1 values which are 10-15%greater than that of Asians or Africans of the similar age, gender, and height (3, 4). However, this variation is not marked in FEV1/FVC ratios which may be normal or slightly lower in Caucasians compared to other ethnic groups. One of the factors responsible for this variation is differences to body build as Caucasians tend to have a higher trunk: leg ratio. Other factors which may account for this variation include differences in nutritional status, physical activity, and environmental pollution.

Prediction equations: The expected normal values for lung function parameters are calculated using prediction equation, also referred to as regression or reference equations. These equations allow prediction of lung function using patient specific information such as age, gender, height, weight, etc.

Prediction equations are developed from pulmonary function tests performed in large samples of carefully selected non-smoking 'healthy' individuals. The selected population should include both men and women in equal numbers and the range of age and height should be wide. The spirometers and the techniques used should meet standard recommendations (1).

Table 1. Representative adult prediction equations from different retions of India

Region	Parameter	Gender/ age group	Prediction equation	SEE
North India (9)	FVC(L)	Men	-3.44-0.013 A-0.00005 A2 + 0.048 H	0.497
		Women	-2.05 – 0.014 A-0.00004 A2 + 0.035 H	0.447
	FEV1(L)	Men	-1.90 –0.025 A +0.00006 A2 + 0.036 H	0.417
		Women	-1.07 –0.030 A + 0.00013 A2 + 0.027 H	0.323
	FEV1/FVC(%)	Men	103 – 0.35 A + 0.002 A2 — 0.07 H	6.6
		Women	111 –0/36 A + 0/003 A2 —0.10 H	5.8
South India (10)	FVC(L)	Men	-6.857 + 0.062 H	0.481
		Women	-2.883 + 0.035 H	0.325
	FEV1(L)	Men	-6.195 – 0.00023 A2 + 0.057 H	0.415
		Women	-1.900 + 0.026 H	0.304
	FEV/FVC(%)	Men	76.695 –0.00613 A2 + 0.080 H	6.638
		Women	94.917 –0.00734 A2 – 0.011 H	5.639
East India (11, 12)	FVC (L)	Men	-3.899 –0.020 A + 0.049 H	0.450
		Women	-0.902 - 0.025 A + 0.027 H	0.310
	FEV1(L)	Men	-3.737 – 0.028 A + 0.047 H	0.380
		Women	-0.354 – 0.027A + 0.021 H	0.284
	FEV1/FVC)%)	Men	94.432 -0.348 A	6.250
		Women	86.100 – 0.241 A	5.680
West India (13)	FVC(L)	Men <30y	-6.058 + 0.019 A + 0.055 H	0.505
		Men>_30y	-4.832 – 0.018 A + 0.054 H	0.462
		Women<30y	-2.284 + 0.006 A + 0.030 H	0.377
		Women>_30y	-3.755 – 0.010 A + 0.043 H	0.341
	FEV1(L)	Men <30y	-3.266 – 0.010 A + 0.039 H	0.392
		Men>_30y	- 2.650 –0.022 A + 0.037 H	0.328
		Women<30y	-1.424 – 0.011 A + 0.025 H	0.341
		Women>	-30y 2.580 – 0.012 A + 0.032 H	0.309
	FEV1/FVC(%)	Men	119.3640 – 0.2457 A – 0.1756 H	7.741
		Women	94.8867 – 0.2146 A – 0.0334 H	11.001

A: Age in years, FEV1: Forced expiratory volume in first second, FVC: Forced vital capacity; H: Height in cm, SEE: Standard error of estimate

Selection of prediction equations

Selection of the appropriate preduction equationis one of the most critical steps in spirometry as the interpretation of the spirometry data will depend on the selected equation. Most standard spirometry software offers a wide selection of prediction equations. The spirometry technicians should select the prediction developed in the population with same ethnicity as that of the subject being tested. The prediction equation used to interpret the study should be mentioned in the spirometry report.

Reference equations for different parts of India are available and should be used (Table 1). Use of Caucasian prediction equations or a fixed percentage of their predicted values (e.g. 90% of predicted) is not suitable for Indians (7). Prediction equations developed in one region of India may not be applicable to all Indians. For example, West Indian and South Indian reference equation may not yield results equivalent to North Indian reference equations (8).

Interpreting pulmonary function parameters using predicted values

Any measured value which is above or below the predicted normal value for a patient is not necessarily abnormal. This is because the normal value is usually considered to be a range rather than a fixed vlue. The lower limit of normal (LLN) and upper limit of normal (ULN) are the limits of the 'normal range 'beyond which the measured values would be considered to be abnormal. In clinical practice, spirometric values which are lower than normal are more commonly encountered than values which are higher than normal. Hence the LLN is more commonly utilised than the ULN.

The common practice of using a fixed percentage of the predicted value to define the LUN (e.g. <80% of the predicted), although simple, is not a valid approach (3). Although this may be acceptable in children, it may result in errors when employed in adults. In spirometry, any value below the fifth percentile is considered to be abnormally low and is used to define the LLN. The fifth percentile LLN can be estimated as predicted value- (1.645 x SEE) where SEE is the standard error of estimate of the prediction equation (3).

Conclusion

Before attempting to interpret spirometry measurements one should take care of the technical and biological factors which may influence the measured values to ensure accurate results. The most appropriate prediction equation suitable for the person being tested should be selelected and applied for reliable interpretation of results (14).

REFERENCES

1. Miller MR, Hankinson J, Brusasco V, Burgos F, Casaburi R, Coates A, et al Standardisation of spirometry. Eur Respir Jour 2005; 26(2): 319-38.
2. Quanjer PH, Hall GL, Stanojevic S, Cole TJ, Stocks J Age and height-based prediction bias in spirometry reference equations. Eur Respir Jour 2912; 40(1): 190-7.
3. Lung function testing: selection reference values and interpretative strategies. American Thoracic Society. Amer Rev Respir Dis 1991; 144(5): 1202-18.
4. Chhabra SK Interpreteatin of Spirometry: Selection of Predicted Values and Defining abnormality Ind J Chest Dis All Sci 2015; 57(2): 91-105.
5. Littleton SW Impact of obesity on respiratory function Respirol (Carlton Vic) 2012; 17(1): 439
6. Salome CM, King GG, Berend N Physiology of obesity and effects on lung function Jour Appl Physiol 2010;,108(1): 206-11.
7. Aggarwal AN, Gupta D, Behera D, Jindal SK Applicability of commonly used Caucasian prediction equation for spirometry interpretation in India Ind Jour Med Res 2005; 127(2): 153 64.
8. Aggarwal AN, Gupta D, Jindal SK Comparison of Indian reference equations for spirometry interpretation Resprirol (Carton Vic) 2007; 12(5): 763-8.
9. Jindal SK Pulmonary function laboratory in the tropics: needs, problems and solution In Sharma SK ed Lung disease in the tropics, New York, marcel Dekker 1991: 523-42.
10. Vijayan VK, Kuppurao KV, Venkatesan P, Sankaran K, Prabhakar R Pulmonary function in healthy young Indians in Madras Thorax 1990; 45(8): 611-5.
11. Chatterjee S, Saha D Pulmonary function studies in healthy non-smoking women of Calcutta Ann Hum Biol 1993; 20(1): 31-8.
12. Chatterjee S, Saha D, Chatterjee BP Pulmonary function studies in healthy non-smoking men of Calcutta Ann Hum Biol 1988; 15(5): 365-74.
13. Udwadia FE, Sunavala JD, Shetye VM, Jain PK The maximal expiratory flow volume curve in normal subjects in India Chest 1986; 89(6): 852-6.
14. Behera D (ed) Spirometry Mumbai, Tree Life Media, Kothari Medicals, 2016.

15
BEDSIDE PULMONARY FUNCTION TESTS

SALIL BHARGAVA

Introduction

Bedside assessment of Pulmonary function is an aspect of pulmonary function testing which has shown major strides in the last few years. This is largely due to an explosion in computer and biomedical technology. This extension of the pulmonary function laboratory to the bedside of the acutely ill patient has many important connotation, e.g.

- A rapid and objective assessment of the physiological characteristics as well as the serial quantification of pulmonary status.
- The rapid assessment of the effectiveness of the ventilatory strategies and pharmacologic interventions.
- Early detection of changes in the pulmonary status, which in turn may prompt an early assessment of these changes, their causes and early remedial measures.

All these tests are invaluable in optimizing clinical management in the ICU.

Clinical Assessment

The Ventilatory aspects of pulmonary function may be assessed clinically at the bedside. However, observer bias and inter-observer variability often limit the utility in long term ongoing evaluation of the acutely ill patient.

Thus, the presence of an obstructive defect of moderate to severe grade is clinically evident at the bedside. The patient adopts a characteristic sitting posture, leaning forwards slightly, bracing the elbows or the hands. He has labored breathing, with expiratory prolongation, wheezing, intercostals and supraclavicular retractions and occasional paradoxical movement of the diaphragm on inspiration. There may be a reduction in tracheal length from cricoid cartilage to the sternal notch and rhonchi and crepitations on auscultation.

However, studies examining the reliability of subjective complaints and physical findings in assessing the severity of obstruction, showed that only retraction of the sternocleidomastoids correlated with the severity of the obstruction. When retractions of the sternomastoids were present, specific conductance (reciprocal of the airway resistance), mid expiratory flow rate and forced expiratory volume in one second were severely reduced, with the forced expiratory volume in one second being less than one litre.

Specific conductance was also found to be correlated with the time required to perform a forced expiration from maximum inspiration and also with increased resonance on percussion (due to hyperinflation secondary to airway obstruction).

During improvement, its sequence is as follows: Sternomastoids retractions, followed by symptoms and lastly the wheezing subsidence. Even with a silent chest and absent wheezing, most spirometric parameters remain abnormal, usually about 60-70% of normal. Hence, while most of the symptoms and signs serve as indicators of obstruction, most correlate poorly with objective measures of obstruction.

Bedside Tests

1. **Respiratory Rate**

   Respiratory rate is essential yet frequently undervalued component of PFT specially while evaluating in weaning and extubation protocols. Increase respiratory rate is found in when there is muscle fatigue , increased work load and weaning fails

2. **Snider's Match blowing test**

   One popular bedside test for the quantifying obstruction is the **match test**. The ability to blowout a match held at 15cm from the open mouth correlates with maximum voluntary ventilation of 60 liter/minute or a forced expiratory volume in one second of 1.6 liter (Snider et al) or alternative with maximum voluntary ventilation of 40 liters/ minute (Olsen et al).

   Procedure: In this test the mouth is kept wide open, the match is held at 15cm distance, chin supported, no head tilting, match stick and mouth are at the same level.

   Results: The observation will be either a person cannot blow out a match or if he is able to blow out a match, his maximum voluntary ventilation is 60 liter/minute or a forced expiratory volume in one second of 1.6 liter.

   Modified Snider's test: In this test the distance between mouth and match stick can vary and the result are interpreted accordingly.

   If the distance is 3 inches MVV > 40 L/min

   – 6 inches MVV > 60 L/min

   – 9 inches MVV > 150 L/min

3. **Forced expiratory time**

   The forced expiratory time (FET) is measured over the trachea from the beginning to the end of maximal expiration from total lung capacity (TLC) is also a useful co-relate of obstruction. Serial measurement of forced expiratory time and subsequent quantification at spirometry shows that most normal subject have a forced expiratory time of 4 seconds and patient with moderate to severe obstruction a forced expiratory time of more than 6 seconds.

4. **Chest Expansion**

   Measure the chest expansion with a tape placed around the chest just below the level of nipples. The normal expands by 5-10 cm following a deep inspiration after a forceful expiration. Chest expansion is decreased in all restrictive diseases. It is also decreased in long standing obstructive disorder.

5. **De Bono's Whistle Test**

   In this test there is a wide bore tube which has a whistle at the end and an adjustable leak hole in the side. The whistle blows when the rate of airflow exceeds a certain limit.

6. **Sebarese's Breath Holding Time**

   Different individuals can hold their breath for variable periods of time depending on the functional status of the lungs, development of respiratory muscles, practice, age and sex. Determination of breath holding time (BHT) is a simple test which can provide of the lungs.

Procedures

1. The subject should sit quietly for a few minutes, breathing normally before the breath holding exercise is started. The procedure should be explained to the subject in clear terms. Use a stop watch and note the time for each determination.

2. Ask the subject to pinch his/her nostrils with the thumb and forefinger, and hold his/ her breath after a quiet inspiration. Note the time for which the breath can be held. Make 3 observation at intervals of 5 minutes

3. Using the same procedure, record the BHT after (a) a quiet expiration, (b) a deep inspiration, (c) a deep expiration, (d) hyperventilation (deep and fast breathing) for 1-2 minutes, (e) re-breathing from a polythene bag for 15-20 seconds with a

nose-clip on (discontinue if there is discomfort), and (f) 8-10 deep breaths of pure oxygen from Benedict-Roth apparatus.

4. Tabulate results as shown below. The highest value for each determination is the BHT for that exercise.

Observation and results

Explain your results from the following data

Breath Holding After	Reading (in seconds)			Maximum Value	Minimum Value
	1st	2nd	3rd		
a. Quiet Inspiration	....	....	....	....	....
b. Quiet Expiration	....	....	....	....	....
c. Deep Inspiration	....	....	....	....	....
d. Deep Expiration	....	....	....	....	....
e. Hyperventilation	....	....	....	....	....
f. Record single recording	....	....	....	....	....
After re-breathing from polythene bag ....sec After 8-10 deep breaths of oxygen ....sec					

5. **Respiratory Endurance Test (40 mmHg test):-** A BP apparatus is required for this test. Disconnect the rubber tube leading from the mercury reservoir to the BP cuff. Ask the subject to take a deep breath pinch his nostrils, and exhale into the tube, raising the mercury to 40 mm level and to hold it there for as long as possible.

   Normal = 40-70 seconds or more.

6. **Expiratory blast test:-** Using the same procedure as above, ask the subject to take a deep breath and then raise the mercury column to as high a and level as possible. A normal person can raise the mercury column to 55-100mm or more during a single forceful expiration.

Thus, while few objectives and subjective co-relates of spirometric abnormalities are available, clinical assessment of pulmonary function is largely an imprecise art often **underestimating the severity** of lung dysfunction. Ongoing objective assessment of respiratory mechanics, ventilatory function, lung perfusion, gas diffusion and oxygenation at the bedside will enable us to detect early changes in pulmonary function and appropriately modify management strategies.

Bedside Measurements

The vital capacity and forced expiratory volume in one second can be measured using a portable spirometer, either electronic or the dry seal variety. The spirometers for bedside use should be carefully selected. They should be portable and sturdy. Both these measurements require good patient co-operation and adequate coaching for reproducible results.

At least three efforts should be made under observation and the best effort values incorporate, taking care that there is less than 10% variability between the three efforts. If the patient cannot perform a forced vital capacity maneuver, then exhaled vital capacity immediately after a 20 second maximum inspiratory pressure determination can be used. It provides comparable results. **Normal forced vital capacity values in supine patients are lower than those obtained in standing or sitting posture due to the effects of upward shift of diaphragm and abdominal contents.** Hence, the **trend of values** carries more information than the initial or any single value. Normal values of vital capacity are 65-75 ml per kg. Value less than 15 ml per kg. implies that there is difficulty in generating an adequate cough and in maintaining adequate ventilation for any period of time.

The **forced expiratory volume** in one second is the volume forcibly expired from maximal inspiration in one second. It is the parameter showing least intrinsic variation. Normal values of forced expiratory volume in one second range from 50-60 ml per kg. value of forced expiratory volume in one second expressed as a ratio of forced vital capacity range from 75-80%.

The **Peak expiratory flow** rate is another useful measurement of ventilatory ability. Being measured at the onset of maximal expiration from full inspiration, it is largely **effort dependent.** Meaning thereby that poor effort, muscular weakness may give spurious low value which may falsely be interpreted as airway obstruction. While normal values may vary with **age, sex,** etc. usually adults have values between 400-600 liters per minute. Proper coaching and observation of patient efforts during test performance are essential for correct interpretation of the test. **Values less than 75-100 liters per minute imply moderate to severe obstruction.** Since different mechanisms, peak expiratory flow rate values vary from one flow meter to the other, serial comparisons of measurement should be made only on readings from a single peak flow meter for correct interpretation of results (Fig.1)..

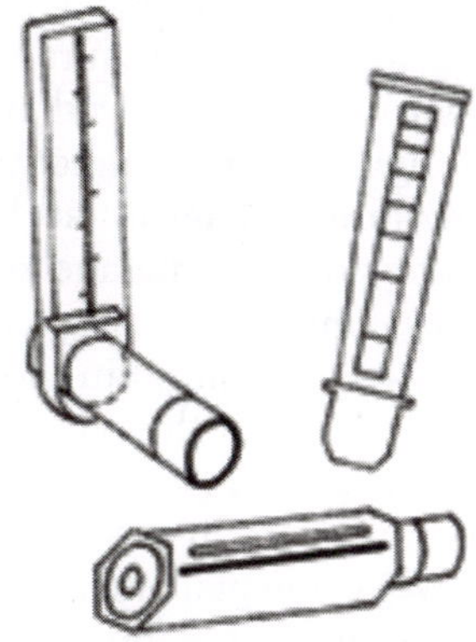

Fig. 1 Different types of peak flow meters

The tidal volume can be measured by a respirometer connected to the endotracheal tube or the face mask.

The minute ventilation can be estimated using a pneumotachometer held at the mouth for 30 seconds. The pneumotech generates an electronic signal in response to respiratory gas flows and this may be used directly to quantify flow rates or the signal may be digitally or electronically integrated with time to display a volume signal. Normal values of minute ventilation are 5-6 liters per minute. Value of more than 10 liters per minute mean that the patient is unlikely to sustain the effort of breathing for any reasonable length of time and respiratory failure is probable.

Mechanical Ventilators

While most of the above parameters are directly measured, several important parameters of lung function may be derived from measurements of airways pressure, flows, volumes etc. in both intubated and non-intubated patients. Most sophisticated mechanical ventilators incorporate software for these calculations which are carried out automatically on activating the relevant software programme.

During mechanical ventilation, tidal volume, respiratory rate, peak gas flow rate, oxygen concentration is set variables. However, ongoing continuous monitoring of the actual delivered tidal volume, minute volume etc., is possible. In addition, peak airway pressure and plateau airway pressures are measured by pressure transducers situated near the endotracheal tube. The peak pressure is determined by both the elastic properties of the lung and resistance to airflow in the conducting air passages. The plateau pressure is measured in the absence of airflow and is related to the elastic properties of the lung. Since there is no airflow, it is not affected by changes in airway resistance. The difference between the plateau pressure and the expiratory pressure (atmospheric or PEEP) is related to the static compliance of the respiratory system compliance being the change in volume per unit change of pressure.

Airway Resistance

While normal resistance values are around 2-3 cm of water/litre/second, the addition of endotracheal tube itself increases airway resistance partly directly and partly due to the reflex bronchospasm it induces. Hence as in compliance, serial changes in airway resistance measurements are of more significance than the initial or any single reading. Airway resistance may be calculated at the bedside also by using the forced oscillation technique.

Perfusion of the lungs affects the V/Q relationships, which in turn affects the gas exchange functions of the lungs. The perfusion stat of the lung cannot be estimated clinically. Radionucleide scanning may help in the determination of the gross abnormalities of perfusion, but they cannot be performed at the bedside. Bedside pulmonary angiography using a portable image intensifier and a video recording system with catetherisation of the pulmonary artery via a sheath passed through the internal jugular vein can be done.

Diffusion measurements using estimation of carbon monoxide diffusion coefficient has been possible even in intubated patient, using the steady state rebreathing technique. Values closely approximate those obtained by the single breath method, and this technique has been used to diagnose reliably lung heamorrhage and differentiate it from other causes of lung infiltrates.

Oxygenation

Oxygenation of the blood is one of the prime functions of an intact respiratory apparatus. Low oxygenation status of the blood is recognized clinically as cyanosis. This is one of the reliable sign since oxygen saturation has to fall to about 70% for cyanosis to be detectable and even at these levels, in artificial lighting, it may not be detectable. Therefore objective measures of oxygenation are required. Information regarding oxygenation may be obtained from values of partial pressure of oxygen (PaO2), oxygen saturation (SaO2) and transcutaneous oxygen measurements (PtcO2), While SaO2 and PtcO2 are non-invasive measures, PaO2 requires indwelling arterial cannula or intermittent arterial puncture ant the subsequent analysis of heparinised blood by the ampermetric method using the clerk electrode. Normal values of PaO2 range from 80-100 mmHg, but this may vary with age, posture etc. a low PaO2 may be due to hypoventilation, diffusion abnormalities, V/Q mismatching or shunt.

The PaO2 measurement is based on the Clark electrode principle where oxygen diffuses across the skin and electrode membrane to react with the electrons provided by the anode, resulting in generation of a current proportional to the oxygen concentration. This is amplified and read in millimeters of mercury. Since it requires heating of skin, skin bums may be a complication. It closely approximates PaO2, but may read false low levels in cases of reduced poor perfusion, thick skin, low cardiac output or low capillary density.

Measurement of oxygen saturation by **Pulse oximetry** represents a significant advance in non-invasive monitoring of oxygenation status, saturation being the percentage of haemoglobin molecules that are saturated with oxygen compared to the total number of haemoglobin molecules present.

The principle of oximetry is based on Beer's Law which states that the concentration of an unknown solute dissolved in a solvent can be determined by light absorption (Fig. 2). When light is passed through the finger, the majority of light is absorbed by the connective tissue, skin, bone and venous blood. The amount of blood absorbed by these substances is constant and does not vary with the cardiac cycle. With each heartbeat, there is an increase in the arterial blood with resultant increase in light absorption. By comparing peak to trough absorbances, the contribution from non arterial sources becomes irrelevant. The light absorbances at two wavelengths is different for oxyHb and reduced Hb and the value of R is determined (R being the ratio of peak and trough absorbances at two wavelengths, usually 660nm and 940nm.).

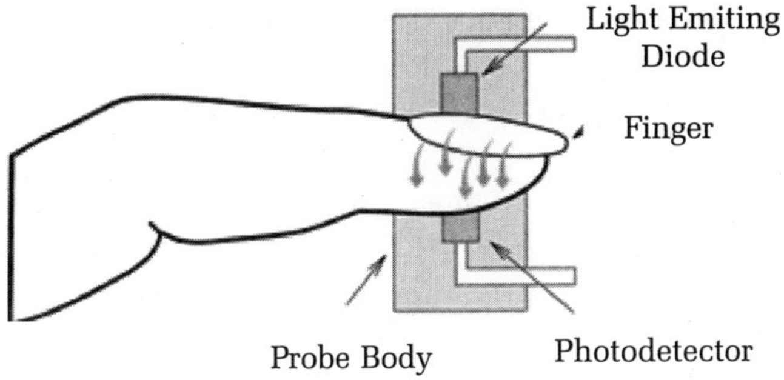

Fig. 2: Principle of Pulse Oximetry

Oxygen saturation is calculated from R based on experimental data. There is no direct mathematical relationship between R and O2 saturation. The manufactures had healthy volunteers to breathe air an oxygen mixtures. The value of R was calculated as also the oxygen saturation determined at each level. A calibration curve was then plotted where values of R were related to oxygen saturation. The oximeter is usually accurate over the range of 75-100%.

Values of oxygen saturation and corresponding partial pressures are as follows:

Saturation (Percent)	Partial Pressure (mm Hg)
100	150
97	90-100
90	60
80	46-48
75	40
50	27

Thus oxygen saturation is a good means to measure the oxygenation status non-invasively, continuously over a period of time. It is possible to monitor comprehensively in an ongoing manner various aspects of lung function. This helps in titrating treatment for optimum outcome and minimal complications.

REFERENCES

1. Pilbeam S Noninvasive gas monitoring in mechanically ventilated patients. Mechanical ventilation – Physiological and Clinical applications. 2nd edition. *Mosby Year Book 1992; 329-357.*
2. Pilbeam S Establishing the need for mechanical ventilation mechanical ventilation-Physiological and Clinical applications. 2nd edition. *Mosby YearBook: 1992: 123-128.*
3. Cullen JA et at: Pulmonary function testing in the critically ill neonate methodology. *Neonatal Network 1994, 13:7-13.*
4. Wragg S et al : Portable measurement of maximum mouth pressure, *European Respir Jour: 1994:398-401*
5. Mori M et al: Lung sound analysis and pulmonary function studies: *RinshoByori 1994: 42:396-400.*
6. Tsubaki et al: A comparative evaluation of commercially available peak flow meters. *Arerugi 1994: 43:571-578.*
7. Tsubaki et al: A comparative evaluation of three commercially use peak flow meters before and after being used a thousand times *Arerugi 1994;43: 1301-1308.*
8. Reiterer F et al. Diagnosis of lung function in intensive care of newborn infants *WeinKlinWochenscher 1994;106: 181-186.*
9. Muma AH et al : Assessment of lung function in the ICU. *Paediatr: Pulmonol 1995;19:118-128.*
10. Kugelman A et al : Comparison of Dynamic and passive measurement of respiratory mechanics in ventilated newborn infants. *Paediatr Pulmonol 1995;20:258-264.*
11. Hamir J et al : Infant lung testing in the ICU. *Intensive Care Medicine 1995;21:744-752*
12. Ghai Textbook of Practical Physiology. Seventh edn. *152-153, 165*

16
CLASSIFICATION OF ABNORMAL PATTERNS OF PULMONARY FUNCTION

BNBM PRASAD

Introduction

Pulmonary function testing plays a valuable role in the evaluation and care of patients with various cardio-respiratory disorders. It is used to evaluate respiratory symptoms, determine the severity of dysfunction, elucidate the pathophysiologic mechanism and assess the response to the therapy. Physiologic response to the presence of disease in the respiratory system conforms to certain patterns of functional impairment or loss of function and can be identified by measuring the ventilatory capacity, lung volumes, transfer factor, mechanical properties of the lung and cardiopulmonary exercise responses. The pattern of abnormal lung function helps to arrive at a functional diagnosis which with clinical, radiological and other supportive data helps to confirm or rule out disorders affecting the respiratory system.

Patterns of impairment

Abnormal patterns of pulmonary functions are classified into following groups:

1. Obstructive impairment
2. Restrictive impairment
3. Combined (obstructive and restrictive)
4. Isolated diffusion defect
5. Respiratory centre unresponsiveness
6. Abnormal blood gases in the absence of other functional abnormalities

Obstructive impairment

Obstructive impairment is characterized by air flow limitation due to diseases of airways and parenchyma. Airway obstruction may be localized or diffuse, fixed or variable, and involve upper or lower airways or both.

(a) **Upper airways obstruction:** Following types of upper airway obstruction are seen and can be identified by analysis of flow volume loop.

- (i) Fixed upper airway obstruction
- (ii) Variable upper airway obstruction
  - Extrathoracic
  - Intrathoracic
- (iii) Combined upper and lower airway obstruction

(i) **Fixed upper airway obstruction:**

It implies that the airway diameter at the site of obstruction does not vary during inspiration or expiration and there is constant flow resistance during both phases of respiratory cycle

Causes: The fixed upper airway obstruction is caused by circumferential lesions of upper airways. Such type of lesions are seen in encircling endotracheal neoplasms, post-intubation cicatricial stenosis of the trachea, encircling goitres, occluded upper airway by inappropriately small endotracheal tube and rarely by stenosis of both main bronchi.

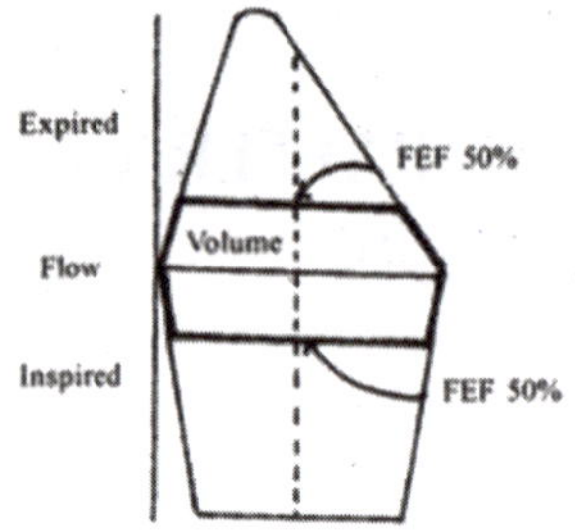

Fig. 1: Fixed airway obstruction

Recognition: Fixed upper airway obstruction can be identified by flow volume curves and spirometry. Flow volume loop shows a plateau in both inspiratory and expiratory limbs, decreased peak flow and almost constant ratio of inspiratory to expiratory flow at mid vital capacity (Fig, 1). The latter which is determined by dividing forced inspiratory flow 50% by forced expiratory flow 50% (FIF 50%/FEF 50%) may not change from the normal value (>1.0). A forced expiratory flow rate equal to or less than 100 L/min, a ratio of forced expiratory volume in one second (FEV1) in ml to peak expiratory flow rate (PEFR) in L/min equal to or greater than 10 and a ratio of FEV to FEV 0.5 equal to or greater than 1.5 are other distinguishing features from lower airway obstruction. Spirometry reveals loss of exponential expiratory curve, almost identical values of forced inspiratory and expiratory volume in one second (FIV=FEV) and similarly of inspiratory and expiratory limbs of spirogram.

(ii) Variable upper airway obstruction

In variable upper airway obstruction, the diameter of the airway at the site of the obstruction varies and it follows the dynamics of flow and pressure during the respiratory cycle. The lesion causing the obstruction is localized rather than circumferential and may be mobile or floppy or even unchanging with respiratory movement. Physiological effects of variable upper airway obstruction is determined by the site of the lesion.

(a) ***Extrathoracic variabile upper airway obstruction***: In extrathoracic variable upper airway obstruction the site of the lesion is in airways more than 2 cm above manubrium. The extrathoracic airway has a negative intraluminal pressure relative to the atmospheric pressure during inspiration. At the site of the obstruction due to phasic changes in airway pressure, the airway diameter decreases during inspiration, thereby resulting in worsening of obstruction, while during expiration, obstruction improves due to dilatation of airway.

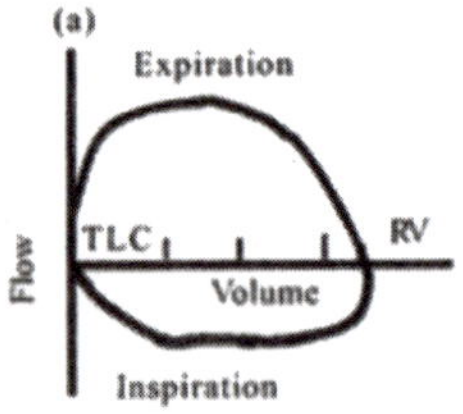

Fig. 2 Flow volume loops in extrathoracic large airway obstruction

Recognition: Flow-volume curve is helpful in diagnosis and is characterized by flow plateau in the inspiratory loop and a normal expiratory loop (Fig.2).

Consequent ot inspiratory flow limitation, the ratio of FIF 50% to FEF 50% is decreased and FEV1, is greater than FIV. Maximum voluntary ventilation (MVV) is reduced disproportionately to that of FEV1 and the ratio of MVV to FEV1, is reduced. Flow volume loop in obstructive sleep apnoea shows typically saw toothing on the inspiratory and expiratory curve due to floppy upper airways.

Causes:

(i) Unilateral or bilateral vocal cord palsy

(ii) Burn injuries

(iii) Trauma and adhesions of vocal cord due to endotracheal intubation

(iv) obstructive sleep apnoea

(ab) Intraathoracic variable upper airway obstruction: The site of obstruciton is in the lower trachea and main bronchi. The airway diameter at the site of obstruction, decreases during expiration and increases during inspiration due to effects of intrathoracic pressure swings on intrathoracic airway. Consequently the obstruction gets worse during expiration.

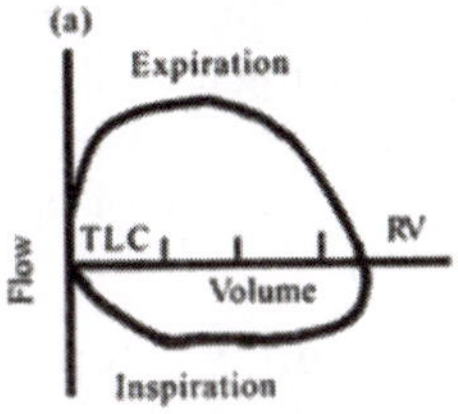

Fig. 3: Flow volume loops in intrathoracic large airway obstruction

Functional impairment in lower tracheal obstruction: The flow volume curve shows fow plateau inthe expiratory loop (Fig.3), flow obstruction, the FEV1 is smaller than FIV1 and the ratio of FIF 50% and FEF 50% is high. Flows at high lung volumes including peak flow are reduced and hence effort dependent portion of Maximal Expiratory Flow Volume (IMEFV1) curve is altered.

Causes:

i) Tumours of lower trachea
ii) Polychonditis of trachea
iii) Tracheomalacia

Functional impairment in main bronchial obstruction: Flow-volume loop reveals well preserved inspiratory and biphasic expiratory flow. The latter, results from superimposition of normal curve of non-obstructed contralateral lung, on an obstructed curve produced by the lung, whose bronchus is obstructed. In combined restrictive and obstructive pulmonary functional impairment, a biphasic expiratory flow loop can be seen, but in this condition the vital capacity is usually smaller than unilateral bronchial obstruction.

Lower airway obstruction: Lower airway obstruction characteristically produces an obstructive ventilatory defect with expiratory flow limitation. Salient functional impairments in obstructive ventilatory defect are given in table 1.

Table.1: Functional impairments in obstructive ventilatory defect

Characteristics of Obstructive defect	Supplementary data confirming obstruction
Normal or Increased RV	Decreased VC
Decreased max. expiratory airflow	Increased airway resistance
Decreased MVV	Abnormal distribution of inspired gas
	Significant response to bronchodilators
	Decreased DLCO
	Decreased lung elastic recoil

Types of lower airway obstruction and their recognition

(i) ***Large airway obstruction***: Airways larger than 2 mm which include first 9 generations and contribute to about 80% of airway resistance. Their obstruction produces a characteristic obstructive ventilatory defect with decreased Peak Expiratory Flow Rate (PEFR), Forced Expiratory Volume in 1 second (FEV1) and ratio of Forced Expiratory Volume in 1 second and Forced Vital Capacity (FEV1/FVC%). In the flow volume loop, the descending limb of expiratory curve loses the normal linearity and becomes concave upwards due to dynamic compression of airways (Fig 4, 5). The loss of linearity correlates with severity of obstruction. The inflection point of expiratory curve is reached.

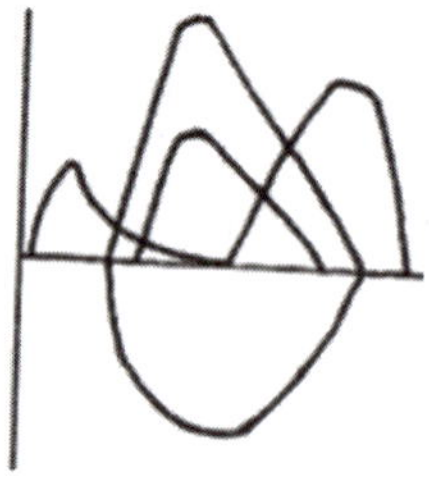

Fig.4 Flow volume curves in;

O= obstructive disease; R (P)=parenchymal restrictive disease; R(E)=extraparenchymal restrictive disease with limitation in inspiration and expiration; T total lung capacity; RV= residual volume

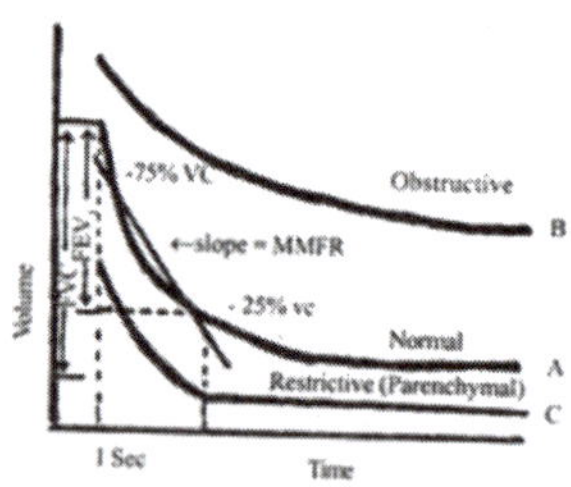

Fig.5 Spirographic tracing of forced expiration

Normal lung tracing (A), and tracings in obstructive (B) and parenchymal restrictive disease (C).

Within 25% of the FVC. Average flow at the effort dependent portion of expiratory curve between initial 200 ml and 1200 ml exhaled i.e FEF 200-1200 FVC or Maximum Expiratory Flow Rate (MEFR) is decreased. Similarly Peak Expiratory Flow which is effort dependent and reflects caliber of large lung airways is also decreased.

(ii) ***Small airway obstruction:*** Small airways, those with size less than 2 mm contribute to about 20% of airway resistance. Considerable degree of small airway disease may go unnoticed as values of PEFR, FEV1/FVC ratio, MVV and airway conductance (Gaw) remain almost normal. However these peripheral airway obstructions, which remain silent otherwise, can be recognised by the following features.

i. Increase in residual volume and closing volume relative to the total lung capacity with resultant increase in ratio of RV and TLC, and closing capacity and total lung capacity (CC?TLC).

ii Slope of the alveolar plateau for nitrogen (Phase III) following a vital capacity breath of 100% oxygen is increased due to poor intrapulmonary mixing of gases(increased SBN2 gradient)

iii Fall in frequency dependent lung compliance $\geq$ 25% of a respiratory of >60 per minute

iv The Forced Expiratory Flow (FEF) between 25% and 75% FVC or Maximal

Mid-expiratory flow rate (MMFR) which reflects effort independent portion of expiratory curve and flow at low lung volumes is decreased

v Laminar flow which occurs in small airways, remain unaffected on breathing helox mixture (80% helium and 20% oxygen mixture)

Small airway obstruction without overt airway obstruction occurs in conditions such as chronic bronchitis, asymptomatic cigarette smokers, asthmatics in remission, bronchiolitis obliterans, exposure to noxious fumes and left ventricular failure.

(iii) ***Combined large and small airway obstruction:*** This occurs in conditions such as chronic bronchitis, bronchial asthma and cystic fibrosis. The following salient features are seen.

(a) Airway resistance (Raw) is increased

(b) Specific airway conductance (SGaw) is increased

(c) FEV1 and FEV1/FVC% are decreased

(d) Peak expiration flow, FEF 35%-75%, FEF 50% and FEF 75% are decreased

(e) Lung volume measurements show features of hyperinflation with elevation of RV, FRC and TLC. The VC and FVC may be normal. In severe obstruction, there is decrease in both VC and FVC with fall in VC often larger than FVC

(f) The MVV which correlates with FRV values is decreased proportional to the degree of obstruction

(g) The capacity ratio which is the ratio of MVV (l/min) and VC (l) is decreased,

(iv) ***Reversible airway obstruction***: The widely accepted criteria for reversibiity of airway obstruction with bronchodilators are;

i. Increase in FEV2 of 15% above base line value,

ii. Absolute increase of at least 200 ml of FEV1 from initial FEV1 value

iii. Increase in FVC of 15% above base line

iv. Increase in isovolume FEF 25%-75%

Reversibility is a *sine qua non* of asthma. Some asthmatics show predominant increase in FVC without increase in flow rates. These cases have severe base line airway obstruction. Such cases are called volume responders. Asthmatic airways are hyperresponsive and are 100 to 1000 times more sensitive to bronchoconstricting effects of various agents compared to normal subjects. Positive test for bronchial hyperresponsiveness is indicated by 20% or more fall in FEV1 and PEFR. 25% fall or more in FEF 25%-75%, 40% or more drop in specific airway conductance (SGaw) and 25% or more increase in FRC following bronchial challenge with non-specific stimuli. The provocation concentration (PC) or provocation dose (PD) of provocative agent which causes 20% fall in FEV1, from baseline (PC 20 or PD 20) is the lowest for bronchial asthma and the magnitude of response to challenge correlates with severity of the disease.

Pulmonary function in syndromes of chronic airflow limitation

Syndrome of chronic airflow limitation occurs usually due to chronic mucus hypersecretion (chronic bronchitis), pulmonary emphysema, airway hyperreactivity (asthma) and changes in small airways including respiratory bronchiolitis. Less commonly it may result from bronchiectasis and syndromes of bronchiolitis, either primary or secondary to rheumatoid arthritis and collagen vascular disease. The differentiation of various common airflow limitation syndrome based on pulmonary function tests are given in the Table 2.

Table 2. Typical functional findings of common chronic airflow limitation syndrome

Function	Asthma	Chronic Bronchitis	Emphysema
Obstuctive Ventilatory			
Defect	Episodic	Persistent	Persistent
Reversibility	Marked	Often present	Can be present
Total lung capacity	Normal or increased	Normal often	Increased
Transfer factor	Normal or increased	Normal	Reduced
KCO (T1/VA)	Normal	Normal	Reduced
Static compliance	Normal	Normal	Reduced
Recoil pressure (below TLC)	Reduced*	Normal	Reduced
Hypoxaemia	Present	Often marked	Present

- During acute episodes

It is to be noted that in both emphysema and interstitial fibrosis the transfer factor is reduced, however the distinction is made using the Total lung capacity and the Static Volume pressure curve. In emphysema a large total lung capacity, a maximal recoil pressure of less than 10 cms of H_2O and a static lung compliance on expiration in excess of 0.4 L/cm H_2O are present.

Restrictive impairment

Restrictive diseases are heterogeneous groups of disorders which are characterized by a decrease in lung volumes, primarily TLC and VC. Features of restrictive ventilatory defect are given in the table 3.

Table 3: Features of restrictive ventilatory defect

Characteristics of restrictive ventilatory defect	Supplementary data confirming restictive pattern
Decreased VC Relatively normal expiratory flow Relatively normal MVV	Decreased TLC Decreased lung compliance flow rate Chronic alveolar hyperventilation Increased (A-a) PO2 Abnormal distribution of inspired gas Decreased DLCO

Flow volume loop in restrictive disorders: Flow volume loop typically is tall and narrow indicating normal expiratory flow rates and reduced VC. This is due to the increase in lung elastic recoil which not only reduces lung volume but also increases driving force of expiratory flow due to outward traction on airways. Therefore, the peak expiratory flows are relatively preserved. In fact, when FEV1 is considered as a percent of FVC, the flow rates are often disproportionately high relative to the size of lungs. The expiratory limb of flow volume loop is linear decreasing rapidly from peak flow to residual volume. The flow volume loop looks like the miniaturised version of normal curve (Fig. 6). In severe restrictive disorders, both VC and TLC are reduced bt usually fall of VC occurs prior to fall of TLC.

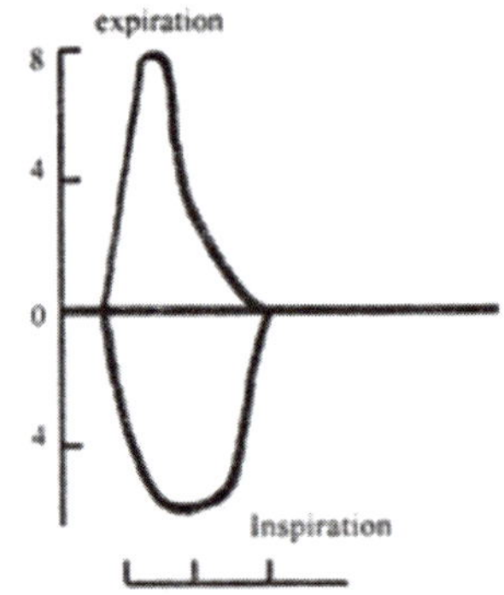

Fig. 6 Flow-volume loop in ventilatory disorder

Patterns of impairment in various restrictive disorders: Depending on the site of the disease process, a restrictive disorder can be divided into following subgroups.

(a) Pulmonary parenchymal restriction
(b) Extra parenchymal restriction

(a) ***Pulmonary parenchymal restriction:***

The salient finding in restrictive disorders due to pulmonary causes is reduced lung compliance due to an increase in the interstitial tissue which can occur due to inflammation (interstitial pneumonia), fibrosis, infiltration or oedema. Reduced lung compliane can also occur due to fibrosis of visceral pleura and sub-pleural tissue. In early stages of the pulmonary restrictive disorders, there is decrease in transfer factor and oxygen tension in the blood with increase in ventilation on exercise. The maximum voluntary ventilation is reduced in far advanced interstitial fibrosis, but the degree of reduction is less than that in lung volume or gas exchange. Consequently, the air velocity index which is the ratio of percent predicted MVV and percent predicted VC, is far above unity. In early stages of interstitial lung disease

(ILD), MVV is generally maintained at normal values and its reduction below normal value indicates presence of concomitant additional factors such as airway obstruction, respiratory muscle involvement or fibrothorax. The functional changes in interstitial lung disease are summarised in the following flow diagram.

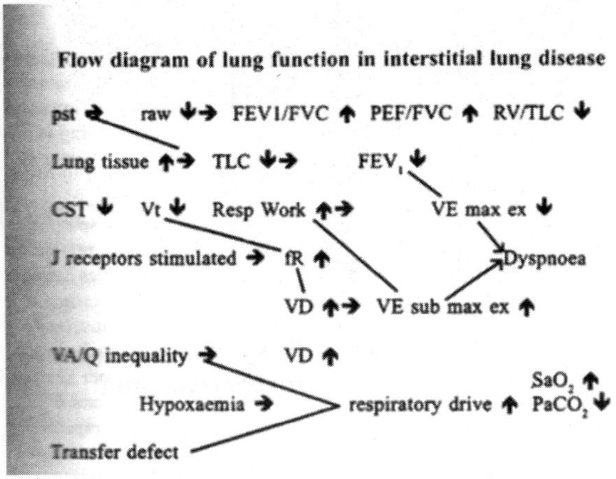

Pst = pressure static: Raw= resistance airways; Cst= compliance static; VA= ventilation; Q= perfusion' VD= physiological dead space' FR= frequency respiration; VE= minute ventilation

Some of the causes of pulmonary parenchymal restrictions are as follows:

- Idiopathic pulmonary fibrosis
- Pneumoconiosis
- Sarcoidosis
- Collagen vascular disease with pulmonary parenchymal involvement
- Extrinsic allergic alveolitis
- Drug or radiation induced lung disease
- Viral pneumonia
- Miliary Tuberculosis
- Pulmonary eosinophilia

(b) ***Extra-parenchymal restriction:***

In the absence of lung diseases, restriction of lung volumes can result from diseases of pleura, thoracic skeleton and chest wall. In all these conditions lung is either normal or is affected secondary to the primary disorder. The functional impairment may occur predominantly in inspiration or in both inspiration and expiration.

In extra-parenchymal restriction with inspiratory dysfunction either due to stiff chest wall (ankylosing spondylitis) or inspiratory muscle weakness, adequate distending forces to overcome the inward recoil of lung at total lung capacity cannot be generated, resulting in a much lower TLC than the predicted value. The residual volume is preserved.

In extra-parenchymal restriction in which there is both inspiratory and expiratory dysfunction, there is elevation of residual volume which can occur even without airway obstruction. At low lung volumes due to the expiratory muscle weakness or stiffness of chest wall (increase in recoil of chest wall), force generated by the expiratory muscles to overcome the outward recoil of chest wall is reduced. This results in an increase in residual volume. Expiratory muscle dysfunction *per se* can cause decrease in the expiratory flow with decreased FRV1 and FVC ratio even without airflow obstruction since the ability to expire rapidly is impaired. The differentiating features of various types of restrictive disorders are shown in the Table 4 and Fig. 4.

Table.4: Functional impairment in restrictive disorders

	TLC	RC	VC	FEV1/FVC
Restrictive pulmonary parenchymal	D	D	D	N to D
Extraparenchymal inspiratory	D	N to D	D	N
Extraparenchymal inspiratory + expiratory	D	D	D	variable

D: decreased; N: normal

The causes of various extraparenchymal restrictive disorders are as follows:

(a) Space-occupying lesions: Tumors, cysts

(b) Pleural diseases: Pneumothorax, haemothorax, pleural effusion, empyma, fibrothorax

(c) Chest wall disorders: Kyphoscoliosis, obesity, ankylosing spondylitis

(d) Extrathoracic conditions: Obesity, ascites, pregnancy

(e) Neuromuscular disorders: Myasthenia gravis, Guillain-Barre syndrome,

Diaphragmatic weakness/paralysis

Respiratory muscle weakness causing restrictive impairment:

The hall mark of respiratory muscle weakness is a hypodynamic (restrictive) type of ventilatory defect with decrease in viral capacity due to reduction in maximal force that can be exerted by the respiratory muscle.

The diagnostic findings of notable respiratory muscle weakness are summarised in the table 5.

Table 5: Diagnostic features of respiratory muscle weakness

Measurement	Positive result
Maximal inspiratory pressure at mouth (PI Max)	<-6 to -8 kPa
Nasopharyngeal pressure (sniff PI, np max)	<-6 kPa
Oesophageal pressure (sniff PI, Oes max)	<-6 kPa
Transdiaphragmatic pressure	<-10kPa in men <-7 kPa in women
Change in vital capacity from sitting to supine position	>30%
MVV and FEV1 ratio, FIV	Decreased
FEV1 and PEV1 ratio	Increased

Combined restrictive-obstructive impairment

Restrictive and obstructive diseases have opposite effect on lung volume. In combined defects the lung volume is inappropriately low for obstructive defect but at the same time inappropriately high for restrictive defect. Often the diagnosis of restrictive disorder may be masked in a patient with combined defect. The spirometric patterns resemble obstructive defect with decreased VC and expiratory flow rate. In such cases lung volume measurement such as TLC is low or inappropriately normal to show evidence of underlying restrictive defect. Following are some of the conditions where combined impairment is seen, due to involvement of both airways and lung parenchyma.

- Pulmonary Tuberculosis
- Sarcoidosis
- Bronchiectasis
- Cystic Fibrosis
- Pneumoconiosis
- Congestive cardiac failure

Consequences of obstructive/ restrictive impairment: The sequence of events which ultimately leads to chronic cor pulmonale in obstructive and restrictive disorders are shown in the following flow diagram.

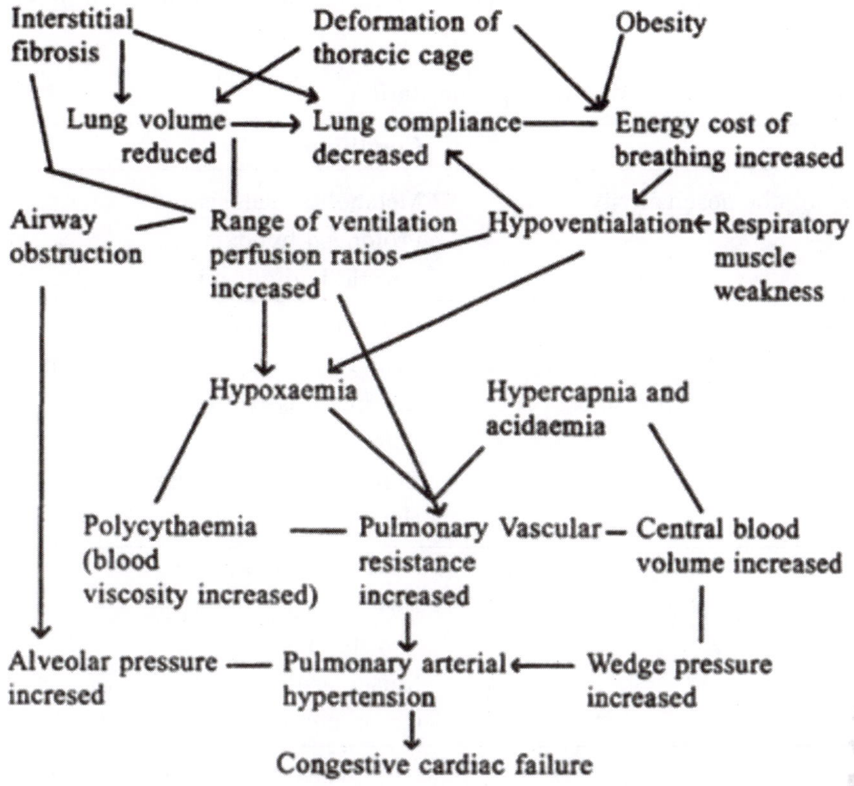

Isolated diffusion defect

Syndrome of defective gas transfer is characterized by reduced transfer factor (DLCO). Often an isolated diffusion defect with normal spirometric values may be the only abnormality detected in certain conditions such as early interstitial fibrosis, stage I sarcoidosis, pulmonary vascular disease, anaemia, carboxyhaemoglobinaemia and *Pneumocystic carinii* Pneumonia. Measurement of DLCO which is reduced in these cases is a sensitive index of early lung involvement in the rpesence of normal clinical and radiological findings. Decrease in transfer factor, hypoxaemia and hyperventilation are frequently observed during exercise in such cases.

Respiratory Centre unresponsiveness

The respiratory centre unresponsiveness is a condition characterised by the diminished responsiveness of respiratory centre to CO2, and/or hypoxia. Yhis results in hypoventilation when there is diminution in alveolar ventilation sufficient to reduce the elimination of carbon dioxide and build up of its tension in the blood. There is hyperbolic relationship between alveolar ventilation (VA) and PaCO2 if the carbon dioxide output (VCO2) is constant as seen from the following equation:

$$VA = \frac{VACO2 \times 0.863}{PaCO2}$$

Alveolar hypoventilation: Alveolar hypoventilation exists when arterial PCO2 increases above normal range of 37 to 43 mm Hg. Various conditions causing chronic alveolar hypoventilation are given in the table 6.

Table 6: Conditions associated with hypoventilation

Defect	Condition
Disorders of chemosensitivity	Metabolic alkalosis Prolonged hypoxia Carotid body dysfunction
Disorders of brain stem integrating and rhythm generating net works induced and brain stem motor neurons	Primary alveolar hypoventilation, Drug respiratory dependence infarction Encephalitis, Trauma Sarcoidosis Demyelinating disorder Haemorrhage
Disorders of spinal cord, Peripheral nerves and respiratory muscles	Motor neurone disease Peripheral neuropathy Myasthenia gravis Muscular dystrophy Chronic myopathy
Disorders of chest wall	Obesity hypoventilation syndromes Fibrothorax Ankylosing spondylitis Kyphoscoliosis

Disorders of lungs and airway disease	Chronic obstructive airway disease Cystic fibrosis Obstructive deep apnoea Laryngeal and tracheal stenosis

In primary alveolar hypoventilation, a disorder of unknown origin, there is no identifiable neurologic disease, respiratory muscle weakness or mechanical ventilatory defects. There is a failure in the automatic or metabolic control of respiration in that the changes in the abnormalities of blood gases and cerebral acid-base status are not sensed and converted into appropriate motor output by central respiratory neurones.The dominant lesion is the loss of central respiratory drive. This causes hypoventilation during sleep when the ventilation is critically dependent on metabolic control. Due to intact behavioural respiratory control, the subjects, can hyperventilate voluntarily. Salient functional findings are hypercapnia, hypoxaemia and chronic respiratory acidosis with normal lung volumes, airflows, MVV , gas transfer and muscle force. In addition the mouth occlusion pressure, ventilatory and diaphragmatic electromyographic response to chemical stimuli namely hypercapnia and or hypoxia are diminished. Polysomnographic studies reveal hypoventilation, frequent episodes of central apnoea or hypopnoea and fragmentation of sleep. Respiratory centre unresponsiveness may be present with chronic obstructive airway disease, obesity and obstructive sleep apnoea.

Abnormal Blood Gases in the absence of other Pulmonary Function abnormalities

Lung plays an important role in the maintenance of acid base balance of the body which is affected by any alterations of total alveolar ventilation and perfusion. Hyperventilation augments CO2 excretion and causes respiratory alkalosis. On the other hand hypoventilation results in CO2 retention and respiratory acidosis. Abnormal changes in blood gases usually occur in association with pulmonary function abnormality. Sometimes abnormality in blood gases can occur with normal pulmonary function tests.

(a) ***Hypoxaemia:*** Low PaO2, with normal lung function (lung volumes, flows,DLCO, MVV and muscle function) or with mild functional impairment not commensurating with degree of hypoxaemia has been observed n certandisorders such as early stage of interstitial lung disease (ILD), small airway obstruction, veno-arterial shunt and chest bellows disorders. In ILD, exercise capacity (DLCO) and PaO2 are normal. in veno-arterial shunt, severe resting hypoxaemia which can not be corrected by inhaling 100% ocygen, with normal pulmonary function test are the features to suggest diagnosis. In small airway obstruction routine pulmonary function tests may be normal yet the disease may cause ventilation-perfusion mismatch and hypoxaemia. In chest bellow disorders, due to reduction in FRC, the premature closure of airways occur at tidal breathing. This results in ventilation-perfusion mismatch and hypoxaemia.

(b) ***Hypercapnia***: Hypercapnia with normal pulmonary function tests is a feature of respiratory centre unresponsiveness.CO2 retention with metabolic alkalosis complicating diuretics, steroids or vomiting may be a clue to the presence of COPD, in cases where the diagnosis is not obvious. Metabolic alkalosis per se does not result in PaCOe values more than 54 mm Hg and a level of PaCO2 above 54 mm Hg is indicative of underlying ventilatory failure. Inadvertent use of sedation and uncontrolled oxygen therapy in such cases will cause further CO2 retention.

Severity of Pulmonary Function Impairment

Severity of pulmonary function impairment is assessed by the decrease in percentage of predicted value and is illustrated in table 7.

Table 7: Severity of pulmonary function impairment (% of predicted normal)

Impairment assessment	VC	FEV1	FEV1 FVC%	FEF 25%-75%	TLC	DLCO
Normal	>80	>80	>70	>65	>80	>80
Mild	66-80	66-80	60-70	50-65	66-80	61-80
Moderate	60-65	50-65	45-59	35-49	50-65	40-60
Severe	<50	<50	<45	<35	<50	<40

Conclusion

By careful analysis of patterns of impairment of pulmonary function, it is possible to draw accurate inference about the site and nature of underlying disorder. Recognition of specific patterns of impairment and their careful interpretation depends on a thorough knowledge of the pathophysiologic basis of the function measured.

REFERENCES

1. Miller RD, Hyatt RE Evaluation of obstructing lesions of trachea and larynx by flow volume loops Am RevRespir Dis 1973; 108: 475-81
2. Miller A, Brown LK, Teirstein AS Dtenosis of main bronchi mimicking fixed upper airway obstruction in sarcoidsois Chest 1985; 88: 744-48
3. Danders MH, Martin RJ, Pennock BE, et al The detection of sleep apnoea in the awake patient The saw tooth sign JAMA 1981; 245: 2414-18
4. Lord UP The expiratory flow volume curve in localized airway obstruction J Maine Med Ass 1969; 60: 1331-34
5. Owens GR, Murphy DMF Spirometric diagnosis of upper airway obstruction by pulmonary function testing Chest 1975: 68: 796-99
6. Aldrich TK, Arora NS, Rochester DF The influence of airway obstructive and inspiratory strength on maximum voluntary ventilation in lung disease Amer Rev Respir Dis 1982; 126: 195-99
7. Hogg JC, Macklem PT, Thurlbeck WM Site and nature of airway obstruction in chronic obstructive lung disease N Engl J Med 1968; 278: 1255-60
8. Jayammanne DS, Epstein H, Goldberg RM Flow-volume curve contour in COPD: correlation with pulmonary mechanics Chest 1980; 77: 749-57
9. Malik SK Chronic bronchitis in North India Chest 1977; 72: 800
10. Miller A patterns of impairment in Miller A (ed) Pulmonary function tests in clinical and occupational lung disease Orlando, Grune & Stratton 1986; 249: 283

11. Pande JN Indirect assessment of lung compliance in chronic lung disease Respiration 1978; 36: 201-206
12. Joshi RC, Madan RN, Eggleston FC Clinical spirometry in normal North Indian males Respiration 1973; 30: 39-47
13. Jindal SK, Wahi PL Pulmonary function laboratory in the tropics: Needs, problems and solutions in Sharma et al (ed) Marcel Dekker 1991; 523-42
14. Bates DV Respiratory function in disease 3 edn, Philadelphia WB Saunders1989
15. Ries AL Measurement of lung volumes Clin Chest Med 1989; 120: 177-86
16. Light RW, Conard SA, George RB The one best test for evaluating effects of bronchodilator therapy Chest 1997; 72: 512-16
17. Mahler DA,Weinberg DH, Wells CK, et al The measurement of dyspnea: contents, interobserver agreement and physiologic correlates of two new clinical indexes Chest 1984; 83: 751-58
18. Braman SS, Corrao WM Bronchoprovocation testing Clin Chest Med 1989;10: 165-76
19. Welch MH Ventilatory function of the lungs *in* Guenter CA, Welch MH eds Pulmonary Medicine, Philadelphia JB Lippincott 1977; 72-123
20. McCarthy DS, Spencer R, Greene R, et al Measurement of closing volume as a simple and sensitive test for early detection of small airway disease Am J Med 1972; 52: 747=53
21. Gelb AF, Gold WM, Wright RR Physiologic diagnosis of subclinical emphysema Am Rev Respir Dis 1973; 107: 50-63
22. Macklem PT, Thurlbeck WM, Fraser RG Chronic obstructive disease of small airways Ann Intern Med 1971; 74: 167-77
23. Seggev J, Mason VG III, Worthen S, et al Bronchiolitis obliterans: Report of three cas with detailed physiologic studies Chest 1983; 83: 169-174
24. Malik SK, Behera D, Jindal SK Reverse smoking and chronic obstructive lung disease Br J Dis Chest 1983; 77: 199-201
25. Pande JN, Jain BP, Gupta RC, Guleria JS Pulmonary ventilation and gas exchange in bronchiectasis Thorax 1971; 26: 727-33
26. Gupta ML, Behera D Pattern of airflow obstruction in bronchial asthma-an observation on home monitoring of peak expiratory flow rate JAPI 1997; 45 94-96
27. Lobowitz MJ The use of peak expiratory flow rate measurements in respiratory diseases Paed Pneum 1991; 11: 166-79
28. Behera D, Malik SK Chronic expiratory disease and ventilatory function impairment in chutta smokers Ind J Chest Dis All Sci 1984; 26: 77
29. Behera D, Malik SK Chronic respiratory disease and ventilatory function in adult rural Oriya females Lung India 1988; 6: 127
30. Weinberger SE, Drazen JM Disturbances of respiratory function *in* Wilson JD Brraunwald E eds Harrison's Principles of Internal Medicine, 12th edn, New York, McGraw Hill 1991; 1033-43
31. Ostrow D, Cherniak RM Resistance to airflow in patients with diffuse interstitial lung disease Am Rev Respir Dis 1973; 108: 205-10
32. Crystal RG, Flmer JD, Roberts WC, et al Idiopathic pulmonary fibrosis: Clinical histologic, radiographic, physiologic, scientigraphic, cytologic and biochemical aspects Ann Intern Med 1976; 85: 769-88

33. Gold WM, Bouschey HA Pulmonary function testing *in* Murray JF, Nadel JA eds Text Book of Respiratory Medicine, Philadelphia, WB Saunders 1988; 611-682

34. Pande JN Interrelationship between lung volume, expiratory flow and lung transfer factor in fibrosing alveolitis Thorax 1981; 856-862

35. Coates JE, Leathart GL Lung function assessment and application in Medicine, 5th edn, Oxford, Blackwell Scientific, 1983

36. Wright PH, Hanson A, Kreel L, et al Respiratory functional changes after asbestos pleurisy Thorax 1980; 35: 51-56

37. Epler GR, Saber FA, Gaensler EA Determination of severe impairment (disability) in interstitial lung disease Am Rev Respir Dis 1980; 121: 647-59

38. Ray CS, Sue DY, Bray G, et al Effects of obesity on respiratory function Am Rev Respir Dis 1983; 128: 501-506

39. Black LE, Hyatt RE Maximal static respiratory pressures in generalized neuromuscular disease Am Rev Respir Dis 1971; 103: 641-51

40. Rochester DF, Arora NS, Braun NMT, et al The respiratory muscles in chronic obstructive pulmonary disease Bull Europ Physiopath Resp 1979; 15: 951-975

41. Arora NS, Rochester DF Muscular weakness and respiratory failure Am Rev Respir Dis 1970; 101: 62-66

42. Braun NMT, Rocheser DF Muscular weakness and respiratory failure Am Rev Respir Dis 1979; 119 (part 2): 123-125

43. Singh T, Finda P, Chatterjee SS, Riding WD, Patel JK Pulmonary function studies before and after closed mitral valvotomy Am Rev Respir Dis 1970; 101: 62-66

44. Pande JN, Guleria JS Comparison of single breath and steady state methods for measurement of pulmonary diffusing capacity for carbon monoxide in non-homogeneous lungs Respiration 1978; 36: 117-126

45. Tow TWY, Miller A, Brown LK, et al DLCOSB in screening for Pneumocystic carinii pneumonia (PCP) in patients with acquired immunodeficiency syndrome (AIDS) Am Rev Respir Dis 1984; 129: 554

46. Ewan PW, Jones HA, Rhodes GG, et al Detection of intrapulmonary haemorrhage with carbon monoxide uptake. Application of Goodpasture's syndrome N Engl J Med 1976; 295: 1391-1396

47. Risk C, Epler GR, Gaensler EA Exercise alveolar arterial oxygen pressure difference in interstitial lung disease Chest 1984; 85: 69-74

48. Pande JN, Gupta SP, Guleria JS Clinical significance of measurement of membrane diffusing capacty and pulmonary capillary blood volume Respiration 1975; 32: 317-24

49. Marks CE Jr, Goldring RM Chronic hypercapnia during methadone maintenance Am Rev Respir Dis 1973; 108: 1088-93

50. Burki NK Measurements of ventilatory regulation Clin Chest Med 1989;10: 215-26

51. Miller A, Teirstein AS, Duberstein J, et al Use of oxygen inhalation in evaluation of respiratory acidosis in patients with apparent metabolic alkalosis Am J Med 1968; 45: 513-19

52. Viswanathan R, Lodi STK, Subramanian S, Radha TG Pulmonary vascular response to ventilation hypercapnia in man Respiration 1976; 33: 165-78

17

EVALUATION OF RESPIRATORY MUSCLE FUNCTION

M. MADHUSUDHAN, ALLADI MOHAN

Introduction

The lungs are situated in the thoracic cavity and are surrounded by a muscles that facilitate breathing. During quiet inspiration, the diaphragm moves downward like a piston over a distance of 1.5 cm to as much as 7 cm when it contracts and accounts for nearly 75% of the change in intrathoracic volume. The external intercostal muscles are the other important inspiratory muscles. Either the diaphragm or the external intercostal muscles alone can maintain adequate ventilation during rest. The scalene and sternocleidomastoid muscles in the neck constitute the accessory muscles of inspiration and help elevating the thoracic cage during deep laboured respiration.

Tests for overall respiratory function

Routine tests of respiratory function include, lung volumes, flows, and indices of gas exchange. These measures are non-specific but provide useful indirect information regarding respiratory muscle performance. Sometimes, the presence of respiratory muscle dysfunction is indicated by the pattern of pulmonary function tests. However, more often, they are of use in assessing the severity, functional consequences, and progress of patients with recognized muscle weakness.

Static lung volumes

Reduction in vital capacity (VC) [1] is the most frequently observed lung volume abnormality in patients with respiratory muscle weakness. In patients with chronic respiratory muscle weakness direct effect of loss of muscle power, reductions in compliance of the lungs [2] as well as the chest wall [3] contribute to the reduction of VC. The rate of decline in VC has been shown to be a predictor of survival in amyotrophic lateral sclerosis [4] and Duchenne muscular dystrophy [5]. However, the VC has poor specificity for the diagnosis of respiratory muscle weakness. In mild weakness, VC is less sensitive to changes than are maximum pressures [6]. Serial measurements of VC is helpful in monitoring progress of patients with acute and chronic respiratory muscle weakness. Measurement of postural change in VC also gives a measure of diaphragmatic weakness relative to the other inspiratory muscles.

Dynamic spirometry and maximum flow

In uncomplicated respiratory muscle weakness, airway resistance is normal [7]. Airway function may appear to be supernormal when volume-corrected indices, such as, forced expiratory volume in the first second (FEV_1) / VC or specific airway conductance are used [2]. The maximum expiratory and maximum inspiratory flow–volume curves reveal a reduction in those flows that are most effort dependent [2,8]. Oscillations of maximum expiratory and/or inspiratory flow (saw-tooth appearance) are evident in patients with weak upper airway muscles and in those with extrapyramidal disorders [9]. However, the "saw tooth" pattern is nonspecific and may be seen in obstructive sleep apnoea (OSA), non-apnoeic snoring, and thermal injury of the upper airways among others.

Maximum voluntary ventilation

Maximum voluntary ventilation (MVV) used to be recommended earlier as a specific test for muscle weakness than volume measurements. However, the proportionate reduction in MVV has been found to be similar to that of VC [10,11]. MVV may be helpful in the assessment and monitoring of patients with extrapyramidal disorders, such as, Parkinson's disease where disproportionate reductions in MVV may be evident [12].

Arterial blood gas analysis

Arterial blood gas (ABG) analysis helps in assessing the functional consequences of respiratory muscle weakness. In Duchenne muscular dystrophy, hypercapnia has been observed to predict shorter survival [5]. However, ABG abnormalities occur late in the course of respiratory muscle weakness and indicate severe impairment.

Measurements during sleep

The utility of sleep measurements in patients with respiratory muscle weakness is presently unclear. In subjects with moderate or severe respiratory muscle weakness, a characteristic dip is seen in arterial oxygen saturation measured by pulse oximetry (SpO_2) during periods of rapid eye movement (REM) sleep [13-15]. Polysomnography (PSG) may be useful in patients with excessive daytime sleepiness and suspected nocturnal hypoventilation. PSG is expensive and not widely available. Overnight pulse oximetry is simple to perform and nocturnal measurements are more sensitive for detecting pulmonary gas exchange abnormalities. However, present evidence suggests that nocturnal hypoxaemia is a less useful prognostic indicator than either VC or awake arterial carbon dioxide tension ($PaCO_2$) [5,16].

Tests for respiratory control

Stimulus response tests (where a receptor is stimulated and the motor output or the consequent downstream mechanical effect are measured) are helpful in assessing the three functional components of respiratory control system, namely, the sensory receptors, central integrating circuits, and motor output to respiratory muscles. However, these tests can not separate the three functional components of the control system and these tests are seldom used for clinical assessment of stable patients. Mouth occlusion pressure during unstimulated breathing may be helpful in assessing respiratory drive and the likelihood of successful weaning in patients with acute respiratory failure.

Carbon monoxide transfer

Single-breath carbon monoxide (CO) diffusing capacity (DLCO) is usually normal or mildly reduced in patients with muscle weakness. The reduction in DLCO is due to inability of the lungs to achieve full distension at TLC and resultant failure of all the alveolar surfaces getting exposed to CO. The pattern of normal or mildly reduced DLCO and raised transfer co-efficient (KCO) is suggestive of extrapulmonary causes, such as, respiratory muscle weakness, rib cage abnormalities and pleural disease.

Exercise testing

Exercise limitation is often evident in patients with muscle weakness,, Sparse variable data reveal that the relation of workload to oxygen consumption and indices of submaximal exercise performance are normal [17]. In subjects with neuromuscular diseases, exercise is limited by weakness of non-respiratory muscles. Further, exercise testing is poorly standardized in these patients.

Tests for respiratory muscle strength

With regard to respiratory system, muscle force is estimated as pressure and shortening is assessed as lung volume change or displacement of chest wall structures. Therefore, quantitative characterization of the respiratory muscle strength has relied on measurements of volumes, displacements, pressures, and the rate of change of these variables with respect to time. Respiratory muscle strength testing by pressure measurement can be done either voluntarily (volitional tests) or involuntarily (non-volitional tests) especially in response to phrenic nerve stimulation.

Volitional tests of respiratory muscle strength

Volitional tests give an estimate of inspiratory or expiratory muscle strength, are easy and simple to perform, and are well tolerated by patients. However, ensuring that the subject is making a truly maximal effort may be difficult [18-21]. Thus, it is difficult to be certain as to whether low mouth pressure measurements accurately represent reduced strength, or merely reflect reduced neural activation.

Maximal static inspiratory and expiratory pressure

Measuring the maximum static inspiratory pressure that a subject can generate at the mouth (PImax) or the maximum static expiratory pressure (PEmax) is helpful in assessing inspiratory and expiratory muscle strength. These pressures reflect the sum of the pressure developed by the respiratory muscles (Pmus), and the passive elastic recoil pressure of the respiratory system including the lung and chest wall (Prs) [22]. As these tests are volitional, a low result may not necessarily indicate reduced inspiratory or expiratory muscle strength. Measurement of maximum static transdiaphragmatic pressure (PIdimax), provides specific information regarding maximal diaphragm strength. However, these tests require passage of balloon catheters and the necessary coordination is difficult for patients [23,24]. These test are used only as a research tools and are carried out in laboratories with specialized expertise.

Sniff Test

A sniff is a short, sharp voluntary inspiratory manoeuvre performed by occluding one or both nostrils. It results in contraction of the diaphragm and other inspiratory muscles. It has been observed that [25] showed that normal subjects generated greater transdiaphragmatic pressure (Pdi) during maximal sniffs than during maximal static inspiratory efforts. The sniff manoeuvre is a useful part of the clinical evaluation of respiratory muscle strength and observations correlates well with response to therapy [27].

Sniffing is a voluntary procedure that requires patient co-operation, and is difficult to perform if there is upper airway distortion especially if the nose is completely obstructed. In clinical practice Pdi,sn,max values greater than 100 cmH2O in males and 80 cm H2O in females are unlikely to be associated with clinically significant diaphragm weakness [23].

Cough tests

Patients with reduced cough pressure are prone to develop chest infections [28,29] and, therefore, this is of clinical importance. In patients in whom measurement of mouth pressure during a static maximal expiratory manoeuvre (PEmax) is technically difficult, measurement of maximal cough gastric pressures is considered to be an alternative [28,29].

Non-volitional tests of respiratory muscle strength

The diaphragm is innervated exclusively by the phrenic nerve. Therefore, phrenic nerve stimulation is useful to investigate the diaphragm independent of other inspiratory muscles. Non-volitional testing of respiratory muscle strength is done by measuring pressures obtained by phrenic nerve stimulation. Four methods phrenic nerve stimulation have been used, especially in healthy volunteers. Two of these methods, needle stimulation [30,31], implanted wire stimulation [32], are invasive methods and are associated with the risk of haematoma and phrenic nerve damage. Currently needle stimulation methods are not recommended. Two other methods, namely, transcutaneous electrical and magnetic phrenic nerve stimulation have been more extensively researched.

Transcutaneous electrical phrenic nerve stimulation

When an electrical field is externally applied, it induces depolarization of phrenic nerve fibers, at mid-distance between the electrode and the cathode. Electrical phrenic nerve stimulation generates a "pure" diaphragmatic contraction. ES can achieve selective supramaximal stimulation of the diaphragm, but requires considerable skill and may be difficult to achieve in an intensive care unit (ICU) setting.

Magnetic phrenic nerve stimulation

Magnetic phrenic nerve stimulation is technically easier to perform and less inconvenience to patients. Cervical magnetic stimulation (CMS) elicits a bilateral diaphragm contraction [33]. However, CMS is less specific than ES, as it activates muscles innervated by the brachial plexus [34-36]. With CMS, achieving and ascertaining supramaximal nerve stimulation can be technically difficult. Sometimes, recording the diaphragm electromyogram can be problematic.. Unilateral anterior-lateral magnetic phrenic nerve stimulation is more specific than CMS, and results are similar to ES. This technique facilitates evaluation of hemidiaphragm function [37, 38].

Twitch transdiaphragmatic pressure

Twitch transdiaphragmatic pressure (Pdi,tw) provides an assessment of diaphragm, or hemidiaphragm, strength. and is a research technique useful to assess the degree of activation of the diaphragm during voluntary efforts (the technique of twitch occlusion) [24].

Clinical uses

With phrenic nerve stimulation, diaphragmatic weakness can be ascertained and quantified, particularly when voluntary manoeuvres have yielded equivocal results. This technique also facilitates pre-operative assessment of patients for possible phrenic pacing [39] after high cervical cord lesions.

Abdominal Muscle Stimulation

Recording of twitch gastric pressure by application of magnetic stimulation over the eighth to tenth thoracic vertebrae posteriorly constitutes a clinically applicable nonvolitional test for assessment of abdominal muscle strength and fatigue [40,41].

Electrophysiologic techniques for the assessment of respiratory muscle function

Electrophysiological methods help in assessing the integrity of the respiratory neuromotor apparatus. There are two common methods of electrophysiologic tests of respiratory muscle function, namely, electromyography (EMG) and stimulation tests.

Electromyography

For assessing respiratory muscle strength, EMG is useful to assess the level and pattern of activation. EMG also helps in detecting and ascertaining neuromuscular pathology. EMG when combined with tests of mechanical function is helpful in assessing the efficacy of contraction. The EMG recording from diaphragm, intercostal, scalene, abdominal, and accessory muscles can be obtained using surface electrodes; oesophageal electrode is used for assessing crural diaphragm.

The surface electrodes have the advantage of being non-invasive and are able to sample a large number of motor units. However, cross-talk from other muscles results in contamination of the signal and is a substantial problem [42-44]. While the oesophageal electrodes offer the advantage of providing more pecific information [45], this method has the disadvantage of being invasive.. EMG frequency domain analysis has been used, as a research tool, to evaluate respiratory muscle fatigue.

In another invasive method intramuscular electrodes are used to selectively record from the diaphragm and intercostal muscles [46]. This method facilitates measurement of motor neuron firing frequency and diagnosis of neuromuscular disorders.

Stimulation tests

The efficiency of neural and neuromuscular transmission can be assessed by stimulation tests. Nerve stimulation can be done with electrical or magnetic stimulators. While electrical stimulation is inexpensive and relatively selective, it is uncomfortable to the patient and is technically difficult. Though magnetic stimulation is technically easier, and is better tolerated by the patient, it is less selective and expensive. The phrenic nerves are stimulated and the diaphragm EMG is recorded for the measuring latencies and compound muscle action potential (CMAP) amplitudes. In demyelination, latencies are prolonged and CMAP amplitude is reduced in traumatic damage to the phrenic nerves.

Cortical stimulation is usually performed with a magnetic stimulator and facilitates the measurement of central conduction times (CCT) for limb muscles and diaphragm [47,48]. CCT is prolonged in multiple sclerosis. However, this technique is not selective, and the application of cortical stimulation to the respiratory system requires specialized skill.

Tests of respiratory muscle endurance

The ability to sustain a specific muscular task over a period of time is termed muscle endurance. Various techniques that have been developed to measure endurance of the respiratory muscles differ largely on the type of task that is being performed.

Pressure-time product

The integration of inspiratory pressure swing over time. Pressure can be oesophageal, Pdi, or mouth pressure (if an external resistance is added to the circuit). Pressure-time product (PTP) is the integration of respiratory pressure over time [1]. Pressure time index (PTI) is the pressure-generating activity of the muscles, independent of a specific breathing rhythm, frequency, or type of load within the limits tested [49]. For example, most normal subjects can sustain a PTI for the chest wall and the synergic inspiratory muscles of up to approximately 0.3 [50].

Work rate of the respiratory system

The ventilatory work rate of the respiratory system (rs) refers to mechanical work performed by the respiratory muscles against the lungs and chest wall during ventilation and is an important determinant of both energy consumption of the muscles and endurance time [51].

Ventilatory endurance tests

Ventilatory endurance testing aims at defining the maximum sustainable ventilation (MSV). Two methods techniques are available to determine MSV, namely, the maximum effort method and the maximum incremental method [52-55]. Standardized normal values of MSV are not available and normal data are defined by each laboratory where the testing is carried out. These tests have been used as research tools.

Endurance of external loads

The most commonly used technique of assessing endurance of external loads is that of threshold loading where the maximum sustainable [56] or the maximum incremental threshold load can be measured. Of these, the incremental threshold loading test [57,58], which uses the same principles as an incremental exercise test, is frequently used. and is helpful to specifically assess the endurance of the inspiratory muscles, relatively independently of lung and chest wall mechanisms.

Repeated maximum inspiratory pressures

In repeated maximum inspiratory pressures testing, the subjects undertake 18 repeated PI,max manoeuvres, each effort lasting 10 seconds with a 5-second period of rest between contractions [59]. Pressure drops to 87% of PI,max in young normal subjects over the period of testing [60].

Maximal sustainable isoflow

Maximal sustainable isoflow is a a method of training the inspiratory muscles as well as documenting their endurance. The subject breathes against a high impedence (air tank) providing a constant flow (1 L/sec) [61,62]. Maximal pressure develops at a duty cycle (TI/Ttot) of 0.40 and declines exponentially to a sustainable level, yielding a PTI of 0.18.

Endurance of the diaphragm

The normal sustainable PTI for the diaphragm (PTIdi) has been documented to be in the range 0.15-0.18 when tidal volume remained at 0.75 L [49,63]. At a duty cycle (TI/Ttot) of approximately 0.4, most normal subjects can sustain approximately 40%-50% of Pdi,max.

ASSESSMENT OF RESPIRATORY MUSCLE FATIGUE

Breathing pattern: tidal volume and breathing frequency

Rapid shallow breathing (high breathing frequency and low tidal volume), develops in progressive respiratory failure or during unsuccessful attempts at weaning from mechanical ventilation and potentially leads to respiratory muscle fatigue. Eventhough, not specific, monitoring breathing frequency and tidal volume is helpful to monitor the development of respiratory muscle fatigue. Further, rapid shallow breathing may be a reflex response to an increase in the respiratory workload [64] rather than the consequence of respiratory muscle fatigue [65].

Thoracoabdominal Motion

Two unusual patterns of muscle recruitment are evident in healthy subjects when subjected to fatiguing inspiratory loads [66]. In the first pattern an increased variability in compartmental contribution to tidal volume is seen, with breaths characterized by rib cage predominance alternating with other breaths where abdominal motion is prominent. In the second pattern, paradoxical movement of one compartment (usually the abdomen) is evident. Abdominal paradoxical movement indicates weak, inefficient or absent contraction of the diaphragm. Occurrence of these patterns in patients during weaning trials from mechanical ventilation indicate diaphragmatic fatigue[67].

Pressure-time index of inspiratory muscles

Pressure-time index of the diaphragm (PTdi) [68] and rib cage muscles (PTrc) [69] other than the diaphragm allow the assessment of the risk of fatigue [70,71].

Volitional maximal pressures

Respiratory muscle fatigue can, be documented by assessing a decrease in volitional maximal respiratory pressures and demonstration of recovery with rest.

Relaxation rate

The relaxation rate of Pes or Pdi can be measured during intermittent contractions against loads [72], during sniffs with [73] or without airway occlusion [74], and during phrenic nerve stimulation [73]. The most useful and simple manoeuvre is the unoccluded sniff, which is easy to perform for most subjects and provides consistent changes in relaxation rate after fatigue [75,76]. Inspiratory muscle relaxation rate has been used as a research tool to detect fatiguing contractions during exercise in patients with COPD [77] or during weaning from mechanical ventilation [78].

Time domain analysis

The time domain EMG assessment provides a means of checking whether observed reductions in respiratory muscle pressure-generating capacity are the result of alterations in action potential transmission or due to intrinsic alterations in peripheral muscle function [79].

Frequency domain analysis

Frequency domain analysis is helpful in demonstrating an EMG spectral power shift in a working muscle [80] and may be helpful in detecting the development of alterations in neuromuscular transmission.

Assessment of chest wall function

Measurement of lung volume displacement, chest wall motion, and pressures are useful in assessing chest wall function..

Assessment of the passive properties of the chest wall

Passive characteristics of chest wall, such as, the relationship between the passive relaxation pressure at the closed mouth and lung volume (Rahn diagram) and has been used as a research tool.

Assessment of the active chest wall

Plotting lung volume against pleural pressure (Campbell diagram) permits calculation of both elastic and resistive respiratory muscle work. The measurement of respiratory work and oxygen consumption facilitates the calculation of muscle efficiency.

Estimation of ventilation by chest wall motion

Plotting rib cage and abdomen diameters (magnetometers) or perimeters (respiratory inductive plethysmograph) (Konno-Mead diagram) allows measurement of tidal volume without the need of a mouthpiece [1].

Inferring respiratory action from oesophageal and gastric pressures

Plotting oesophageal against gastric pressure (Macklem diagram) allows categorization whether breaths are achieved by rib cage muscles or diaphragm [1].

Assessing activation and electromechanical effectiveness of the diaphragm from EMG

Assessing activation and electromechanical effectiveness of the diaphragm from EMG has also been used to assess chest wall function [1].

Imaging respiratory muscle function

Several radiographic techniques are used to assess respiratory muscle function (Table 1). Ultrasonography is frequently being used to assess the diaphragm (Table 2). Volumetric computed tomography (CT) [81-85] and magnetic resonance imaging (MRI) [86-88] are helpful in determining the shape of diaphragm and configuration of the thoracic cavity [81,82,84-86,89-91].

Table 1: Radiographic techniques are used to assess respiratory muscle function

Radiographic technique	Information provided	Diagnostic use
Standard postero-anterior lateralchest radiograph at TLC	Position of diaphragm domes at TLC	Unilateral/bilateral and diaphragmaticparalysis, emphysema
Fluoroscopy during tidal breathing and sniffs	Movement of right and left domes: paradoxic motion exaggerated by brisk contraction of normal dome of diaphragmduring sniffs	Unilateral or bilateral diaphragm paralysis
Obtaining set of radiographs at different lung inflation between RV and TLC	Relationship between diaphragm length and function	Emphysema pre- and post-lung volume reduction surgery

TLC = total lung capacity; RV = residual volume

Adapted from reference 1

Table 2: Uses of ultrasonography in the assessment of function of diaphragm and other function

Ultrasonography method	Information provided	Diagnostic use
Diaphragm Dome ultrasound (M-mode) Ultrasound probes with adequate penetration (3 or 3.5 MHz) are placed over abdomen or over lateral rib cage	Movement of domes of diaphragm	Unilateral or bilateral diaphragmatic paralysis
Zone of apposition ultrasound* High-resolution probe with less penetration (7.5 MHz) are placed over intercostal space, usually in anterior axillary line (B- or M-mode)	Thickness at different lung volumes Detects contraction during tidal breathing or inspiratory efforts	Effects of pulmonary or neuromuscular disease, training and disuse
Linear probe in craniocaudal plane over lateral rib cage (B-mode)	Length at different lung volumes	Estimates of diaphragm length and swept volume
Other respiratory muscles Ultrasonography of neck, rib cage and abdominal muscles (B-mode)	Thickening during respiratory manoeuvres	Contraction during tidal breathing or inspiratory efforts
High-resolution probe (7.5 MHz) is placed over appropriate muscles intramuscular electrodes	Distance from overlying skin	Placement of intramuscular Electrodes

* both measurements are usually made on the right side

Adapted from reference 1

Single-photon emission computed tomography (SPECT) and positron emission tomography (PET) are being evaluated regarding their potential usefulness in assessing respiratory muscle function.

Tests for upper airway function

The skeletal muscles surrounding the upper airway exhibit respiratory-related activity [92-95] which is distinctly different from those of the respiratory pump muscles. Numerous techniques have been developed to assess respiratory related upper airway structure and function, ranging from measurements of upper airway resistance to MRI. However, these tests are not used in routine clinical practice and are used for research purposes.

Laryngeal narrowing can result from laryngospasm or vocal cord paralysis, among others. Indirect laryngoscopy, fiberoptic imaging, EMG, flow-volume loops are helpful in detecting upper airway narrowing. In patients with obstructive sleep apnea (OSA), upper airway narrowing occurs in the pharynx and is characterized by the suppression of upper airway muscle activity during sleep. Polysomnography, though not considered to be a specific test of upper airway function, is helpful to diagnose the repetitive closure of the pharyngeal airway during sleep.

REFERENCES

1. American Thoracic Society/European Respiratory Society. ATS/ERS Statement on respiratory muscle testing. Am J Respir Crit Care Med 2002;166:518-624.
2. Gibson GJ, Pride NB, Newsom Davis J, Loh C. Pulmonary mechanics in patients with respiratory muscle weakness. Am Rev Respir Dis 1977; 115:389-95.
3. Estenne M, Heilporn A, Delhez L, Yernault J-C, De Troyer A. Chest wall stiffness in patients with chronic respiratory muscle weakness. Am Rev Respir Dis 1983;128:1002-7..
4. Fallat RJ, Jewitt B, Bass M, Kamm B, Norris FH. Spirometry in amyotrophic lateral sclerosis. Arch Neurol 1979;36:74-80.
5. Phillips M, Smith PEM, Carroll N, Edwards RHT, Calverley PMA. Does nocturnal oxygen desaturation predict survival in childhood onset muscular dystrophy? Thorax 1997;52:A18.
6. Black LF, Hyatt RE. Maximal static respiratory pressures in generalized neuromuscular disease. Am Rev Respir Dis 1971;103:641-50.
7. Wesseling G, Quaedvlieg FCM, Wouters EFM. Oscillatory mechanics of the respiratory system in neuromuscular disease. Chest 1992;102:1752-7.
8. De Troyer A, Borenstein S, Cordier R. Analysis of lung volume restriction in patients with respiratory muscle weakness. Thorax 1980;35:603-10.
9. Vincken WG, Cosio MG. Flow oscillations on the flow-volume loop: clinical and physiological implications. Eur Respir J 1989;2:543-9.
10. Serisier DE, Mastaglia FL, Gibson GJ. Respiratory muscle function and ventilatory control. I. In patients with motor neurone disease; II. In patients with myotonic dystrophy. Q J Med 1982;51:205-26.

11. Braun NMT, Arora NS, Rochester DF. Respiratory muscle and pulmonary function in polymyositis and other proximal myopathies. Thorax 1983;38:616-23.

12. Tzelepis GE, McCool FD, Friedman JH, Hoppin FG. Respiratory muscle dysfunction in Parkinson's disease. Am Rev Respir Dis 1988;138:266-71.

13. Bye PTP, Ellis ER, Issa FG, Donnelly PM, Sullivan CE. Respiratory failure and sleep in neuromuscular disease. Thorax 1990;45:241-7.

14. White JES, Drinnan MJ, Smithson AJ, Griffiths CJ, Gibson GJ. Respiratory muscle activity and oxygenation during sleep in patients with muscle weakness. Eur Respir J 1995;8:807-14.

15. Smith PEM, Calverley PMA, Edwards RHT. Hypoxaemia during sleep in Duchenne muscular dystrophy. Am Rev Respir Dis 1988;137:884-8.

16. Gay PC, Westbrook PR, Daube JR, Litchy WJ, Windebank AJ, Iverson R. Effects of alterations in pulmonary function and sleep variables on survival in patients with amyotrophic lateral sclerosis. Mayo Clin Proc 1991;66:686-94.

17. Carroll JE, Hagberg JM, Brooks MH, Shumate JB. Bicycle ergometry and gas exchange measurements in neuromuscular disease. Arch Neurol 1979;36:457-61.

18. Gandevia SC, McKenzie DK. Activation of the human diaphragm during maximal static efforts. J Physiol 1985;367:45-56.

19. Bigland-Ritchie BR, Furbush FH, Gandevia SC, Thomas CK. Voluntary discharge frequencies of human motor neurones at different muscle lengths. Muscle Nerve 1992;15:130-7.

20. Allen GM, Gandevia SC, McKenzie DK. Reliability of measurements of muscle strength and voluntary activation using twitch interpolation. Muscle Nerve 1995;18:593-600.

21. De Troyer A, Legrand A, Gevenois P-A, Wilson TA. Mechanical advantage of the human parasternal intercostal and triangularis sterni muscles. J Physiol 1998;513:915-25.

22. Agostoni E, Mead J. Statics of the respiratory system. In: Fenn WO and Rahn H, editors. Handbook of physiology: respiration, Vol. 1, Section 3. Washington DC: American Physiology Society; 1964. p.387-409.

23. Mier-Jedrzejowicz A, Brophy C, Moxham J, Green M. Assessment of diaphragm weakness. Am Rev Respir Dis 1988;137:877-83

24. Bellemare F, Bigland-Ritchie B. Assessment of human diaphragm strength and activation using phrenic nerve stimulation. Respir Physiol 1984;58:263-77.

25. Miller JM, Moxham J, Green M. The maximal sniff in the assessment of diaphragm function in man. Clin Sci 1985;69:91-6.

26. Laroche CM, Mier AK, Moxham J, Green M. The value of sniff esophageal pressures in the assessment of global inspiratory muscle strength. Am Rev Respir Dis 1988;138:598-603.

27. Polkey MI, Green M, Moxham J. Measurement of respiratory muscle strength. Thorax 1995;50:1131-5.

28. Loring SH, Yoshino K, Kimball WR, Barnas GM. Gravitational and shear-associated pressure gradients in the abdomen. J Appl Physiol 1994;77:1375-82.

29. Yernault J. Lung mechanics. I. Lung elasticity. *In*: Quanjer PH, ed. Standardized lung function testing, Chapter 4. Bull Eur Physiopathol Respir 1983;19(Suppl 5):28-32.

30. Aubier M, Farkas G, De Troyer A, Mozes R, Roussos C. Detection of diaphragmatic fatigue in man by phrenic stimulation. J Appl Physiol 1981;50:538-44.

31. Mier A, Brophy C. Measurement of twitch transdiaphragmatic pressure: surface versus needle electrode stimulation. Thorax 1991;46:669-70.

32. Hubmayr RD, Litchy WJ, Gay PC, Nelson SB. Transdiaphragmatic twitch pressure: effects of lung volume and chest wall shape. Am Rev Respir Dis 1989;139:647-52.

33. Similowski T, Fleury B, Launois S, Cathala HP, Bouche P, Derenne JP. Cervical magnetic stimulation: a new painless method for bilateral phrenic nerve stimulation in conscious humans. J Appl Physiol 1989; 67:1311-8.

34. Wragg S, Aquilina R, Moran J, Ridding M, Hamnegard C, Fearn T, Green M, Moxham J. Comparison of cervical magnetic stimulation and bilateral percutaneous electrical stimulation of the phrenic nerves in normal subjects. Eur Respir J 1994;7:1788-92.

35. Laghi F, Harrison MJ, Tobin MJ. Comparison of magnetic and electrical phrenic nerve stimulation in assessment of diaphragmatic contractility. J Appl Physiol 1996;80:1731-42.

36. Similowski T, Duguet A, Straus C, Boisteanu D, Attali V, Derenne J-P. Assessment of the voluntary activation of the diaphragm in man using cervical and cortical magnetic stimulation. Eur Respir J 1996;9:1224-31.

37. Mills GH, Kyroussis D, Hamnegard CH, Wragg S, Moxham J, Green M. Unilateral magnetic stimulation of the phrenic nerve. Thorax 1995;50:1162-72.

38. Bellemare F, Bigland-Ritchie B, Woods JJ. Contractile properties of the human diaphragm in vivo. J Appl Physiol 1986;61:1153-61.

39. Similowski T, Straus C, Attali V, Duguet A, Jourdain B, Derenne J-P. Assessment of the motor pathway to the diaphragm using cortical and cervical magnetic stimulation in the decision making process of phrenic pacing. Chest 1996;110:1551-7.

40. Kyroussis D, Polkey MI, Mills GH, Hughes PD, Moxham J, Green M. Stimulation of cough in man by magnetic stimulation of the thoracic nerve roots. Am J Respir Crit Care Med 1997;156:1696-9.

41. Kyroussis D, Mills GH, Polkey MI, Hamnegaard C-H, Koulouris N, Green M, Moxham J. Abdominal muscle fatigue after maximal ventilation in humans. J Appl Physiol 1996;81:1477-83.

42. De Troyer A, Peche R, Yernault JC, Estenne M. Neck muscle activity in patients with severe chronic obstructive pulmonary disease. Am J Respir Crit Care Med 1994;150:41-7.

43. De Troyer A, Estenne M, Ninane V, Van Gansbeke D, Gorini M. Transversus abdominis muscle function in humans. J Appl Physiol 1990;68: 1010-6.

44. De Troyer A, Farkas GA. Linkage between parasternals and external intercostals during resting breathing. J Appl Physiol 1990;69:509-16.

45. McKenzie DK, Gandevia SC. Phrenic nerve conduction times and twitch pressures of the human diaphragm. J Appl Physiol 1985;58:1496-1504.

46. Estenne M, Ninane V, De Troyer A. Triangularis sterni muscle use during eupnea in humans: effect of posture. Respir Physiol 1988;74:151-62.

47. Barker AT, Jalinous R, Freeston IL. Noninvasive stimulation of the human motor cortex. Lancet 1985;1:1106-7.

48. Gandevia SC, Rothwell JC. Activation of the human diaphragm from the motor cortex. J Physiol 1987;384:109-18.

49. Bellemare F, Grassino A. Effect of pressure and timing of contraction on human diaphragm fatigue. J Appl Physiol 1982;53:1190-5.

50. Zocchi L, Fitting JW, Majani U, Fracchia C, Rampulla C, Grassino A. Effect of pressure and timing of contraction on human rib cage muscle fatigue. Am Rev Respir Dis 1993;147:857-64.

51. Collett PW, Perry C, Engel LA. Pressure–time product, flow, and oxygen cost of resistive breathing in humans. J Appl Physiol 1985;58:1263-72.

52. Keens TG, Krastins IRB, Wannamaker EM, Levison H, Crozier DN, Bryan AC. Ventilatory muscle endurance training in normal subjects and patients with cystic fibrosis. Am Rev Respir Dis 1977;116:853-60.

53. Belman MJ, Mittman C. Ventilatory muscle training improves exercise capacity in chronic obstructive pulmonary disease patients. Am Rev Respir Dis 1980;121:273-80.

54. Mancini DM, Henson D, LaManca J, Levine S. Evidence of reduced respiratory muscle endurance in patients with heart failure. J Am Coll Cardiol 1994;24:972-81.

55. Mancini DM, Henson D, La Manca J, Donchez L, Levine S. Benefit of selective respiratory muscle training on exercise capacity in patients with chronic congestive heart failure. Circulation 1995;91:320-9.

56. Nickerson BG, Keens TG. Measuring ventilatory muscle endurance in humans as sustainable inspiratory pressure. J Appl Physiol 1982;52: 768-72.

57. Martyn JB, Moreno RH, Pare PD, Pardy RL. Measurement of inspiratory muscle performance with incremental threshold loading. Am Rev Respir Dis 1987;135:919-23.

58. McElvaney G, Fairbarn MS, Wilcox PG, Pardy RL. Comparison of two minute incremental threshold loading and maximal loading as measures of respiratory muscle endurance. Am Rev Respir Dis 1989;96:557-63.

59. McKenzie DK, Gandevia SC. Influence of muscle length on human inspiratory and limb muscle endurance. Respir Physiol 1987;67:171-82.

60. McKenzie DK, Gandevia SC. Strength and endurance of inspiratory, expiratory and limb muscles in asthma. Am Rev Respir Dis 1986;134:999-1004.

61. Bellemare F, Wight D, Lavigne CM, Grassino A. Effect of tension and timing of contraction on blood flow of the diaphragm. J Appl Physiol 1986;54:1597-606.

62. Clanton TL, Ameredes BT. Fatigue of the inspiratory muscle pump in humans: an isoflow approach. J Appl Physiol 1988;64:1693-9.

63. Field S, Sanci S, Grassino A. Respiratory muscle oxygen consumption estimated by the diaphragm pressure–time index. J Appl Physiol 1984;57:44-51.

64. Tobin MJ, Perez W, Guenther SM, Semmes BJ, Mador MJ, Allen SJ, Lodato RF, Dantzker DR. The pattern of breathing during successful and unsuccessful trials of weaning from mechanical ventilation. Am Rev Respir Dis 1986;134:1111-8.

65. Mador MJ, Tobin MJ. The effect of inspiratory muscle fatigue on breathing pattern and ventilatory response to CO2. J Physiol (Lond) 1992;455:17-32.

66. Roussos C, Fixley M, Gross D, Macklem PT. Fatigue of inspiratory muscles and their synergic behavior. J Appl Physiol 1979;46:897-904.

67. Respiratory Muscle Fatigue Workshop Group. Respiratory muscle fatigue: NHLBI Workshop Summary. Am Rev Respir Dis 1990;142:474-80.

68. Bellemare F, Grassino A. Effect of pressure and timing of contraction on human diaphragm fatigue. J Appl Physiol 1982;53:1190-5.

69. Zocchi L, Fitting JW, Majani U, Fracchia C, Rampulla C, Grassino A. Effect of pressure and timing of contraction on human rib cage muscle fatigue. Am Rev Respir Dis 1993;147:857-64.

70. Bellemare F, Grassino A. Force reserve of the diaphragm in COPD patients. Appl Physiol 1983;55:8-15.

71. Vassilakopoulos T, Zakynthinos S, Roussos C. The tension–time index and frequency–tidal volume ratio are the major pathophysiologic determinants of weaning failure and success. Am J Respir Crit Care Med 1988;158:378-5.

72. Esau SA, Bellemare F, Grassino A, Permutt S, Roussos C, Pardy RL. Changes in relaxation rate with diaphragmatic fatigue in humans. J Appl Physiol 1983;54:1353-60.

73. Esau SA, Bye PTP, Pardy RL. Changes in rate of relaxation of sniffs with diaphragmatic fatigue in humans. J Appl Physiol 1983;55:731-5.

74. Koulouris N, Vianna LG, Mulvey DA, Green M, Moxham J. Maximal relaxation rates of esophageal, nose, and mouth pressures during a sniff reflect inspiratory muscle fatigue. Am Rev Respir Dis 1989;193: 1213-7.

75. Mador MJ, Kufel TJ. Effect of inspiratory muscle fatigue on inspiratory muscle relaxation rates in healthy subjects. Chest 1992;102:1767-73.

76. Kyroussis D, Mills G, Hamnegard CH, Wragg S, Road J, Green M, Moxham J. Inspiratory muscle relaxation rate assessed from sniff nasal pressure. Thorax 1994;49:1127-33.

77. Kyroussis D, Polkey MI, Keilty SEJ, Mills GH, Hamnegard CH, Moxham J, Green M. Exhaustive exercise slows inspiratory muscle relaxation rate in chronic obstructive pulmonary disease. Am J Respir Crit Care Med 1996;153:787-93.

78. Goldstone JC, Green M, Moxham J. Maximum relaxation rate of the diaphragm during weaning from mechanical ventilation. Thorax 1994;49:54-60.

79. Stephens JA, Taylor A. Fatigue of maintained voluntary maximal contraction in man. J Physiol (Lond) 1972;220:1-18.

80. Moxham J, Edwards RHT, Aubier M, De Troyer A, Farkas G, Macklem PT, Roussos C. Changes in EMG power spectrum (high/low ratio) with force fatigue in man. J Appl Physiol 1982;53: 1094-9.

81. Pettiaux N, Cassart M, Paiva M, Estenne M. Three dimensional reconstruction of human diaphragm with the use of spiral computed tomography. J Appl Physiol 1997;82:998-1002.

82. Cassart M, Pettiaux N, Gevenois PA, Paiva M, Estenne M. Effect of chronic hyperinflation on diaphragm length and surface area. Am J Respir Crit Care Med 1997;156:504-8.

83. Margulies SS, Lei GT, Farkas GA, Rodarte JR. Finite-element analysis of stress in the canine diaphragm. J Appl Physiol 1994;76:2070-5.

84. Krayer S, Rehder K, Vettermann J, Didier EP, Ritman EL. Position and motion of the human diaphragm during anesthesia-paralysis. Anesthesiology 1989;70:891-8.

85. Whitelaw WA. Shape and size of the human diaphragm in vivo. J Appl Physiol 1987;62:180-6.

86. Gauthier AP, Verbanck S, Estenne M, Segebarth C, Macklem PT, Paiva M. Three-dimensional reconstruction of the in vivo human diaphragm shape at different lung volumes. J Appl Physiol 1994;76:495-506

87. Gierada DS, Curtin JJ, Erickson SJ, Prost RW, Strandt JA, Goodman LR. Diaphragmatic motion: fast gradient-recalled-echo MR imaging in healthy subjects. Radiology 1995;194:879-84.

88. Kanematsu M, Imaeda T, Mochizuki R, Yamawaki Y, Goto H, Sone Y, Doi H. Dynamic MRI of the diaphragm. J Comput Assist Tomogr 1995;19:67-72.

89. Cassart M, Gevenois PA, Estenne M. Rib cage dimensions in hyperinflated patients with severe chronic obstructive pulmonary disease. Am J Respir Crit Care Med 1996;154:800-5.

90. Cassart M, Verbandt Y, de Francquen P, Gevenois PA, Estenne M. Diaphragm dimensions after single-lung transplantation for emphysema. Am J Respir Crit Care Med 1999;159:1992-7.

91. Cassart M, Hamacher J, Verbandt Y, Wildermuth S, Ritscher D, Russi EW, de Francquen P, Cappello M, Weder W, Estenne M. Effect of lung volume reduction surgery for emphysema on diaphragm dimensions and configuration. Am J Respir Crit Care Med 2001;163:1171-5.

92. Van Lunteren E, Strohl KP. The muscles of the upper airways. Clin Chest Med 1986;7:171-88.

93. Bartlett D Jr. Respiratory functions of the larynx. Physiol Rev 1989; 69:33-57.

94. Bartlett D Jr. Upper airway motor systems. *In*: Fishman AP, Cherniack NS, Widdicombe JG, Geiger SR, editors. Handbook of physiology: the respiratory system, Section 3, Vol. II. Bethesda, MD: American Physiological Society; 1986.p.223-45.

95. Mathew OP, Sant-Ambrogio G, editors. Respiratory function of the upper airway. *In:* Lenfant C, ed. Lung biology in health and disease, Vol. 35. New York: Marcel Dekker; 1988.

18
EXERCISE TESTING

DHIMAN GANGULY

Introduction

Dyspnea on exertion is a common presenting symptom to a practicing physician – and one that raises the possibilities of a cardiac, respiratory, impaired exercise capacity (deconditioning), or a combination of any two, or all three of these in a given instance. Utility of Cardiopulmonary Exercise Testing (CPET) lies in its sensitivity to differentiate between multiple coexistent disease states as the cause of exercise limitation (1).

Exercise performance

To be able to rationally approach this problem, we need to have some idea of the basic science of exercise performance. Exercise is a remarkable example of integrative and adaptive capacities of the body. Diseases may impose limitations on the capacity of body to acquire, transport and utilize oxygen. Performance of exercise (daily living, manual labor, recreations, sports) involve both mechanical power (muscle strength) and metabolic power. The first one (external power) is the actual biomechanical performance (running, jumping, throwing) that is visible, and the second one is the internal power generated in the muscle cells by aerobic and anaerobic mechanisms(2) that produce high energy phosphate compound adenosine triphosphate (ATP). For continued muscle cell activity ATP must be resynthesized, as the concentration of ATP molecules at a given point of time is too low to sustain muscle activity beyond a few seconds. In the context of clinical exercise testing we will leave out the mechanical part and concentrate on the metabolic part that would enable us to understand and interpret exercise testing(3).

Definition

Definition of certain terms, that we use frequently to discuss exercise physiology and testing are shown in table 1.

Table 1. Basic Definition

Exercise	**Any or all physical activity, resulting from forces generated by active skeletal muscles**
Power	**Mechanical – rate at which work is performed** **Metabolic - rate at which energy is released in muscles**
Newton (N)	**Force that accelerates 1 kg by 1 m/sec^2 (100,000 dynes)**
Work	**Force x Distance, Joule (J) work performed when a force of 1 N (Newton) acts through 1 m**
Watt	**Unit of measurement of power (work per unit of time) Work of 1 J per second Haemodynamic factors**

For effective resynthesis of ATP, there are three prerequisites, oxygen for aerobic metabolism, fuel to oxidize (fat and carbohydrate, the higher the intensify of exercise higher is the relative contribution of carbohydrate) and adequate level of the enzyme system in the mitochondria to run the oxidative process(4).

In normal individuals, maximum exercise is limited by haemodynamic factor, particularly the level to which the cardiac output can be elevated and the ability of the muscles to generate sufficient metabolic energy. No limitations are imposed by either ventilator capacity or pulmonary gas exchange.

Low level exercise results in an increase in cardiac output, widening of arterial mixed venous oxygen difference and a rise in O_2 consumption and CO_2 output. The minute ventilation increases to keep the alveolar ventilation at a level that will remove the extra CO_2 produced, consequently, the $PaCO_2$ remains normal. The alveolar – arterial O_2 tension gradient $P(A\text{-}a)O_2$ may decrease slightly, because of improvement in ventilation-perfusion relationship.

As the intensity of exercise is increased, the aerobic metabolism (as assessed by oxygen uptake VO_2) becomes greater and reaches maximal aerobic power (VO_2 max). When a certain high level of aerobic metabolism is attained (usually for non athletic subject at 50-60% of predicted VO_2 max) anaerobic glycolysis begins to make a contribution. This form of glycolysis has two disadvantages. Firstly, it is less cost effective metabolically. There is a net gain of 36 molecules of ATP by oxidation of 1 molecule of 6-carbon sugar by aerobic glycolysis, whereas anaerobically the same sugar produces only 2 molecules of ATP, and secondly, blood lactate concentration increases in a progressively steeper rate(5). Lactic acid is buffered by bicarbonate to produce CO_2 in excess of that produced by aerobic metabolism making CO_2 production (VCO_2) versus Vo_2 relationship steeper. This has been labelled as "anaerobic threshold" (AT- also known as lactate threshold, gas exchange threshold or ventilatory threshold)(5), and is an index of aerobic fitness and cardiac function. At this juncture ventilation increases inordinately, accompanied by reduction in blood pH and bicarbonate (metabolic acidosis).

Incremental exercise

Ventilatory anaerobic threshold (VAT) can be determined by analyzing the slope of VCO_2 versus VO_2 (plotted on equal scales) relationship, where VAT is the point of transition of VCO_2 versus VO_2 slope from less than one (aerobic metabolism alone) to greater than one (anaerobic plus aerobic metabolism). In response to this non-oxidative CO_2 production, minute ventilation (VE) rises disproportionately to the VO_2- a signal showing that the anaerobic threshold (AT) has been reached(6). AT is referenced to VO_2 at which this change occurs and its expressed as a percentage of predicted value VO_2 max. At higher exercise level the pH falls sufficiently to drive VE out of proportion to CO_2 production causing a fall in $PaCO_2$.

It is now known that well a trained athlete can raise his minute ventilation from around 6L/minute at rest to about 180L/minute at maximum exercise. Similarly, the cardiac output in such an individual can be raised from 5L/minute at rest to about 36L/minute at peak exercise.

Exercise being a stress on cardiovascular and respiratory system, measurement of physiological parameters in resting state may not be useful. Incremental exercise gives us an insight into the precise mechanism explaining the problem of dyspnea on exertion. There are broadly speaking, four possible reasons to undertake an exercise testing:

a) To quantitate the degree of functional impairment
b) To indicate the limiting factor for exercise in the individual – pulmonary/cardiac/poor conditioning / poor effort
c) To monitor response to therapy

d) To provide a basis for development of rational reconditioning programmes.

The oxygen required to perform various tasks is shown in Table 2(7). It is important to realize that propulsion of a wheel chair takes much less oxygen that walking at 2.5 mph, therefore, more people with severe exercise limitations might benefit from this device.

Table - 2. Oxygen requirements for average-sized adults during various activities

Activity	Consumption (ml/min)
Rest, supine	200
Sitting	240
Standing relaxed	280
Eating	280
Conversation	280
Typing	360
Dressing, undressing	460
Propulsion, wheelchair	480
Driving car	560
Peeling potatoes	580
Walking 2.5 mph	720

Table 3 gives the relationship between oxygen consumption, WATT and multiples of resting O_2 consumption (metabolic equivalents or METS).

Table -3. Relationship between O_2 consumption and other measure of work

O_2 Consumption (ml/min)	WATTS	METS
900	50	04
1500	100	07
2100	150	10
2800	200	13
3500	250	16
4200	300	19
5000	350	22

The series of physiological changes that, occur with increase in exercise load has already been outlined. We will now take a closer look at changes in pulmonary function during exercise. The importance of respiratory system in maintaining oxygen supply to exercising muscles is that the ventilator pump (consisting of chest wall, respiratory muscles and the centres that control them) has been regarded as unlikely to limit maximal exercise performance in normal. Maximum exercise ventilation is substantially less than the potential maximum capacity of the pump, (maximum voluntary ventilation - MVV). This pump under resting condition works at about 5% of MVV through the life time (8).

During light-to-moderate exercise the increase in ventilation is mostly achieved by an increase in the tidal volume (VT) until it reaches 50% of vital capacity.

During heavy exercise the breathing frequency progressively increases and the VT remains constant or increases only slightly. At maximal exercise while the frequency(f) increases to about 50 breaths per minute in normal subjects, VT may decrease. Obviously, the major factor would be a choice of f and VT that would achieve adequate alveolar ventilation to eliminate the CO_2 load, and maintain homeostasis of arterial blood gases and H+ion concentration, minimizing the work of breathing within the constraints of mechanical properties of lung . By using predominant increase in VT upto a moderate power output, flow resistive work is minimized. At VT > 75% of VC elastic work is increased, hence, at very high power output f increases and VT shows no further change (9).

Performance of exercise testing

Self-paced walking tests such as the 12-minute or 6-minute test have the advantage of being very natural tests of exercise capacity, and the procedure is very simple too. However, they give information only on overall exercise tolerance and allow no physiologic measurement during exercise.

Cardiopulmonary exercise testing (CPET) has become an important clinical tool to evaluate exercise capacity and predict outcome in patients with heart failure and other cardiac conditions. This test increasingly being used assessment of reduced effort tolerance (10).

During ergometer or treadmill exercise tests will depend on the information desired from the test. In general, there are four stages of exercise testing (11). In state 1, the patient is exercised at increasing work load until exhaustion, with monitoring of heart rate and ventilation. As VO_2 can be estimated from the workload, these tests can determine if the patient's exercise capabilities are within normal limits. An estimate of the VO_2 can be obtained from the nomograms that relate the power output or the treadmill grade and speed to the VO_2 (12). Cardiovascular dysfunction is suggested by a stage 1 test demonstrating a heart rate that is high, relative to the workload and an early onset of the anaerobic threshold as evidence by non-linear increases in ventilation. A ventilator limitation is suggested when the maximum ventilation reaches 35 times the FEV_1 and the anaerobic threshold and the maximum predicted heart rates not achieved.

In stage 2 exercise testing, mixed expired gases are also collected and analyzed.

The additional information provided include the VO_2 and the VCO_2 the VE/CO_2, and VE/VO_2. Therefore, the aerobic capacity can be accurately determined (VO_2max.). In addition, cardiac outputs and stroke volumes can be determined if a rebreathing procedure is used to obtain the mixed venous PCo_2. These measurements are useful in defining exercise limitations further, but are unnecessary if exercise capacity is normal.

In stage 3 exercise testing arterial blood gas analysis is also done. This permits detection of hypoxaemia, hypercapnea, and respiratory or metabolic acidosis during exercise. In addition VD/VT can be calculated. Detection of hypoxaemia alone is possible non-invasively with a pulse oximeter, but it must be kept in mind that some pulse oximeters consistently overestimate the SaO_2 during hypoxaemia while exercising. In state 4, a Swan-Ganz catheter is used in addition.

Measurements and Calculations

There are only four basic measurements:

1. VO_2 max.
2. Breathing factors
3. Pulmonary gas exchange
4. Anaerobic threshold (AT)
5. VO_2 max

VO_2 max

VO_2 max is the best available index for assessment of exercise capacity. A reduced VO_2 max. reflects defects in either O_2 delivery (heart/lungs/systemic/pulmonary circulation) or peripheral utilization (muscle).Reduced VO_2 max may also reflects poor effect. A value of 84% of VO_2 max predicted is often used as lower limit of normal exercise capacity (13).

With exercise the cardiac output increases, initially by increase in stroke volume, and at higher work loads almost exclusively by increase in heart rate (HR) (14). The HR-VO_2 relationship is linear. A near maximal HR at relatively low values of VO_2 is seen in a variety of clinical situations. In patients with CVS disease (low stroke volume) cardiac output goes up through increase in HR. Higher HR at submaximal level of VO_2 results in an upward (or leftward) displacement of the HR-VO_2 relationship (15). Patients with reduced O_2 delivery due to reduced O_2 content (hypoxia, anaemia, COHb) may have upwardly shifted and steep HR-VO_2 relation with near attainment of max. HR. Deconditioning often resembles and accompanies cardiovascular disease and is associated with upward HR-VO_2 relation but usually, with a normal slope. The distinction between deconditioning and genuine CVS disease is accomplished by monitoring improvement in HR. Finally, patients with

COPD often have an upward displacement of HR-VO_2 relationship, but usually with a normal slope and low maximally achieved HR (16)

The third inter-relationship examined with VO_2 is the VE-mVO_2. Abnormal ventilator response patterns include excessive ventilation (increased VE at submaximal VO_2) which may be found in most patients with cardiorespiratory disease, and is therefore, nondiagnostic. Patients with both COPD and mitral valve disease have reduced VE max. and higher ventilator requirements. Excessive ventilation may be seen in some metabolic conditions including hyperthyroidism and conditions associated metabolic acidosis (17).

Breathing factors

Patients with respiratory disease most often show a rapid shallow breathing pattern in which the increase in VT is much reduced with significantly greater increase in f, A tachypnoeic breathing pattern in seen in cardiovascular diseases as well.

The VT max ((maximal exercise tidal volume)/ VC ratio of maximal exercise has been used in differential diagnosis of exercise intolerance in a variety of cardiopulmonary diseases. Current knowledge suggests that the use of peak VT and VT max./VC may have limited differential diagnostic ability (18).

Pulmonary gas exchange

Although arterial blood gas data are most reliable in identifying abnormal ventilation-perfusion relationship, VE/CO_2 data are useful as estimators of dead space ventilation and provide a non-invasive assessment of the appropriateness or efficiency of minute ventilation during exercise (17).

The ratio of VD/VT (physiologic dead space/ tidal volume) provides a valuable estimate during exercise of ventilation perfusion inhomogeneity within the lung.

The difference between arterial and end tidal PCO_2 is another measurement to assess V/Q inhomogeneity. Normally this value P (a-ET) CO_2 is slightly positive at rest but negative during exercise (17).

PaO_2 usually increases or remains the same during incremental exercise. A spectrum of responses of P (A-a)O_2 (i.e. increase, remaining the same or decrease), has been reported in normal people(19). A fall in arterial oxygen (SaO_2) of greater than or equal to 4%, a SaO_2 of less than 88%, or a PaO_2 of less than or equal to 55mm of Hg is usually considered clinically significant (20).

Anaerobic threshold

This is one measurement that provides a non-invasive estimate of the adequacy of cardiovascular function in response to an exercise stimulus. Although O_2 delivery is the most clinically relevant determinant of AT, the other mechanisms occurring less frequently and involving impairment of skeletal muscle O_2 extraction and utilization should also be considered (i.e. mitochondrial respiratory chain defect) (21, 22). It is generally agreed that less than 40% VO_2 max value is the lower limit of normal for AT.

Clinical considerations

The characteristics of exercise test results, in patients with obstructive ventilator dysfunction, exercise induced asthma, restrictive ventilator dysfunction, pulmonary hypertension, cardiovascular dysfunction; poor physical condition and poor effort are summarized below.

Obstructive ventilatory dysfunction

These patients are at a disadvantage on two counts. Firstly, their ventilator capacity is limited by their airway and lung disease, and secondly and more importantly, their ventilator requirement for a given workload is increased as their wasted ventilation is increased (VD/VT). The cardiovascular response to exercise in patient with COPD is relatively normal (23). The typical results seen are as follows:

a) Stops exercising due to shortness of breath rather than leg fatigue
b) VO_2 max is reduced, and VE at exhaustions at least 35 times the FEV_1 or 70% of the MVV
c) The VD/VT at rest is usually elevated and does not decrease with exercise, and the VE/ VCO_2 is above 30.
d) For a given VO_2 the heart rate is higher than normal, but the maximum HR is reduced because VO_2 max is so low
e) The anaerobic threshold is not reached frequently, owing to the ventilator limitation

Exercise-induced asthma

If this condition is suspected spirometry should obtained before the exercise test and at 5 minute intervals after completion of the exercise test. The exercise should be for 6-8 minutes at an intensity of 85-90% of the predicted maximal heart rate. The diagnosis is established if the FEV_1 falls more than10% after exercise (24).

Restrictive ventilatory dysfunction

The exercise capacity of patients with interstitial lung disease is limited by reduced ventilator capacity. The reduced FVC results in a relatively low maximal tidal volume, necessitating a very high respiratory rate. This limitation coupled with a decreased efficiency of gas exchange (increased VD/VT), leads to decreased exercise tolerance. Arterial blood gases during exercise reveals hypoxaemia and endurance exercise can be prolonged with supplemental oxygen (25).

Pulmonary hypertension

The exercise tolerance as reflected by the VO_2 max of patients with primary pulmonary hypertension is markedly reduced. The limiting factor is the cardiac output. The AT occurs at a relatively low workload. The PaO_2 tends to decrease in these patients with exercise. Although the ventilation at any given workload is higher than in normal (due to increased VD/ VT and early onset of anaerobic metabolism), there is no evidence that these patients are ventilator limited (26).

Cardiovascular dysfunction

Here again, the limiting factor is the cardiac output. The typical results of an exercise test are as follows (12):

a) The VO_2 max. is reduced but the VE is less than 35 times the FEV_1 and less than 70% of the MVV.
b) The VD/VT is near normal and the $VENCO_2$ is below 30
c) The heart rate is elevated relative to VO_2 (owing to the low stroke volume) and the anaerobic threshold is reached at a low VO_2
d) Arterial blood gases reveal a normal PaO_2 but a reduced $PaCO_2$ and a metabolic acidosis.

Deconditioning

The result of exercise tests in this group is similar to that of cardiovascular dysfunction problems. VO_2 max is low, the AT is reached at a low VO_2 because of the poor distribution of the cardiac output. The maximum heart rate is normal and the VE is below 35 times the $FEV_{1.}$ Deconditioning is often difficult to distinguish from early or mild heart disease (27).

Obesity

A spectrum of exercise response may be seen, depending mostly on the severity of obesity VO_2 max may be reduced, when expressed per kilogram of body weight. VO_2 is increased for a given work rate. The excessive metabolic requirement reflects the high energy lost of moving the weight of the legs. It has been postulated that obese patients might have relatively less efficient cardiac performance, relying on grated tissue extraction during exercise compared with normal subjects (27).

Poor effort and maligering

Individuals complaining of exercise intolerance may not show any abnormality at the initial assessment. It is important to find out whether they are actually impaired, particularly when litigation or compensation is involved. When subjected to a maximal exercise test, such individuals may not give maximum effort. Therefore, they will have decreased VO_2 max. But their VE will be less than 35 times their FEV_1, their maximal heart rate will be reduced, though VO_2 for a given heart rate will be normal; they will be fail to reach their AT and their blood lactate levels will be less than 8 mm/L and arterial blood gases will remain normal(28).

Lastly, there are patients who have mild or moderate impairment on the basis of their pulmonary function tests, but complain shortness of breath while working. Exercise testing for these people is useful, because there is no close relationship between tests of pulmonary function and VO_2 max. The following rating of impairment is recommended.

1. If the VO_2 max. is greater than 25 ml/kg/min., the subject will be capable of continuous exertion throughout an 8 hour shift, in all but the most physically demanding of jobs.
2. If the VO_2 is between 15 and 25ml/kg/min; and 40% of the observed VO_2 max. is greater than the average metabolic work requirement of the subject's job, then the subject should be able to perform the job comfortably.
3. If the VO_2 max. is less than 15 ml/kg/min., the subject will be uncomfortable even travelling to the place of employment.

Table 4: Basic Patterns Observed On Cardiopulmonary Exercise Testing (29).

	Disease Category				
Variable	**Normal Patient**	**Cardiovascular Disease**	**Obstructive Lung Disease**	**Pulmonary Vascular Disease/ILD#**	**Neuromuscular Disease**
$VO_{2\,max}$	Normal*	Decreased	Decreased	Decreased	Decreased
Heart Rate Reserve	Absent to small Reserve (<20 bpm)	Absent to small reserve (<20bpm)	Large (<30 bpm)	Small (<20-30 bpm)	Large (> 30 bpm)
V_E.max/MVV (Ventilatory Reserve)	< 0/.8	<0/.8	> 0.8	< 0.8	< 0.8
Ventilatory Threshold	Present	Present	Absent	Present	Usually present
Dead Space (V_D/V_T)	Decreases	Decreases	Decreases	Remains stable Or increases	Decreases
Oxygen Saturation	Stable	Stable	Decreases	Decreases	Stable
End-TidalCO_2 (in late Exercise)	Decrease	Decrease or stable	Increase	Decrease or stable	Increase
Reason for Stopping	Leg Fatigue	Leg Fatigue	Dyspnea	Dyspnea, leg fatigue	Fatigue

Note :
*"Normal" or "decreased" refers to how the variable changes relative to age, gender and size matched individual.

Interstitial lung disease patients demonstrate a patterns very similar to the pulmonary vascular patterns and can only be differentiated based on their PFTs and chest imaging.

REFERENCES

1. Gay SE, Weisman IM, Flaherty KR, Martinex FJ, Cardiopulmonary exercise testing in unexplained dyspnea. In: Weisman IM, Zeballos RJ, editors. Clinical exercise testing. Basel: Karger; 2002; 81-88.
2. Knuttgen, HG. The science of exercise physiology: What is exercise? Phys. Sports Med 2003; 31 : 31-49
3. Knuttgen, HG. Strength training and aerobic exercise: comparison and contrast. J. Strength Cond. Res. 2007; 21(3):973-978
4. Ries AL, Exercise. In: Bordow RA, Moser KM (eds.) Manual of clinical problems in pulmonary medicine. 3rd ed. Boston, Little Brown 1991; 20-22.
5. Hill AV, Long CNH, Lupton H. Muscular exercise , lactic acid and the supply and utilization of oxygen. Proc. R Soc Lond 1924, 96:438-475.
6. Binder RK, Wonisch M, Corra U, et al. Methodological approach to the 1st and 2nd lactate threshold in incremental cardiopulmonary exercise testing . Eur J Cardiovasc Prev. Rehab 2008;15:726-734.
7. Gordon FE, Energy costs of activities in health and disease. Arch Int Med 1958; 101:702.
8. Otis AB. The work of breathing. Physical Rev 1954;34:449-458.
9, Lorring SH, Mead J. Action of diaphragm on the rib cage inferred from a Core-Balance Anaysis J.Appl Physiol 1982;52: 700-704.
10. Mezzania A, Agostoni Alain P, et al Standards for the use of cardiopulmonary exercise testing for the functional evaluation of cardiac patients : a repotr from the Exercise Physiology Section of the European Association for Cardiovascular Prevention and Rehabilitation. Eur J Cardiovasc Prev. Rehab 2009; 16(3): 249-67.
11. Jones NL, Campbell EJM. In : Clinical exercise testing. 2nd ed. Philadelphia, EB Saunders, 1981
12. Albouaini K, Egred M, Alahmar A et al. Cardiopulmonary exercise testing and its application. Postgrad Med J 2007 (985); 83: 675-82
13. Wasserman K, Hansen JE, Sue DY, et al. Principles of exercise testing and interpretation Ist ed. Philadelphia, Lea and Febige 1987.
14. Astrand PO, Rodahl K, Text Book of Work Physiology, 3rd ed. New York, McGraw-Hill, 1986.
15. Francis GS. Haemodynamic and neurohumoral responses to dynamic exercise; normal subjects versus patients with heart disease. Circulation 1987;76:1-11.
16. Wasserman K, Whipp BJ. Exercise physiology in health and disease. Am. Rev. Resp. Dis. 1975;112:219-249

17. Weissman IM, Zeballos RJ. An integrated approach to the interpretation of cardiopulmonary exercise testing. Clin. Chest Med 1994; 215:421-442.

18. Gowda KS, Zintel T, McParland C, et al. Diagnostic value of maximal exercise tidal volume Chest 1990;98:1351-1354.

19. Zeballos RJ, Weisman IM, Johnson B, Moreno A, p(A-a)O2 during exercise in healthy young blacks with sickle cell trait (SCT) and controls. Fed Proc 1985;44:1368.

20. American Association for Respiratory Care ; Clinical practice guideline: Exercise testing for evaluation of hypoxaemia and / ordesaturatlon. Resp Care 1992;37: 907-912.

21. Bogaard JM, Scholte HR, Busch HFM, et al Anaerobic threshold as detected from ventilator and metabolic exercise responsesin patients with mitrochondrial respiratory chain defect. Adv Cardiol 1986; 35:135-145.

22. Nery LE, Wasserman K, Andrews JD, Huntsman DJ, Hansen JE, Whipp BJ. Ventilatory and gas exchange kinetics during exercise in chronic airways obstruction. J Appl Physiol 1982;53:1594–1602.

23. Jones NL, Jones G, Edwards RH. Exercise tolerance in chronic airway obstruction. Am Rev Respir Dis1971;103:477–491.

24. Mahler DA. Exercise-induced asthma. Med Sci Sports Exerc 1993; 25: 554-561.

25. Bye PB, Anderson SO, Woolcock AJ, et al. Bycycle endurance performance of patients with interstitial lung disease breathing air oxygen. Am. Rev Respir Dis 1982;126: 1005-1012.

26. D'Alonzo GE, Gianotti LA, Pohil RL, et al. Comparison of progressive exercise performance of normal subjects and patients with primary pulmonary hypertension. Chest 1987;92: 57-62.

27. ATS/ACCP statement on Cardiopulmonary Exercise Testing. Am J Respir Crit Care Med 2003; 167: 211-77.

28 Magarian GJ. Hyperventilation syndromes: infrequently recognized common expressions of anxiety and stress. Medicine (Baltimore) 1982;61:219–236.

29. Luks AM, Glenny R, Robertson HT Introduction to Cardiopulmonary Exercise Testing 2nd edn Division of Pulmonary and Critical Care Medicine, University of Washington, 2010.

19

PREOPERATIVE ASSESSMENT OF PULMONARY FUNCTION TESTS

S.K. JINDAL

Introduction

In spite of limitations, pulmonary function tests (PFTs) are heavily relied upon for preoperative evaluation of a patient for surgery. It is a general practice to seek pulmonary clearance and lung function testing for patients awaiting surgery. Almost 50 percent of requests for lung function tests are received from the surgical units in most PFT Laboratories in India (1).

Why do we need pre-operative PFT?

There are a number of changes in pulmonary physiology and defence mechanisms which happen during the postoperative period (Table 1). These changes are often responsible to make the patient prone to pulmonary complications especially infections. Altered lung mechanics lead to significantly reduced mucociliary clearance which contributes to the retention of secretions.

Table 1. Postoperative changes in pulmonary physiology and defense mechanisms

i. Physiological changes

a. Moderate-to-severe reduction in Vital Capacity (VC) and smaller reductions in Functional Residual Capacity (FRC)

b. Reductions in other lung volumes, including Total Lung Capacity (TLC), Inspiratory capacity (IC), Expiratory Reserve Volume (ERV), and Residual Volume (RV)

c. Diaphragmatic dysfunction

d. Postoperative hypoxemia: ventilation-perfusion mismatch, alveolar hypoventilation, anesthetic-induced inhibition of hypoxic pulmonary vasoconstriction, right-to-left shunting, and depressed cardiac output.

e. Micro-thromboemboli

ii. Changes in lung defense mechanisms

a. Ciliary damage (endotracheal intubation and inhalation of dry gases)

b. Reduced tracheal mucus velocity

c. Ineffective cough reflex (due to postoperative pain)

d. Excessive use of narcotics

Some of these alterations are responsible for a high risk of atelectasis and hypoxia, especially in the first 24 hours. Reduction in lung function is seen more often with thoracic and upper abdominal procedures; it gradually recovers within three weeks. These changes can often be attributed to the postsurgical pain and associated muscle splinting, and the diaphragm dysfunction which impair lung mechanics.

Indications for pre-operative PFT assessment

*It is important to have a general assessment of lung function to make an appropriate decision. However, n*ot all patients require PFT prior to surgery. Following are the main indications for PFT assessment:

1. to make a decision whether a patient can tolerate surgery,
2. to predict the occurrence of post operative respiratory complications,
3. to assess the post-operative respiratory disability, and
4. to detect unrecognized pulmonary problem

I. Preoperative Pulmonary Evaluation

It is not always possible to give a blanket "yes" or "no" decision for most patients for whom the preoperative clearance for thoracic surgery has been asked for. The decision also depends upon the "indication" for surgery and the presence of respiratory (or other) risks. There are situations when any possible risk is to be brushed aside if the indication for the surgical procedure is urgent or life-saving. On the other hand, it will be unwise to opt for surgery which can wait in the presence of a risk factor which can be removed. Clinical judgement for all such patients is made on the basis of risk benefit ratio after considering all the probabilities. Lung function assessment is of great help in making this decision (2). There are several risk factors which are required to be assessed to decide the fitness of a patient for surgery (Table 2). They are also important to predict the possibility of postoperative complications in patients due to undergo thoracic or non-thoracic surgery (3, 4).

i. **Primary surgical problem**
Site of the primary problem and the surgery being considered are of great importance. For example, respiratory fitness is more critical for patients requiring abdominal (especially upper abdominal), brain or thoracic surgery. Duration and type of anaesthesia as well as of surgery are also important in determining pulmonary risk.

ii. **Pulmonary factors**
Current smoking history and recent respiratory infections are important risk factors. Presence of a concurrent lung disease such as bronchial asthma, pulmonary tuberculosis, bronchiectasis and chronic obstructive lung disease is not a contraindication for any surgery unless the complicating disease is severe, advanced or uncontrolled. Lung function assessment will help to define the extent of abnormality and preoperative risk determination.

iii. **Non pulmonary factors**
Lung function is likely to be impaired in a patient with history of chronic smoking, obesity or advanced age. Smoking and obesity have been shown to bear a significant relationship with increased morbidity and postoperative complications. Similarly, kypho-scoliosis and presence of neuromuscular diseases are important indications for preoperative pulmonary evaluation. Other co-morbidities such as hypertension, ischemic heart disease, diabetes, connective tissue disorders, malignancies, hypothyroidism and others, which may also contribute to impairment of lung function in one or other manner important for overall pre-operative assessment.

II. Prediction of Postoperative Complications

It is difficult to predict the occurrence of postoperative problems merely on the basis of lung function assessment. Most of the risk factors which are required to be looked into have been listed earlier. The poorer the lung function, the more likely is the development of a problem. Yet it is not possible to exclude the chances of even serious complications on the basis of normal lung function. For example, acute respiratory distress syndrome, pulmonary embolism or respiratory infections can develop in a patient with entirely normal preoperative lung function tests. On the other hand, preoperative presence of reduced lung function or airway obstruction does indicate that the respiratory disability and/or infections are more likely.

III. Preoperative Assessment of Postoperative Respiratory Function

This is an important issue to dwell upon especially in case of thoracic surgery when lung resection is envisaged. Resection of a diseased and non-functional lobe or lung, for example due to bronchiectasis or other fibro-cavitary diseases may not make much difference in lung function before and after resection. But resection of a healthy or even a partially functional lobe, such as in the presence of a lung tumour, is going to reduce the postoperative function and cause functional disability. It is therefore, important to take care that a patient is not made a respiratory cripple following resection.

In general, surgical resection is not recommended if the predicted postoperative FEV is less than 0.8 L. This is however not considered as an absolute contraindication at most centres (5).

Patient evaluation

The minimal respiratory evaluation of preoperative patient for any type of surgery includes a good history-taking, physical examination and chest roentgenography. Lung function test assessment is required for those who have got either a high risk (Table 2) or require thoracic/ upper abdominal surgery. Tests required for this assessment can be classified as screening and specialized tests depending upon the type of indication and the level of risk factor.

Table 2. Factors important to decide the fitness for non-thoracic surgery

- **i. Related to primary disease and treatment**
  - a. Site and number of organ involvement
  - b. Type of surgery and anaesthesia
  - c. Duration of surgery-prolonged anaesthesia
  - d. Pulmonary resection
- **ii. Pulmonary risk-factors**
  - a. Smoking history (esp. more than 1 pack per day)
  - b. Obesity; 30% over ideal weight
  - c. Age (> 70 years

Screening tests

1. Spirometry: Spirometric measurement of lung volumes and expiratory flows is the simplest and cheapest method to assess lung volumes. This gives a fair degree of information on the presence of both restrictive and obstructive lung diseases. It also helps to decide whether a patient can withstand the stress of anaesthesia and surgery. More importantly, it is helpful to monitor and gauze the preoperative preparation and postoperative recovery of the patient.

It is important that each spirometric parameter is assessed with respect to age, sex, height, ethnicity and race of the individual. Nomograms for prediction of different spirometric parameters are now available for different populations including those from India. In general, the Indian values have been reported to be lower by about 10 to 15 percent for those Western values (1). Within India, the northern population is closer to that of the West as far as lung function is concerned. People of the hilly regions such as Bhutan had much better parameters (6).

Spirometric variations due to diurnal, hormonal and seasonal effects within the same individual should be considered while interpreting the results. The other biological variations important in the measurement and interpretation of lung function relate to the place of residence, environmental pollution, physical activity, socioeconomic status, body muscularity, past and present health etc (7). Measurement errors due to technical factors and/or calibration problems must be excluded before interpreting the results.

It is difficult to set absolute values for different sprometric indices to decide fitness (or otherwise) for surgery. As per generally accepted guidelines, the values which indicate an increased risk of morbidity and mortality are as follows (1, 2):

FVC< 50% predicted

FEV_1<2 L or < 50% predicted

Maximum Voluntary Ventilation (MVV) < 50% predicted.

An FVC of 1.5 L or FEV1< 1.0L indicate a high risk patient.

MVV is a better parameter to rely upon especially because it involves and assesses the components of patient's cooperation, motivation, understanding and stamina (8). But MVV is less reproducible than FEV_1 and more dependent on muscle strength and effort.

2. Arterial Blood Gas Measurement

Analysis of partial pressures of O_2 and CO_2 in arterial blood is done only if there is moderate or greater degree of spirometric abnormality or if lung resection is planned. It is the presence of hypercapnia (e.g Arterial PCO_2 > 45 mmHg) which is a more reliable index for a high risk patient than hypoxemia. Oximetry is a simple and cheap measure of gas exchange. Being relatively insensitive, it cannot be relied upon for preoperative assessment. This is a test of great use for postoperative monitoring. Hypoxaemia, attributed to the presence of right to left shunt in lung lobe with obstructed bronchus (e.g. due to bronchogenic carcinoma) which is proposed to be resected, is fallacious while deciding surgery. Such hypoxaemia shall in fact, improve after resection. Therefore, it is important to consider the cause of hypoxaemia before using this parameter to decide operability.

3. Exercise testing: Postoperative disability may not only relate to pulmonary but also cardiovascular factors. Therefore, exercise testing may give a better assessment of overall risk and postoperative function than spirometry alone. A lower incidence of postoperative complications is reported in patients with a maximal O_2 uptake of more than 20 mL/Kg/min vis-a-vis higher rates in patients with maximal O_2 uptake of < 15 mL/Kg/Min. But it is not an absolute test to evaluate most patients with chronic airflow obstruction. Even Peak VO2 is only one of several criteria. Patients with an anaerobic threshold of <11 ml/min/Kg are at risk for major surgery.

Cardiopulmonary exercise testing (CPET) is now considered an important tool to predict post-operative outcome and risk-stratification in patients undergoing intra-abdominal surgery such as renal transplantation, colorectal, upper abdominal and bariatric surgery (9). A large multicentre study with a prospective, cohort design is in progress to measure Exercise Tolerance before major non-cardiac surgery to predict postoperative morbidity and mortality (10).

Specialized Tests

More specific and specialized tests are required when either lung resection surgery is planned or the diagnosis for the presence of an underlying lung disease is required to be established. PFTs in these situations should be interpreted along with other important investigations such as chest radiography and broncho-endoscopy. PFTs are required both to determine whether a patient can tolerate the anticipated resection and retain adequate postoperative lung function.

1. **Tests for Lung Mechanics:** Besides spirometry measurement of residual volume (RV), total lung capacity (TLC) and their ratio (RV/TLC) shall indicate the presence of airways obstruction. Hyperinflation with RV/TLC ratio >50% is considered an index for high risk surgery. Measurements of airway resistance and compliance are not routinely done except when the presence of an underlying early lung disease is suspected. Such measurements are sometimes required in chronic smokers or in some patients for cardiac surgery.

2. **Diffusion capacity:** Pulmonary diffusion capacity (DLCO) of less than 40% predicted indicates significant involvement of lung interstitium. This is an indicator of higher morbidity. DLCO is recommended only in patients with restrictive disorders.

3. **Regional Lung Function Tests:** Differential broncho spirometry or split lung function testing was frequently used to study regional lung function. Computed tomography, magnetic resonance imaging and nuclear scans are now available at most places where lung surgery is done. A fair degree of information about regional lung problems can be obtained with their help.

4. **Balloon occlusion of pulmonary artery:** Whenever a patient is considered for lung resection in the presence of pulmonary hypertension, pulmonary arterial pressure measurement is made after occlusion of the unilateral pulmonary artery of the lung to be resected. This is done to determine whether the patient would have an adequate pulmonary circulation after resection. Pulmonary arterial pressure of less than 30 mm Hg after occlusion of artery is generally acceptable as criterion for operability. However, most surgeons do not consider this test as essential.

Disease specific assessment

Preoperative assessment in patients with pulmonary disorders such as chronic obstructive pulmonary disease (COPD) and lung cancer needs specific consideration.

1. **Chronic obstructive pulmonary disease:** PFT assessment in COPD is important for diagnosis, staging of severity, monitoring the disease progress and preoperative risk categorization, for example in patients for lung volume reduction surgery or resection of a lung nodule (11). Patients undergoing surgery are shown to benefit by preoperative pulmonary evaluation and rehabilitation.

   The Society of Thoracic Surgeons (STS) generally employs a risk-assessment model to predict postoperative outcome after cardio-thoracic surgery. It did not find any additional benefit on adding individual PFT parameters or different COPD classifications to predict complications, thereby pointing to the limited clinical utility (12).

2. **Lung Cancer Surgery:** Lung resection which remains the treatment of choice for early stage non-small cell lung cancer treatment is bound to affect the postoperative lung function. Most of these patients have got impaired lung function due to the effects of lung cancer with or without the presence of concomitant illnesses (e.g. COPD). The aim of PFT assessment in these patients is twofold i.e. i, to decide about the fitness for surgery and ii, to predict the postoperative pulmonary functions. Preoperative assessment is done as for any other patient for thoracic surgery for assessment of cardiopulmonary reserve (13,14).

   Use of stair climbing as a surrogate marker of maximal O_2 consumption has been also found to be useful in making decision in such cases (13). Various other tests which help in predicting the post- resection lung function include various PFT measures such as FEV1 and DLCO (2).

   In addition to decide fitness, it is important to predict postoperative residual lung function. Patient s with even severe impairment can however be undertaken for surgical resection at specialised centres with low morbidity and mortality.

3. **Cardiac Surgery**: Routine PFT assessment before coronary artery bypass graft (CABG) surgery is advisable for several reasons, one of which is the likelihood of an unsuspected lung dysfunction or disease due to a common factor of smoking. Patient undergoing CABG from left internal mammary artery may have temporary left

diaphragmatic dysfunction causing difficulty in weaning from the ventilator. It has been also shown that patients spending longer periods in Intensive Care Units have preoperative pyrometer abnormalities. Since $PaCO_2$ of over 45 mmHg is associated with higher preoperative mortality. It may also be assessed preoperatively in patients with concomitant history of heavy tobacco smoking or a lung disease.

Post-operative monitoring with PFT

Regular postoperative assessment of PFT is helpful to monitor certain types of pulmonary complications. This is important in patients with multiple trauma, multiple blood transfusion, acute pancreatitis, burns and septicaemia. Serial blood gas measurements and chest roentgenography shall help in early detection and treatment of complications. PFT monitoring is required for postoperative management of patients with underlying lung diseases such as asthma, chronic obstructive lung disease or interstitial lung disease.

In summary, pre-operative PFT assessment helps to decide about the fitness and risk-stratification for patients undergoing both thoracic and non-thoracic surgery. Spirometry is also helpful to evaluate the residual postoperative lung function and respiratory disability. It is however important to interpret the result in conjunction with other pre-operative assessment and surgical-indication.

REFERENCES

1. Jindal SK, Wahi Pl. Pulmonary Function Laboratory in the Tropics: Needs, Problems and solutions. In: Sharma OP, Lung Disease in the Tropics, New York, Marcel Dekker Inc. 1990:523-42
2. Celli BR. What is the value of preoperative pulmonary function testing. Med Clin N Amer 1993; 77: 309-25.
3. Yoshimi K, Oh S, Suzuki K, Kodama Y, Sekiya M, Seyama K, Fukuchi Y. Impact of Airflow Limitation on Comorbidities and Postoperative Complications in Patients Undergoing Thoracic Surgery: A Retrospective Observational Study. Ann Thorac Cardiovasc Surg. 2016; 22:146-52.
4. Lakshminarasimhachar A, Smetana GW. Preoperative Evaluation: Estimation of Pulmonary Risk. Anesthesiol Clin. 2016; 34:71-88.
5. Eerfolio RJ, Allen MS, Trastek VF, Deschampa C, Scanlon PD, Pairolero PC. Lung resection in patients with compromised pulmonary function. Ann Thorac Surg 1996; 62:348-51.
6. Giri BR, Sharma BK, Jindal SK. Normal spirometry in healthy natives of Bhutan. J Ass Phy India 1996; 44:320-22.
7. Becklake MR. Concepts of normality applied to the measurement of lung function Am J Med 1986; 80; 1158-64.
8. Older P, Hall A. Clinical review: how to indentify high- risk surgical patients. Crit Care 2004; 8: 369-72.
9. Moran J, Wilson F, Guinan E, McCormick P, Hussey J, Moriarty J. Role of cardiopulmonary exercise testing as a risk-assessment method in patients undergoing intra-abdominal surgery: a systematic review. Br J Anaesth. 2016;116:177-91.
10. Wijeysundera DN, Pearse RM, Shulman MA, Abbott TE, Torres E, Croal BL, Granton JT, Thorpe KE, Grocott MP, Farrington C, Myles PS, Cuthbertson BH; METS Study Investigators. Measurement of Exercise Tolerance before Surgery (METS) study: a protocol for an international multicentre prospective cohort study of cardiopulmonary exercise testing prior to major non-cardiac surgery. BMJ Open. 2016; 6(3):e010359.
11. Cooper CB. Assessment of pulmonary function in COPD. Semin Respir Crit Care Med 2005; 26:246-52.
12. Ivanov A, Yossef J, Tailon J, Worku BM, Gulkarov I, Tortolani AJ, Sacchi TJ, Briggs WM, Brener SJ, Weingarten JA, Heitner JF. Do pulmonary function tests improve risk stratification before cardiothoracic surgery? J Thorac Cardiovasc Surg. 2016;151(4):1183-9.e3.
13. Bolliger CT, Koegelenberg CF, Kendal R. Preoperative assessment for lung cancer surgery. Curr Opin Pulm Med 2005; 11:301-6.
14. Mazzone PJ, Arroliga AC. Lung cancer: preoperative pulmonary evaluation of the lung resection candidate. Am J Med 2006; 118: 578-83.

20

LUNG FUNCTION STUDIES DURING SLEEP

HARMANJIT SINGH HIRA

Spirometry

Traditional methods of measuring ventilation depended upon breathing through a mouthpiece with the nose occluded by a nose clip connected to a spirometer or penumatochograph. However, since ventilation is subject to behavioural influences, extraneous stimuli from such apparatus may interfere with the pattern of breathing and with assessment of the neural control of breathing. In his original description of the spirometer in 1944, John Hutchinson cautioned that errors might arise with the employment of instruments requiring the use of the mouthpiece (1). It is also unable for long-term monitoring of ventilation during sleep. This problem has induced investigators to attempt to measure ventilation indirectly by recording motion of the chest wall, which reflects change in thoracic gas volume and under the usual circumstances is equivalent to tidal volume measured by spirometry.

The contribution of the rib cage and abdomen to tidal breathing varies with posture. In the erect position, most subjects breathe predominantly with rib cage expansion, approximately two-thirds rib cage and one-third abdominal expansion, whereas the contribution is reversed in the supine position (Fig.1). Recording of motion of rib cage and abdomen provides a measure of ventilatory performance and pulmonary function.

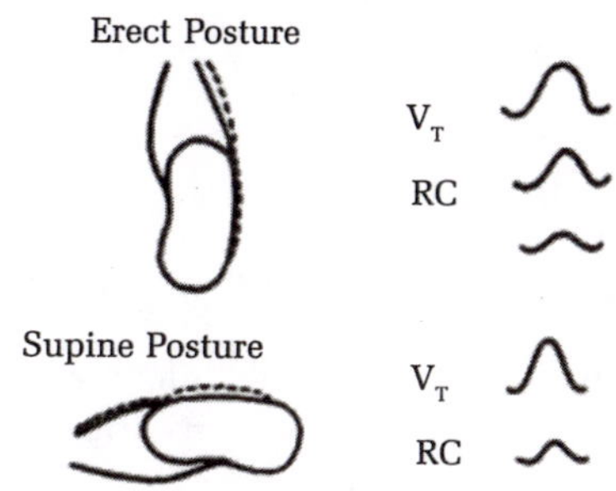

Fig 1: Variation in rib cage (RC) and abdominal (AB) contribution to tidal volume (TV) during erect and supine postures.

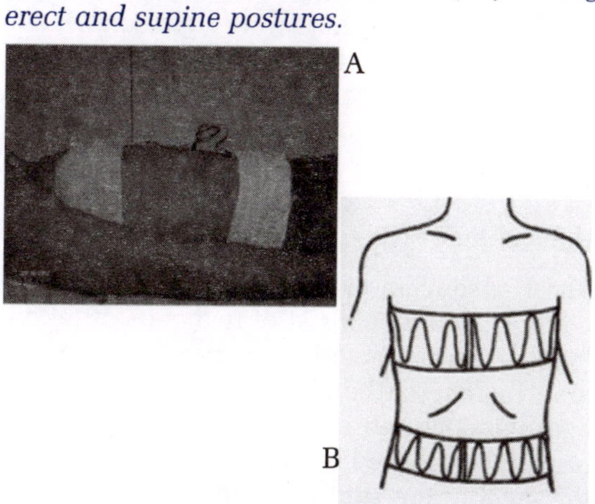

Fig 2A and B shows transducer bands of Respiratory Inductive Plethysmography (RIP), RC Respiband is placed around rib cage below armpits, and another AB Respiband centred on umbilicus.

During sleep, indirect non-invasive methods of performing pulmonary functions are used. The major methods that have been employed are;

1. Visual observation
2. Chest measurer
3. Stethometer
4. Bellows pneumograph
5. Mercury-in-silastic strain gauge
6. Impedance pneumograph
7. Jerkin plethysmograph
8. Linear differential transducers
9. Magnetometers
10. Respiratory inductive plethysmograph (RIP)

Respiratory inductive plethysmography

This technique has become the most widely accepted method of measuring ventilation non-invasively during sleep. The original respiratory inductive plethysmograph consisted of insulated wire stitched in a zig-zag pattern of about 2 cm pitch into a vest consisting of elastic material. The vest encompassed the complete tarso from upper chest to pubis, and there were eight continuous complete turns of the wire. Later this device was modified into two separate coils and remains the basis of the currently employed system (2).

Operational Principles (3)

The transducers of the respiratory inductive plethysmograph consist of two coils of teflon-insulated wire sewn in a zigzag pattern on to elastic-fabricated bands measuring approximately 10 cm in height (Fig. 2). One band is positioned to encircle the rib cage, at the level of the sternum with the upper edge just under the axillae, whereas the other band is worn midway between the lower ribs and the iliac crests at the level of umbilicus. The hands are held in place by an elastic net garment, or if a prolonged study is anticipated as during sleep, it is often helpful to tape the fabricated bands to the skin surface using adhesive tape so as to prevent slippage. The wires in the hands are connected to one or two small oscillator modules, which in turn are attached to the bands. The oscillator cycles at frequencies of about 300 kHz and puts out frequency-modulated signals of about 20 kHz. The frequencies of the oscillator signals are proportional to alteration in the self-inductance of the coil. The self-inductance of the coil, and so the frequencies of its oscillator, are proportional to the cross-sectional area enclosed by the coil.

The signals from the oscillator are sent through wires to a demodulator calibrator unit which provides patient isolation with optocouplers. The signals from the optocouplers are then sent to phase-locked loops which demodulate the signals from the oscillator and provide DC output signals. These signals are sent through a band-pass filter, with an upper frequency limit of 15 Hz. In addition, there is an optional low-pass filter with a time constant of 100 seconds, which may be used in order to restore the signal outputs to a fixed baseline. This latter mode is the AC-couple version. The DC coupled version is usually employed for research studies as it allows measurement of changes in the end-expiratory level (FRC) and there is less distortion of signals during both slow and rapid vital capacity maneuvers than with the AC-coupled version. If a study over a prolonged time period is planned, the AC-coupled version is generally used, as it restores the signals to a fixed baseline. The outputs from the filters go to sealing amplifiers and then to a recording device.

Calibration: Calibration of the respiratory-inductive plethysmograph is based on the assumption that the respiratory system possesses two degrees of freedom, rib cage and abdominal motion (4). A number of different methods, some of which can be performed by hand and others requiring the assistance of a computer can derive the rib cage and abdominal calibration factors.

The least squares method of calibration is the currently preferred method of calibrating the respiratory inductive plethysmograph (5) and is a mathematical equivalent of the simultaneous equation technique. Calibration is again based on the assumption that the respiratory system possesses two degrees of freedom of motion, so that volume change from a spirometer (SP) is equal to the sum of the volume change of the rib cage (RC) and abdomen (AB).

RC + AB = SP

This equation can be rearranged by dividing across by volume (SP) giving the following equation.

$$RC/SP + AB/SP = 1$$

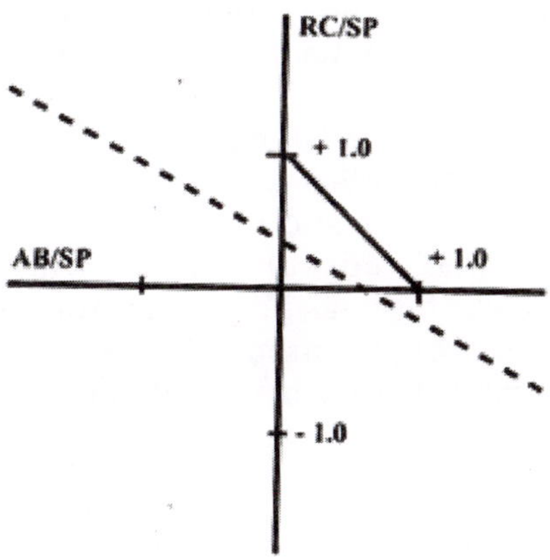

Fig 3: Least squares method of calibrating the rib cage (RC) and abdominal (AB) signals. The continuous line is the ideal calibrated line with intercepts of one on both axes SP is volume change from a spirometer

When this equation is plotted with RC/SP on the V axis and AB/SP on the X axis, the equation, shown by a continuous line in Fig. 3 should have a slop of -1and intercepts at one on both axes. Thus, if volume change is solely due to abdominal displacement, the AB/SP ratio should be 1.0 and, if volume change is due to rib cage motion, the RC/SP ration should be 1.0. For other relative contributions of the rib cage and abdomen, their ratios to spirometry should fall on the continuous line when the respiratory inductive plethysmograph is correctly calibrated.

Analysis of breathing patterns on RIP

Over the same period that technology for non-invasive measurement of ventilatiion inspired, significant advances occurred in analytical approach to breathing patterns. From a traditional point of view, minute ventilation (Vmin) has been analysed in terms of its classic components, tidal volume (VT) and respiratory frequency (f).

Vmin = VT x f

Milic-Emili and Grunstein proposed a further mathematical analysis of the breathing cycle (6) (Fig.4). The traditional equation of minute ventilation is rearranged as

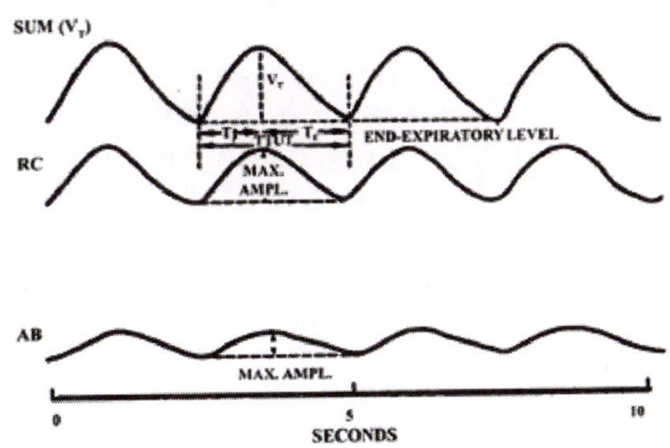

Fig 4: Schematic recording of the respiratory cycle depicting the points of reference for computation of various breathing pattern parameters. SUM (VT) represents the sum of rib cage (RC) and abdominal (AB) excursions and represent inspiratoryTI and TE expiratory times respectively. TTOT is time for total breath. MAX AMPL is the maximum amplitude from to peak amplitudes of rib cage and abdominal excursions respiratory cycle (TTOT) or single breath.

Vmin = VT x 601 TTOT

Conceptually, 60 can be deleted and the equation reduce to

Vmin =VT x II TTOT

dividing by inspiratory time (TI) while multiplying by TI

Vmin =VT/TI x TII TTOT

The first parameter (VT/TI has been termed mean inspiratory flow rate, and the second parameter, TII TTOT has been called the fractional inspiratory time.

Since the neural impulses controlling inspiratory drive are independent of reflex activity once inspiration has begun. VT/TI reflects central inspiratory drive as it is the mechanical transformation of the neural activity (7). This variable relates to standard indices of respiratory centre output, such as mouth pressure generated at 0.1 second after the onset of inspiration against an occluded airway (PO.I) and alteration in minute ventilation during CO2 stimulation. An elevated VT/TI reflects increased respiratory centre drive and *vice versa*. An advantage of VT/TI is that it provides a measure of respiratory drive during resting breathing, unlike most published information on respiratory centre derive which has been derived from studies with hypercapnea, hypoxia, and exercise. Furthermore, VT/TI can be measured non-obtrusively.

The fractional inspiratory time, TI/TIOT indicates the relationship between the ratio of inspiration and expiration. Patients with obstructive lung disease typically display prolonged expiration on physical examination, and II/TTOT has been shown to be a significant, although weak, predictor of airway obstruction (8). This ratio also reflects respiratory phase switching and has been called the effective ratio. When viewed in an engineering framework, TI/TTOT has been termed the 'duty cycle', as it indicates that portion of the respiratory cycle when respiratory muscles are active. Thus a prolonged TI/TTOT predisposes to respiratory muscle fatigue, and is of equal importance to the tension developed by the muscle as determinant of a diaphragmatic fatigue. Prolonged TI/TTOT also indicates restrictive lung disease.

Examining the phase relationship (PR) between rib cage and abdominal motion may also provide important information on respiratory muscle fatigue. Hoover is usually credited with describing the presence of asynchronous respiratory movements in patients with obstructive lung disease (9). Inadequate diaphragmatic contraction is thought to result in paradoxical abdominal motion because the negative pleural pressure generated by the other inspiratory muscles pulls up the diaphragm and with it, the anterior abdominal wall, or the negative pressure is transmitted across the flaccid diaphragm causing a fall in abdominal pressure resulting in inward displacement of the abdominal wall. The presence of rib cage abdominal synchrony has important prognostic importance and in a prospective study of COPD patients on admission to hospital, its presence was the best single factor in predicting subsequent requirement of mechanical ventilation (10, 11).

In addition to obtaining information on the presence and degree of asynchronous movements, quantitative recording of rib cage and abdominal motion measures the contribution of each compartment to volume change. An increase in the rib cage contribution to tidal volume in a supine subject suggests recruitment of the intercostal/accessory muscles. Respiratory alterans was fluctuations between predominant rib cage and abdominal expansion, reflecting respective employment of intercostal/accessory muscles and the diaphragm has been proposed as another marker of respiratory muscle fatigue (12).

Separate recording of rib cage-abdominal motion (PR, Phase relation) during sleep is also important in the diagnosis of type of sleep apnoea syndrome (13, 14). Motion of the rib cage and abdomen ceases during a central apnoeic episode, whereas there is complete paradoxic motion of the two compartments during an obstructive episode. The nocturnal hypoxemia, breathing abnormalities and arrhythmias in patients of kyphoscoliosis, chronic obstructive pulmonary disease, and bronchial asthma during sleep, oxygen saturation, breathing pattern and arrhythmias in patients of chronic obstructive pulmonary disease and bronchial asthma during sleep (14-17).

After understanding the functioning of respiratory inductive plethysmography discussed above, readers shall be able to appreciate the following various parametes of pulmonary function during sleep.

VT (Tidal volume): It is measured as average volume from beginning to end of inspiration. Normal values for adult is 200-350 ml (semi-quantitative)-%CV=45%.

Vmin (minute ventilation): It is the volume of air breathed in one min and measured by mean tidal volume multiplied by frequency of breathing. normal value for adult is 4.0-8.5 litres/min(semi-quantative).

VT/TLC (Mean inspiratory flow): It is computed as mean breath by breath tidal volume divided by time of inspiration. It reflects respiratory centre drive. A normal value is 150-350 ml/se (semi-quantitative). Presence of increased value than normal indicates increased respiratory central drive and *vice versa*.

TI (inspiratory time): It is a mean time from beginning to end of inspiration calculated on a breath by breath basis. It is a crude indicator of respiratory centre drive. The normal value is 1.20-2.45 sec. Value less than 1.0 sec reflects elevated centre drive.

TI/TTOT (fractional inspiration time): It is the ratio of inspiratory time divided by time of total breath calculated on breath basis. It is a crude indicator of airways obstruction. Normal value for adult is 0.36-0.47; decreased value suggests airways obstruction while increased value suggests restrictive lung disease.

% RC (percent rib cageNT): It is calculated as percent of rib cage contribution to tidal volume. It is an indicator of intercostal (RC) and diaphragmatic (AB) muscular activity. Normal adult value ranges between 30-50% (supine) and 50-70% (upright posture). Its diminished or negative value suggests upper airway obstruction (snoring, intubation with narrow endotracheal tube), and REM sleep; while its increased value >100% suggests bilateral diaphragmatic paralysis and respiratory muscle fatigue.

TCDNT (total compartmental displacement/ Tidal volume): It is a ratio of total excursions (motion) of the rib cage and abdominal compartment during inspiration irrespective to direction of the movement divided by tidal volume. The normal value is 1.00-1.20.

In fully synchronous respiration, TCD and VT are equal, so the ratio is to be 1.00. With asynchronous or paradoxical breathing, one compartment subtracts from the other such that TCD becomes greater than VT and hence ratio is <1.00. Its elevated value reflects paradoxical motion between RC and AB as

1.20-1.50: Common in stable COPD patients

1.50-2.24 found in COPD with respiratory failure and

>2, 50: usually found with obstructive apnoea and hypopnoea

Apnoea/Hypopnoea (A/H): It is computed by cessation of breathing from end of inspiration for at least 10 sec or tidal volume less than 100 ml and/or 25% of baseline VT for at least 10 sec. It is denoted by flat or nearly flat sum tracing on plot during A/H followed by PR% and duration in seconds at top of plot.

Hypopnoea (H): It is calculated as tidal breathing ranging from 25-45% of baseline VT for at least 10 sec. It is denoted as small v bars during hypopnoea followed by H at the top of plot.

PR (Phase relation): It is the percent of time during apnoea/hyponoea that rib cage (RC) and abdomen (AB) are moving in the same direction (in phase). Values of 98-99 suggests a central apnoea and <97 suggests an obstructive and/ or mixed apnoea.

Apart from above parameters varieties of instruments are being used to measure ventilation during sleep e.g. airflow and oxyhemoglobin saturation.

Airflow: It can be measured with pneumatachography, carbon dioxide analyzer and thermistor. A thermistor detects airflow by measuring the difference in temperature between expired and inspired air. It is well tolerated by sleeping subjects because it is small, light, and able to be attached unobtrusively. It produces small signals when there is no air flow. Nasal and oral airflow may be monitored separately by taping one thermistor to the skin above the upper lip and just below the nasal orifice, and another besides the mouth.

Oxyhemoglobin saturation: Arterial oxygen saturation can be measured non-invasively during sleep by pulse oxymetry.

HR (heart rate): Mean heart rate is recorded in beats per minute from pulse oximeter.

Snoring: Vibratophone is taped in place at side of patient's larynx. Its display indicates presence of snoring or other laryngeal sounds.

Percent activity: Actigraph is fastened on patient's wrist or ankle. Percent activity represents portion of time activity detected during mean epoch. It is printed out below % rib cage/VT display.

REFERENCES

1. Hutchinson J Lecture on vital statics, embracing an account of a new instrument for detecting the presence of disease in the system Lancet 1844; 2: 594-6
2. Cohn MA, Rao AS, Broudy M, Brich H The respiratory inductive plethysmograph: a new non-invasive monitor of respiration Bull Eur Physiopathol Resp 1982; 18: 643-58
3. Konno K, Mead J Measurement of he separate volume changes of rib cage and abdomen during breathing J Appl Physiol 1962; 22: 407-22
4. Tobin MI Noninvasive evaluation of respiratory movement. *in* Nochomovitz ML, Cherniack NS eds Non-invasive respiratory monitoring 1st edn, New York, Churchill Livingstone 1980; 39-57
5. Chadha TS, Watson H, Birch S, Jenouri G, Schrieder A, Cohn MA, Sackner MA Validation of respiratory inductive plethysmography using different calibration procedures Am Rev Respir Dis 1982; 125: 644-47
6. Milic-Emili J, Grumstein MM Drive and timing components of ventilation Chest 1976; 70: 131-33
7. Renners JE Analysis of ventilatory response Chest 1976; 70: 134-7
8. Tobin MJ, Chadha TS, Jenouri G, Birch SJ, Gazeroglu MD, Sackner MA Breathing patterns. 1 Diseased subjects Chest 1983; 64: 202-205

9. Hoover CF The diagnostic significance of inspiratory movements of he costal margins Am J Med Sci 1920; 159: 633-37

10. Ashutosh K, Gilbert R, Auchincloss JH, Peppi D Asynchronous breathing movements in patients with chronic obstructive pulmonary disease Chest 1978; 67: 555-57

11. Hira HS, Arora S, Chauhan MR Oxygen saturation, breathing pattrn and arrhythmias in patients of chronic obstructive pulmonary disease and bronchial asthma Lung India 1994; 17: 186-91

12. Roussos C, Fixley M, Gross D, Macklem PJ Fatigue of inspiratory muscles and their synergic behaviour J Appl Physiol 1979; 46: 897-904

13. Tobin MJ, Jenouri G, Birch S, lind B, Gonzales H, Ahmed T, Sackner MA Effect of positive end-expiratory pressure on breathing patterns of normal subjects and intubated patents with respiratory failure Crit Care Med 1983; 11: 859-67

14. Hira HS, Arora S Sleep apneasyndrome: An Indian experience Ind J Chest Dus All Sci 1995; 37: 119-125

15. Hira HS., Sharma R. Nocturnal Hypoxemia, Breathing abnormalities and Arrhythmias in patients of Kyphoscoliosis during sleep. JAPI 1997; 45 :12 - 14.

16. Hira HS, Arora S, Chauhan MR. Oxygen saturation, breathing pattern and arrhythmias in patients of chronic obstructive pulmonary disease and bronchial asthma during sleep. Lung India 1994; 12:186-191

17. Hira HS, Sharma RK. Study of oxygen saturation , breathing pattern and Arrhythmias in patients of interstitial lung disease during sleep. Ind J Chest Dis & Allied Sci 1997; 39 :157-162.

21
ARTERIAL BLOOD GASES

MAYUR H PATEL

Introduction

In humans, the acid-base homeostasis is tightly balanced by a series of interactions involving the lungs, the kidneys, and a complex system of buffers. Metabolic systems and bodily functions are optimal when pH is in the range of 7.35–7.45. Multiple homeostatic responses are activated if the pH deviates from the normal to restore normal acid-base status (1). To begin with, the buffer system will make an attempt to neutralize the derangement. If that fails the lungs make ventilatory adjustments and, finally kidneys will make alterations in acid excretion.

Arterial blood gases (ABG) is an important and frequently requested laboratory test in the critically ill patients. ABG is safe and easily obtainable at bedside (2), and it furnishes vital information regarding oxygenation, ventilation and acid-base status, which are closely interrelated physiological parameters, to maintain the pH homeostasis (3).

ABGs are invaluable in assessing the nature, progression and severity of respiratory and metabolic disturbances. Correct interpretation of ABG requires knowledge of patients' clinical status, therapy applied, and other data (e.g. mixed venous blood gas data, haemoglobin concentration, and cardiac output). A simple, consistent, stepwise approach can nearly always unravel acid-base disorders in the most complex of situations (4).

The measurement of ABG depends on various gas laws by Henry which pertain to laws governing rate of diffusion and dissolution of gases in liquids, pressures exerted by gases and relation of gas volumes with change of temperature respectively (5).

What are the indications for ABG?

ABG study in any of the following situations:

- In patients with an acute onset dyspnea
- In patients with unexplained changes in mental status
- For documenting and assessing the severity of respiratory failure
- For monitoring patients on mechanical ventilation and to assist in weaning
- In "high-risk" patients undergoing major surgery.

How to collect ABG?

The ideal artery for sampling for ABG should be large enough, superficial, situated away from important structures, and should be easily accessible with good collateral circulation. The radial artery meets all these criteria and is therefore preferred. It is better to cannulate the artery, if frequent sampling is required or if the patient has coagulopathy. The recommended radial artery technique is as follows (6) (Fig. 1):

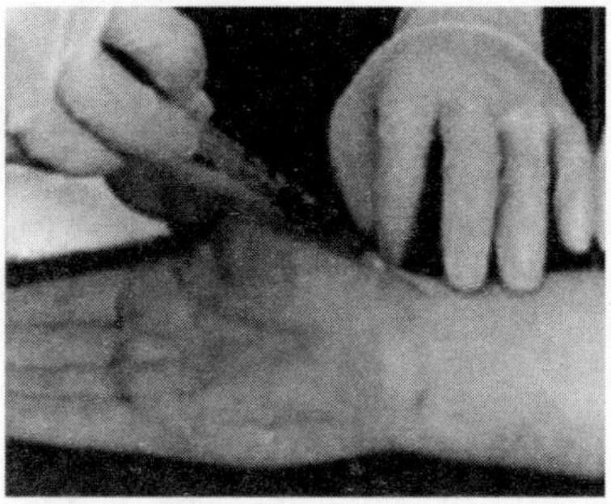

Fig. 1. Taking radial arterial blood sample.

1. Use local anaesthesia over the radial artery before puncture.
2. Use a 22-gauge needle with a preheparinised syringe.
3. Express the heparin from the syringe before taking the sample; adequate heparin will remain in the 0.2 ml dead space of the barrel and needle.
4. At least 3 ml of blood is required to avoid a dilution effect from the heparin.
5. Sample with more than fine air bubbles should be discarded. Air bubbles result in gas equilibration between the air and the arterial blood, lowering PCO_2 and increasing PO_2.
6. If the sample cannot be analysed quickly it should be cooled to 5°C immediately.

Currently, ABGs can be done by using 0.2 ml of nonheparinised blood into a cartridge (7), which when put into the ABG module gives results in 2 minutes. It is very useful in a busy ICU where multiple ABGs are necessary. In a whole-blood ABG analysis, oxygen saturation, bicarbonate and base excess or deficit are calculated numbers based on the measured pH, PO_2, and PCO_2, respectively (8).

By convention, ABG specimens are analysed at 37° C or any temperature that is entered corresponding to the patient's body temperature. As temperature drops, PCO_2 decreases while pH increases and vice versa. The recommendation is to utilize uncorrected values measured at 37 °C to guide management while keeping in mind the expected values that would correspond to the patient's temperature (8).

Analysis of ABG

Proper analysis of ABG gives valuable information in assessing, diagnosing and managing various critical illnesses. Following distinct processes should be evaluated on ABG:

1. Oxygenation
2. Alveolar ventilation
3. Acid-base status

Oxygenation

The function of cardiopulmonary system is to provide adequate oxygen to the tissues. The arterial oxygen tension (PO_2) can be affected by several factors:

a) As the age advances, the PO_2 decreases. A value below 80 mmHg at sea level in an adult patient breathing room air is defined as Hypoxemia, whereas Hypoxia is decrease in oxygen tension at tissue level.

b) The PO_2 is influenced by barometric pressure (Pb) and therefore by altitude.

c) The PO_2 proportionately increases with increase in fraction of inspired oxygen concentration (FiO_2). The rule of thumb is as follows: $PO_2 = FiO_2 \times 5$ (e.g. if a patient is breathing 50% FiO_2, then expected PaO_2 will be 50x5=250 mmHg). A PO_2 below this value suggests that the patient will be hypoxemic when he is breathing room air.

d) Haemoglobin (Hb) level. Oxygen is transported in combination with Hb and the relationship between PO_2 and Hb saturation with oxygen is defined by the oxyhemoglobin curve. If PO_2 falls below 60 mmHg, the Hb may still be 90% saturated. But with a drop from 60 to 40 mmHg, saturation falls steeply below 75% (9). This relationship is responsible for a fundamental goal in treating hypoxemia to get PO_2 above 60 mmHg.

Hypoxemia makes tissue hypoxia a distinct possibility. Hypoxemia is classified as (Table 1):

Table 1. Classification of Hypoxia

Value	Grade	Symptoms
PAO_2 60-79mmHg	Mild	May be asymptomatic
PAO_2 45-59mmHg	Moderate	Hypoxia is possible, leading to tachycardia, hypertension and cool extremities
PAO_2 mmHg	Severe	Hypoxia is <45 certain, leading to arrhythmias, brain damage

Once hypoxemia is diagnosed, probable causes should be considered, ruled out and correct therapy should be instituted. Common causes of hypoxemia are:

a) A decrease in FiO_2/Pb as in high altitude.

b) Hypoventilation is characterized by a rise in PCO_2 levels on ABG. It's common in patients with chronic obstructive pulmonary disease (COPD), disorders of central ventilatory control or respiratory neuromuscular disease. With supplemental oxygen, hypoxemia will be relieved but ventilation will not improve.

c) Ventilation-perfusion (V/Q) mismatch is characterized by increased perfusion relative to ventilation (Low V/Q). Seen commonly in patients with asthma, COPD or pulmonary fibrosis.

d) Shunt. Hypoxemia can also result if the venous blood bypasses the ventilated lung and reaches the systemic circulation without getting exposed to oxygen e.g. severe pneumonia, atelectasis or right-to-left intracardiac shunt. If such patients are given 100% oxygen, there will be a small rise in PO_2 indicating the presence of a shunt.

e) Diffusion defect.

Alveolar-arterial oxygen gradient (A-a gradient)

There are 2 types of respiratory failure: type I - hypoxemia without carbon dioxide retention and type II - where there is hypercapnia. Calculating the gradient in type II respiratory failure will determine whether the patient has associated lung disease or just reduced respiratory effort.

$(A\text{-}a)PO_2 = PAO_2/ - PaO_2$

$PAO_2/ = (Pb - PH_2O) \times FiO_2 - PAO_2//R$

Where Pb is barometric pressure (760 mmHg at sea level), PH_2O is water pressure, and R respiratory quotient (0.8 normally).

The $(A\text{-}a)PO_2$ is normal in patients who have hypoxemia secondary to decreased Pb or hypoventilation. Widened gradient is seen in patients who have structural lung disorders which reduces oxygen transfer.

Characteristically, patients with hypoventilation or V/Q mismatch show a 3-5 mmHg rise in PCO_2 for each 1% increment in FiO_2, whereas patients with a shunt show < 2 mmHg rise for each 1% increment in FiO_2. Ratio of $PAO_2//P_AO_2$ is an useful alternative to $(A\text{-}a)PO_2$ calculation as it is not affected by changes in FiO_2 (Table 2) (10).

Table 2. Guidelines for assessing hypoxemia

$(A\text{-}a)PO_2$ PAO_2/PAO_2		
5-20 0.75	Normal	
30-50	Low V/Q	0.65
>60 <0.55	Shunt	

Alveolar ventilation

Carbon-dioxide is a waste product of metabolism and is excreted by lungs, which is reflected by arterial CO_2 tension (PCO_2). The equation $PCO_2 = 0.86 \times VCO_2 / V_A$ expresses the quantity of CO_2 produced in body and its excretion through the lungs, where VCO_2 is the carbon-dioxide production per minute and V_A is the alveolar ventilation. The equation indicates an inverse relationship of $PaCO_2$ to V_A. Thus, PCO_2 is an ideal index for the assessment of alveolar ventilation. High PCO_2 (> 45 mmHg) indicates alveolar hypoventilation and low PCO_2 (< 35 mmHg) implies alveolar hyperventilation (3). Hypo or hypercapnia can be a feature in a patient who is mechanically ventilated. It could be due to improper setting of tidal volume and respiratory rate. Under this circumstances, ventilatory setting can be changed to achieve desired PCO_2 as per the following equation:

$$\text{Desired minute volume} = \frac{\text{Present minute vol x present } PCO_2}{\text{Desired } PCO_2}$$

Acid-base status

Correct interpretation of acid-base status is challenging. Various methods adopted in interpreting the acid-base status are simplistic explanations of dynamic complex processes going on in the body making all the calculations subject to error and merely approximations.

There are three methods of quantifying acid–base disorders: a) the physiological approach, b) the base-excess (or Copenhagen) approach, and c) the physicochemical approach (or the Stewart method)(11). The physiological approach is simple and follows step-wise method in the assessment.

All cellular and extracellular functions are altered if there is deviation of pH from the normal (7.35-7.45). Values less then <7.35 are termed Acidemia, whereas values more than >7.45 are referred to as Alkalemia. Disorders that lowers the pH to <7.35 is called acidosis, while disorders that increases the pH >7.45 is called alkalosis. The Henderson-Hasselbalch equation provides the basis for the relationship between the blood pH with metabolic and respiratory components (12):

$pH = 6.1 + \log ([HCO_3]/(0.03xPCO_2))$.

When the disorder is primarily due to a change in PCO_2, it is called 'respiratory' and if it is due to variation in HCO_3 levels, it is called 'metabolic'.

Clinical evaluation

Careful clinical evaluation can provide clues regarding the underlying acid–base disorder. Patient may present with symptoms like diarrhea and vomiting. Detailed history should be obtained regarding chronic medical conditions such as diabetes, heart, lung, liver, and kidney diseases. Also enquire regarding the current medications consumed by the patient (e.g. laxatives, diuretics, or metformin) which can affect acid-base status. Look for signs of intoxications causing acid-base disturbances (e.g. acetone foetor in diabetic ketoacidosis or alcohol, visual disturbances in methyl alcohol) (11).

On examination, it is necessary to look for signs of shock, signs of infection, altered mental status, tachypnoea, acidotic breathing, clubbing, cyanosis, etc.

Step-wise approach

Step 1 a. To validate the report check the pH

- Rationale – since pH, PCO_2 and PO_2 are directly measured and HCO_3 is a derived variable, it is possible that one of the electrodes is giving wrong reading.
- Check for the validity of ABG by the modified Henderson equation.

$$24 = \frac{H^+ \text{ x } HCO_3}{PCO_2}$$

- The hydrogen ion is calculated by subtracting the two digits after the decimal point of pH from 80, e.g., if the pH is 7.23 then $[H^+] = 80 - 23 = 57$
- Concentration of H^+ ion can be calculated from the following table 3:

Table 3. pH value and corresponding H+ ion concentration.

pH	H+	pH	H+
6.70	200	7.4	40
6.75	178	7.45	35
6.80	158	7.5	32
6.85	141	7.55	28
6.90	126	7.60	25
6.95	112	7.65	22
7.00	100	7.70	20
7.05	89	7.75	18
7.10	79	7.80	16
7.15	71	7.85	14
7.20	63	7.90	13
7.25	56	7.95	11
7.30	50	8.00	10
7.35	45		

Step 1 b. Check the pH

If pH is < 7.35, it indicates acidemia and if pH is > 7.45 it indicates alkalemia. A normal pH may actually be a clue to the existence of a mixed disorder and proceed to the next step.

Step 2. Check the PCO_2 and HCO_3

This step identifies the primary derangement and compensatory response.

A low pH associated with reduced PCO_2 and HCO_3 is consistent with metabolic acidosis.

A low pH associated with high PCO_2 and HCO_3 is consistent with respiratory acidosis.

A high pH associated with elevated PCO_2 and HCO_3 is consistent with metabolic alkalosis.

A high pH with reduced PCO_2 and HCO_3 is consistent with respiratory alkalosis.

In simple acid-base disorders (Table 4) (13), deviations in PCO_2 and HCO_3 are in the same direction.

Table 4. Simple acid-base disorders

Disorder	pH	PCO_2	HCO_3	Clinical examples
Metabolic acidosis	< 7.35	↓	↓	Lactic acidosis, renal failure, diabetic ketoacidosis, renal tubular acidosis
Respiratory acidosis	< 7.35	↑	↑	Laryngeal oedema, bronchospasm, emphysema, hypoventilation
Metabolic alkalosis	> 7.45	↑	↑	Vomiting, diuretics, Conn's syndrome, Cushing syndrome
Respiratory alkalosis	> 7.45	↓	↓	Congestive cardiac failure, raised intracranial pressure, sepsis

In mixed acid-base disorders deviations are in opposite directions (Table 5) (13).

Table 5. Mixed acid-base disorders

Disorder	pH	PCO_2	HCO_3	Clinical examples
Respiratory and metabolic acidosis	Very low	↑	Lower than expected	Cardiopulmonary arrest, cerebrovascular accident andrenal failure
Respiratory and metabolic alkalosis	Very high	↓	Higher than expected	Congestive cardiac failure and vomiting, diuretic therapyand liver failure
Metabolic acidosis and respiratory alkalosis	7.45	Lower than expected	↓	Salicylate overdose, septic shock, sepsis and renal failure
Metabolic alkalosis and respiratory acidosis	7.45	Higher than expected	↑	Diuretic therapy or vomiting and mphysema
Metabolic acidosis and metabolic alkalosis	7.45	→	→	Lactic acidosis or diabetic ketoacidosis and vomiting
Triple disorder: mixed metabolic acidosis and alkalosis plus respiratory alkalosis or acidosis	Variable	Variable	Variable	Renal failure, vomiting and congestive cardiac failure

Step 3. Calculate the compensation

The purpose of calculating the compensation is twofold: to identify mixed acid–base disorders, and to define the acuity of the disorder in the case of respiratory derangements.
Table 6 shows the adaptive responses to acid-base disorders (1, 13).

Table 6. Adaptive responses to acid-base disorders

Disorder	Rule of compensation	Limit of compensation
Metabolic acidosis	$PCO_2 = 1.25 \times HCO_3$ $PACO_2 = 1.5(HCO_3) + 8 \pm 2$	PCO_2 - 10–15 mmHg.
Metabolic alkalosis	$PCO_2 = 0.6 \times HCO_3$ $PCO_2 = 0.9(HCO_3) + 9 \pm 2$	PCO_2 - 55 mmHg.
Respiratory acidosis		
Acute	- HCO_3 increases 1 mEq/L (0.25–1.75) for every 10mmHg increase in PCO_2. - pH decreases 0.08 for every 10 mEq/L increase in HCO_3.	HCO_3 - 30 mmol/lTime to completion →5 - 10 min

Chronic	HCO_3 increases 4 mEq/L for every 10 mmHg increase in PCO_2 (±4).	HCO_3 - 45 mmol/lTime to completion → 3 - 5 days
Respiratory alkalosis		
Acute	HCO_3 drops 1 to 3.5 mEq/L for every 10 mmHg drop inPCO_2.	HCO_3 - 17-18 mmol/lTime to completion → 5 - 10 min
Chronic	HCO_3 drops 2–5 mEq/L for every 10 mmHg drop in PCO_2.	HCO_3 - 12-14 mmol/lTime to completion → 2 - 3 days

Step 4: Calculate the anion gap (AG).

The AG helps in evaluating the metabolic component of an acid–base disorder. To maintain electroneutrality, the sum of total circulating cations and anions must be equal. The AG is useful to uncover the actual anions elevated in the blood. The three ions with the highest plasma concentrations are used to calculate the excess of "unmeasured anions" that constitutes the "anion gap," and is calculated by the following formula (11):

Na – (Cl + HCO_3). A normal AG is 8-12 mEq.

Albumin is the major source of an unmeasured anion. For every drop in albumin by 1gm, AG increases by 2.5. Adjusted AG for drop in albumin or

Corrected AG = AG + 2.5 (4.5-Albumin) (8).

Deviations in the AG

Reflect either errors in the measurements of its constituents or changes in the concentrations of unmeasured cations and/or anions (14).

Low or Negative AG

Low AG most commonly indicate laboratory error or hypoalbuminemia but can denote the presence of a paraproteinemia or intoxication with lithium, bromide, or iodide.

A negative AG is caused by pseudohyperchloremia in bromide or iodide intoxication (11).

Delta Gap (Gap)

Delta gap is the comparison between change () in the AG and the change () in bicarbonate (HCO_3).

Gap = AG- (HCO_3)

Delta ratio, defined as **AG: HCO_3** is usually 1:1 in patients with an uncomplicated high AG acidosis. A value below 1:1 suggests a combined high and normal AG acidosis. A value above 2:1 suggests a combined metabolic alkalosis and a high AG acidosis (14).

Limitations of AG

- There is variability in the Ä AG/ Ä HCO_3 undercutting the ability to use this ratio alone to detect complex acid-base disorders
- Needs adjustment for hypoalbuminemia
- AG is less sensitive to pick up Lactic Acidosis (14).

Osmolar Gap

Osmolality = 2 x S. Na x glucose/18 + BUN/2.8

If the calculated osmolality differs from the measured osmolality by 15 mosm/kg H_2O, this is called as osmolar gap. High osmolar gap metabolic acidosis is seen in methanol and ethylene glycol intoxication. High serum osmolar gap without acidosis is seen in mannitol infusion and ethanol ingestion (15).

Metabolic Acidosis

Results due to following mechanisms: Increased Acid (H^+) Generation, Increased Loss of HCO_3 and Diminished Renal Acid (H^+) Excretion.

Depending on the AG, metabolic acidosis can be divided into 2 types:

1. High Anion Gap Metabolic Acidosis - (HAGMA)
2. Normal Anion Gap Metabolic Acidosis - (NAGMA)

HAGMA

An elevated AG is a relatively common occurrence, particularly among critically ill patients. It can happen due to increased acid production, decreased acid excretion or the combination of the two. The causes of HAGMA can be remembered by mnemonic - GOLDMARK (16):

G - Glycols
O - 5 Oxyproline
L - L- Lactate
D - D-Lactate
M - Methanol
A - Aspirin
R - Renal failure
R - Rhabdomyolysis
K - Ketoacidosis

NAGMA

Also called hyperchloremic metabolic acidosis. It occurs when the decrease in HCO_3 ions corresponds with an increase in chloride ions to retain electroneutrality. NAGMA can occur in following conditions: a) gastrointestinal loss of HCO_3 (e.g., because of diarrhea or ureteral diversion), b) renal loss of HCO_3 (renal tubular acidosis), and c) iatrogenic due to infusion of large volumes of normal saline (11). NAGMA can further classified as per serum potassium levels (Table 7).

Table 7. Classification of normal AG metabolic acidosis (13).

With hypokalaemia	With normo- or hyperkalaemia
Diarrhoea	Early uremic acidosis
Renal tubular acidosis type 1 and 2	Aldosterone deficiency or resistance
Ureteral diversion to intestine	Obstructive uropathy
Recovery phase of ketoacidosis	Hyperalimentation (lysine, histidine, arginine HCl)
Carbonic anhydrase inhibition	Ingestion/infusion of HCl, NH_4Cl

Urine Anion Gap (UAG)

UAG = (Na+K-Cl)

Urine AG is an indirect estimate of the urine NH_4 excretion.

It is typically negative in patients with NAGMA secondary to diarrhoea.

It is positive in renal failure, distal renal tubular acidosis, or hypoaldosteronism (17).

UAG is unreliable when patient is polyuric, urine pH is > 6.5 and when U Na is < 20 mEq as acidification of urine needs distal delivery of Na (11).

Metabolic Alkalosis

Results from an increase in bicarbonate production, a decrease in bicarbonate excretion, or a loss of hydrogen ions. Any history of excessive vomiting or diarrhoea, recently added or increased dosages of diuretics, recent history of surgery that required nasogastric tube insertion may lead the clinician to a diagnosis of metabolic alkalosis. A bicarbonate level higher than 30 mmol/L in association with hypokalemia is pathognomonic for metabolic alkalosis (18).

Urine chloride concentration (U Cl) is a useful tool in the diagnosis of metabolic alkalosis. In chloride-responsive (U Cl < 10), the alkalosis is corrected by volume expansion using saline. Table 8 lists the causes of metabolic alkalosis (18).

Table 8. Causes of metabolic alkalosis

Chloride depletion syndrome	***Mineralocorticoid excess***
Gastrointestinal fluid losses Vomiting Nasogastric suctionCongenital chloridorrhea Villous adenomasHigh-volume ileostomy losses **Renal losses** Diuretic administration Impairment of Chloride-linked sodium transport Bartter syndrome Gitelman syndrome	Primary hyperaldosteronism Glucocorticoid-remediable aldosteronism Secondary hyperaldosteronism (high renin syndrome) Renal artery stenosis Accelerated hypertension Renin-secreting tumor
Apparent mineralocorticoid excess Syndromes	***Other causes***
Liddle syndrome 11b-Hydroxysteroid dehydrogenase deficiency Fludrocortisone administration	Alkali intake or administration Milk alkali syndrome Severe potassium depletion

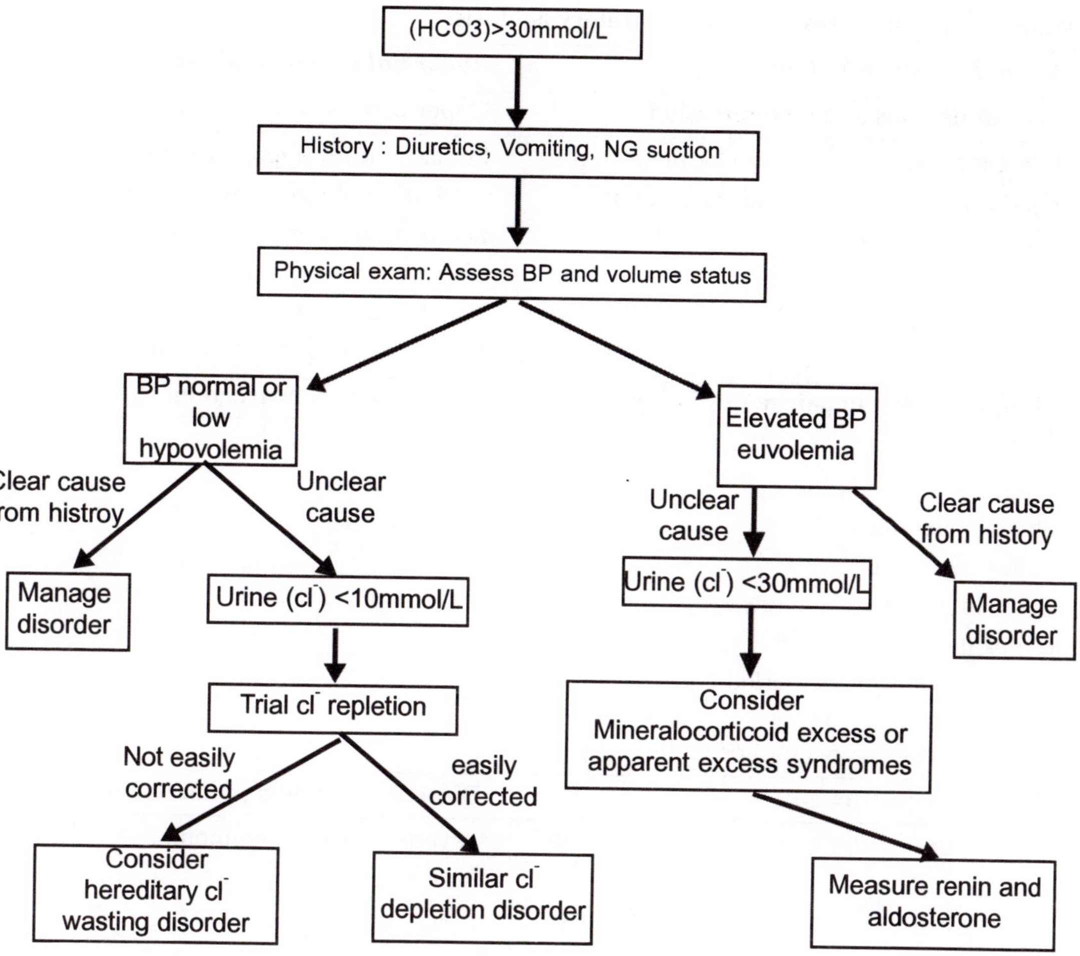

Fig. 1. An algorithmic approach to the workup and metabolic alkalosis. BP, blood pressure; NG, nasogastric (18).

Respiratory Acidosis

Respiratory disorders are common in ICU and can make the interpretation of ABG complex due to co-existing metabolic disorders. It is initiated by an increase in PCO_2 and reflects a decrease in alveolar ventilation. Increased production of CO_2 can cause respiratory acidosis in patients with marked limitation in pulmonary reserve or those receiving constant mechanical ventilation.

The major threat to life from CO_2 retention in subjects breathing room air (FiO_2, 21%) is the associated obligatory hypoxemia, as indicated by the alveolar gas equation:

$P_AO_2 = 150 - 1.25 \times PCO_2$, where PAO2 is alveolar oxygen tension. Thus, in the absence of supplemental oxygen, it is not possible for PCO_2 to reach values much higher than 80 mm Hg while the level of PO_2, is still compatible with life. Extreme hypercapnia can only be seen in subjects receiving oxygen supplementation (19).

Respiratory acidosis elicits adaptive increments in plasma HCO_3 concentration that attenuate the impact of hypercapnia. The secondary physiologic response to respiratory acidosis can be acute or chronic as described above in Table 6. Table 9 and 10 lists the causes of respiratory acidosis (19).

Table 9: lists the causes of acute respiratory acidosis:

Normal airway and lungs	*Abnormal airway and lungs*
Central nervous system depression	**Upper airway obstruction**
General anesthesiaSedative overdose Head trauma Cerebrovascular accident Central sleep apnea Encephalitis Cerebral edema Brain tumor	Coma induced hypopharyngeal obstruction Aspiration of foreign body or vomitus Laryngospasm or angioedema Obstructive sleep apnea Inadequate laryngeal intubation Laryngeal obstruction post intubation
Neuromuscular impairment	**Lower airway obstruction**
High spinal cord injury Guillain-Barre syndrome Status epilepticus Botulism, tetanus Crisis in myasthenia gravis Hypokalemic myopathy Familial hypokalemic periodic paralysis Drugs or toxic agents (curare, succinylcholine, aminoglycosides,organophosphates)	Generalized bronchospasm Severe asthma Bronchiolitis
Ventilatory restriction	**Disorders involving pulmonary alveoli**
Rib fractures with flail chest Pneumothorax Hemothorax Impaired diaphragmatic function	Severe bilateral pneumonia Acute respiratory distress syndrome Severe pulmonary edema
Iatrogenic events	**Pulmonary perfusion defect**
- Misplacement or displacement of airway cannula during anesthesia or mechanical ventilation - Bronchoscopy associated hypoventilation or respiratory arrest - Increased CO_2 production with constant mechanical ventilation	Cardiac arrest Severe circulatory failure Massive pulmonary thromboembolism Fat or air embolism

Table 10 lists the causes of chronic respiratory acidosis:

Normal airway and lungs	*Abnormal airway and lungs*
Central nervous system depression	**Upper airway obstruction**
Sedative overdose Methadone/heroin addiction Primary alveolar hypoventilation Obesity-hypoventilation syndrome Brain tumor Bulbar poliomyelitis	Tonsillar and peritonsillar hypertrophy Paralysis of vocal cords Tumor of the cords or larynx Airway stenosis post prolonged intubation Thymoma, aortic aneurysm
Neuromuscular impairment	**Lower airway obstruction**
Poliomyelitis Multiple sclerosis Muscular dystrophy Amyotrophic lateral sclerosis Diaphragmatic paralysis Myxedema Myopathic disease	Chronic obstructive lung disease (bronchitis, bronchiolitis, bronchiectasis, emphysema)
Ventilatory restriction	**Disorders involving pulmonary alveoli**
Kyphoscoliosis, spinal arthritis Obesity Fibrothorax Hydrothorax Impaired diaphragmatic function	Severe chronic pneumonitis Diffuse infiltrative disease Interstitial fibrosis

Respiratory Alkalosis

Respiratory alkalosis is initiated by a reduction in PCO_2 and reflects an increase in alveolar ventilation. It elicits adaptive decrements in plasma HCO_3 concentration, which attenuates the impact of hypocapnia. The secondary physiologic response to respiratory alkalosis can be acute or chronic as described above in Table 6. Table 11 lists the causes of respiratory alkalosis.

Table 11: lists the causes of respiratory alkalosis.

Hypoxemia or tissue hypoxia	Central nervous system stimulation
Decreased inspired O_2 tension High altitude Bacterial or viral pneumonia Aspiration of food, foreign body, or vomitus Laryngospasm Drowning Cyanotic heart disease	Voluntary Pain Anxiety Psychosis Fever Subarachnoid hemorrhage Cerebrovascular accident

Severe anemia Left shift deviation of HbO_2 curve Hypotension Severe circulatory failure Pulmonary embolism	Meningoencephalitis Tumor Trauma
Stimulation of chest receptors	**Drugs or hormones**
Pneumonia Asthma Pneumothorax Hemothorax Flail chest Infant or adult respiratory distress syndrome Cardiac failure Noncardiogenic pulmonary edema Pulmonary embolism Interstitial lung disease	Nikethamide, ethamivan Doxapram Xanthines Salicylates Catecholamines Angiotensin II Vasopressor agents Progesterone Medroxyprogesterone Dinitrophenol Nicotine
	Miscellaneous
	Pregnancy Sepsis Hepatic failure Mechanical hyperventilation Heat exposure Recovery form metabolic acidosis

PEARLS

- Recognition and appropriate management of acid-base disorders requires a systematic approach.
- Information obtained from the history and physical examination is essential for correct interpretation of laboratory data.
- The stepwise approach comprises the following:
  - Check the pH: pH <7.35 indicates acidemia; pH >7.45 indicates alkalemia; normal or near normal pH may indicate mixed acidosis and alkalosis
  - Check for the primary disorder and compensatory response by examining the PCO_2 and HCO_3, deviations are in the same direction in simple disorders, but in opposite directions in mixed disorders
  - Check the serum electrolytes and anion gap; calculate the delta ratio if Ä AG and Ä HCO_3 appear discordant
  - Define the acid-base disorder and request further testing if required, e.g. toxic screen, osmolal gap, lactate, ketones.
- Measurement of urine electrolytes and calculation of anion and osmolal gaps may be helpful in the differential diagnosis of metabolic alkalosis and normal anion gap metabolic acidosis.

REFERENCES

1. Alshehri AA, Alyahya MA, Alsolamy SJ. Acid-Base Disturbance: A Comprehensive Flowchart-based Diagnostic Approach. Emergency Med 2015; 4:245. doi:10.4172/2165-7548.1000245.
2. Petty TL, Bigelow B, Levine B. The simplicity and safety of arterial puncture. JAMA 1966; 195:185.
3. Barthwal MS. Analysis of Arterial Blood Gases — A Comprehensive Approach. JAPI 2004; 52: 573.
4. Ansari KA, Patel MH. Arterial Blood Gas Analysis. In Pulmonary Function Tests in Health and Disease. P S Shankar (Ed), Second edn, Mumbai The National Book Depot 2007; 250.
5. Geha DG. Blood gas monitoring. In "Monitoring in Anesthesia and Critical Care Medicine". Ed. Blitt CD. New York, Churchill Livingstone. 1985; 291.
6. Williams AJ. Assessing and interpreting arterial blood gases and acid-base balance. BMJ 1998; 317:1213.
7. www.abbottpointofcare.com/en-in/
8. Al-Khadra E. Disorders of the Acid–Base Status. In Pediatric Nephrology in the ICU. Kiessling SG, Jens G, Michael JGS (Eds.). 2009; 19.
9. Miller RD, Pardo MC. Basics of Anesthesia. Philadelphia: Elsevier. 2011; 519:56.
10. Peris LV, Boix JH, Salom JV, et al. Clinical use of the arterial/alveolar oxygen tension ratio. Crit Care Med. 1983; 11:888.
11. Berend K, Devries APJ, Gans ROB. Physiological Approach to Assessment of Acid–Base Disturbances. N Eng J Med. 2014; 371:1434.
12. Ayers P, Warrington L. Diagnosis and treatment of simple acid-base disorders. Nutr Clin Pract. 2008; 23:122.
13. Oosthuizen NM. Approach to acid-base disorders – a clinical chemistry perspective. CME. 2012; 30:230.
14. Kraut JA, Madias NE. Serum anion gap: its uses and limitations in clinical medicine. Clin J Am Soc Nephrol 2007; 2:162.
15. Lynd LD, Richardson KJ, Purssell RA, et al. An evaluation of the osmole gap as a screening test for toxic alcohol poisoning. BMC Emerg Med. 2008; 8:5. doi:10.1186/1471-227X-8-5.
16. Mehta AN, Emmett JB, Emmett M. GOLD MARK: an anion gap mnemonic for the 21st century. The Lancet. 2008; 372:892.
17. Reddy P, Mooradian AD. Clinical utility of anion gap in deciphering acid-base disorders. Int J Clin Pract 2009; 63:1516.
18. Soifer JT, Kim HT. Approach to Metabolic Alkalosis. Emerg Med Clin N Am.2014; 32: 453.
19. Madias NE, Adrogué HJ: Respiratory Alkalosis and Acidosis. In: The Kidney: Physiology and Pathophysiology. DW Seldin, G Giebisch (eds). Third edin, Philadelphia, Lippincott Williams &Wilkins 2000: 2131-2166.
20. Stewart PA: Modern quantitative acid–base chemistry. Can J Physiol Pharm 1983; 61:1444.
21. Adrogué HJ, Gennari FJ, Galla JH, Madias NE. Assessing acid-base disorders. Kidney Int 2009; 76:1239.

22
ALVEOLAR-ARTERIAL GRADIENT

ANAND SARAF / SALIL BENDRE

Definition

Alveolar-arterial (A-a)gradient is a measure of difference between the alveolar concentration of oxygen and arterial concentration of oxygen. It helps to assess the integrity of alveolar capillary unit. Also it is used to diagnosed the source of hypoxemia.(1). Alveolar oxygen is termed as PAO2 and arterial oxygen is termed as PaO2.

A normal A-a gradient for young adult non - smoker is 5-10 mm Hg. However it increases with age. For every 10 years person has lived, expected to increase in A-a gradient by 1 mmHg. Estimate of normal A-a gradient less than [age in years /4] +. 4... hence for example a 50 years old should have an A-a gradient less than 16.5.

After calculating the A-a gradient and determining if it is elevated or normal, we can evaluate several causes of hypoxia.(2).

For example,

1) In condition of high altitude or hypoventilation in which the lung parenchyma is normal, the A- a gradient should be within normal limits. Pao2 low is only because PAo2 is low.

2) In contrast in person with diffusion defects, ventilation(V)-perfusion(Q) mismatch, or right to left shunting, oxygen is not effectively transferred from the alveoli to blood and results in an elevated A-a gradient.

The alveolar to arterial difference of oxygen depends on variables like ventilation, cardiac output ,respiratory exchange ratio and arterial PO2. The arterial PO2 itself depends on ventilation to perfusion ratio, pulmonary shunt, and metabolic status of the patient. When the alveolar –ventilation is normal, the A-a gradient reflects gas exchange abnormalities and when alveolar –ventilation is increased ,A-a gradient can increase because of decrease in PaCO2. The factors that alters A-a oxygen difference were investigated in pulmonary diseases such as pulmonary embolism, lung fibrosis and chronic obstructive lung disease (3).

Equation(5)

The equation for calculating the A-a gradient is:
A-a gradient = PAO2 – PaO2

Where, PAO2 =alveolar PO2 (which is calculated from the alveolar gas equation)

PAO2= FiO2 (P atm – P H2O) – PaCO2/0.8
FiO2 (Patm – P H2O) is termed as PiO2 which is inspired partial pressure of oxygen.

If patient is breathing room air at sea level the equation can be simplified to:

PAO2 = (760 MMHG-47 MMHG) X 0.21-PaCO2/0.8
= 150MMHG –PaCO2/0.8(at sea level)

[Remark - at sea level, on room air, the (P atm – P water) x Fio2 is 149.7 mmHg (approx 150mmgh), we don't need to calculate this every time].

In above equation 0.8 is a respiratory quotient, which is defined as the ratio of volume of carbon dioxide evolved to that of oxygen consumed by an organism, tissue, or cell in given time. When RQ is used In mathematical calculation there are only 3 options to use as there are only couple of different fuel sources. 2 options are fatty acid and glucose. If cells are using exclusively glucose for energy production,1 molecule of CO2 is created for each oxygen burn, so RQ is 1. If cells are using fatty acids for energy production, -for every 10 oxygens consumed ,cells make 7 CO2 ,so RQ is 0.7. At some circumstances, cells are uses mix of glucose and fatty acids at the time. Hence 8 CO2 produced for every oxygen consumed, and RQ is 0.8.

Hence for calculations,

1) If patient is receiving an IV glucose solution, we will use RQ as 1.0
2) If the patient is hypoglycemic, or diabetic and relying on fatty acid metabolism, we will use RQ as 0.7.
3) And if there is nothing ,assume that the RQ is 0.8.

hence in equation if we use above values,

$PAO2 = FiO2 \ (Patm - PH2O) - PaCO2/RQ$
$= 149.7 - [40/0.8] = 99.7$ MMHG

And PaO2 is calculated from the ABG. There will be a decline in PaO2 with increase In age. This decrease in PaO2 with increase in age is most likely due to increase in V/Q mismatch.

Hence in its expanded form,

A-a gradient

= (FiO2 (P atm-P H2O)-PaCO2/0.8)- PaO2.
= 99.7 – PaO2

Causes of hypoxia

Causes of hypoxia differentiated by A-a gradient

A) Increased A-a Gradient

a) Right to left intrapulmonary shunt (due to fluid filled alveoli)
  1) Congestive cardiac failure
  2) Adult respiratory distress syndrome (ARDS)
  3) Lobar pneumonia

b) V/Q mismatch (due to lung dead space)
  1) pulmonary embolism
  2) atelectasis
  3) pneumonia
  4) Obstructive lung disease (Asthma, COPD)
  5) pneumothorax

c) alveolar hypoventilation
  1) interstitial lung disease

B) Normal A-a gradient

a) Hypoventilation
  1) Neuromuscular disorders
  2) Central nervous system disorder

b) Low inspired FIO2 (e.g. high altitude)

Limitations

- Gradient varies with age and FiO2:
  - FiO2 (0.21) –7 mmHg in young ,14 mmHg in elderly
  - FiO2 (1.0) –31 mmHg in young ,56 mmHg in elderly
- For every decade a person has lived, their A-a gradient is expected to increase by 1 mmHg - a conservative estimate of normal A-a gradient is < [age in years/4] + 4.
- An exaggerated FiO2 dependence in intrapulmonary shunt and even more so in V/Q mismatch.

Alveolar air equation

It is the method for calculating partial pressure of alveolar gas (PAO2).

Equation to calculate.

Significance

Partial pressure in O2 in alveoli, used to determine alveolar O2 tension to calculate.

PA-a02 gradient, a/A ratio and % shunt (7).

Uneven distribution of Gas in acute respiratory distress (8)

The study is used to assess the volume of gas being poorly ventilated or non ventilated in lungs of patient with acute respiratory distress syndrome.

Method -A study was performed of 25 sedated and paralysed ARDS patients, mechanically ventilated with a positive end-expiratory pressure (PEEP) of 5 cmH_2O in intensive care unit of hospital. The volume of poorly ventilated or non-ventilated gas was assumed to correspond to a difference between the ventilated gas volume, determined as the end-expiratory lung volume by rebreathing of Sulphur hexafluoride ($EELV_{SF6}$), and the total gas volume, calculated from computed tomography images in the end-expiratory position ($EELV_{CT}$). The methods used were validated by similar measurements in 20 healthy subjects in whom no poorly ventilated or non-ventilated gas is expected to be found. Study found that $EELV_{SF6}$ was 66% of $EELV_{CT}$, corresponding to a mean difference of 0.71 litre. $EELV_{SF6}$ and $EELV_{CT}$ were significantly correlated. In the healthy subjects, the two methods yielded almost identical results. So the conclusion is about one-third of the total pulmonary gas volume seems poorly ventilated or non-ventilated in sedated and paralysed ARDS patients when mechanically ventilated with a PEEP of 5 cmH_2O. Uneven distribution of ventilation due to airway closure and/or obstruction is likely to be involved.

REFERENCES

1) Logan, Carolynn M.; Rice, M. Katherine (1987). Logan's Medical and Scientific Abbreviations. Philadelphia: J. B. Lippincott Company. p. 4. .

2) Riley RL, Lilienthal JL Jr, Proemmel DD, et al: On the determination of the physiologically effective pressures of oxygen and carbon dioxide in alveolar air.

3) Fenn WO, Rahn H, Otis AB: A theoretical study of the composition of alveolar air at altitude. Am J Physiol 1946; 146:637-653

4) Maya Martinez M, Carrion Valero F, Diaz Lopez J, Marin Pardo J. [Barometric pressure and respiratory quotient for estimating the alveolar-arterial oxygen gradient]. An Med Interna. 2000;17(5):243-6

5) Kanber GJ, King FW, Eshchar YR, et. al. The alveolar-arterial oxygen gradient in young and elderly men during air and oxygen breathing. Am Rev Respir Dis. 1968;97(3):376-81.

6) Mellemgaard K. The alveolar-arterial oxygen difference: its size and components in normal man. Acta Physiol Scand. 1966 ;67(1):10-20.

7) Rodenstein DO, Stanescu DC: Reassessment of lung volume measurement by helium dilution and by body plethysmography in chronic air-flow obstruction. Am Rev Respir Dis 1982; 126: 1040-1044.

8) Story DA. Alveolar oxygen partial pressure, alveolar carbon dioxide partial pressure, and the alveolar gas equation.Anesthesiology. 1996 ;;84(4):1011.

9) Stein PD, Goldhaber SZ, Henry JW. Alveolar-arterial oxygen gradient in the assessment of acute pulmonary embolism. Chest. 1995 ;107(1):139-43.

23

BRONCHOPROVOCATION TESTS

V. K. VIJAYAN

Introduction

Bronchial hyperresposiveness (BHR) is an exaggerated bronchoconstrictive reaction of airway smooth muscles resulting in airway narrowing on exposure to various stimuli that do not provoke such a reaction in normal subjects (1-3). Both genetic and environmental factors are involved in the pathogenesis of bronchial hyperresponsiveness (4). In addition to allergens and certain industrial chemicals, viral infections of the respiratory tract play an important role in the development, maintenance and exacerbation of bronchial hyperresponsiveness. Bronchial hyperresponsiveness has been found to be associated with airway inflammation (1). Inflammatory cells such as macrophages, eosinophils and mast cells play an important role in the pathogenesis of BHR. Although many mediators have been implicated, platelet activating factor (PAF) is the only mediator known to cause a sustained increase in bronchial hyperresponsiveness (2). Neural control that includes cholinergic, adrenergic and non-adrenergic non-cholinergic (NANC) mechanisms also contributes to bronchial hyper-responsiveness (2). In the general population, bronchial hyperresponsiveness to histamine or methacholine has been reported in 15.9 to 33% of children and in 10.5 to 39.4% of adults (1).

Airway hyperresponsiveness is the fundamental abnormality in patients with asthma and chronic airflow obstruction. Studies have demonstrated that there is an increased bronchial hyperresponsiveness in family members of asthmatic subjects even if they do not demonstrate overt clinical disease **(5).** Airway hyperresponsiveness also has a deleterious effect on airflow obstruction especially in smokers. Although the severity of asthma and chronic airflow obstruction is generally assessed from history taking, physical examination and severity of airflow obstruction measured by forced expiratory volume in one second (FEV1), measurement of airway hyperactivity may be an useful adjunct to estimate the severity of disease and the necessity for treatment.(3).

Bronchoprovocative tests

Bronchoprovocative tests (BPT) is used in research studies and in clinical diagnosis of patients with variable airways obstruction (7). BPT as a diagnostic procedure in asthma is required in those patients with atypical symptoms without otherwise documented variable airway obstruction (8). Since airway hyper-responsiveness is also associated with chronic obstructive pulmonary disease (COPD), a positive BPT cannot be used to differentiate it from asthma (9) and currently there are no challenging agents that can differentiate asthma from COPD. Serial measurements of BPT are also useful to monitor any aggravation of responsiveness following exposure to sensitizing agents and also to document improvement after the treatment (10, 11).

Bronchial hyper-responsiveness is measured by observing the change in airway caliber after inhalation of a broncho-constrictor stimulus. Bronchial challenge tests (BCTs) have been found to be accurate, safe and reproducible and can be done in children and adults (12). BCTs are performed by the inhalation of a broncho-constrictor substance followed by noting the changes in lung function especially forced expiratory volume in one second (FEV1). The fall in FEV1 from the basal measurement is calculated and the test is terminated when there is a fall in FEV1 between 15 and 20% from the baseline. The concentration or dose is calculated to obtain Provocative Concentration (PC) or Provocative Dose (PD).

There are certain oral/inhaled medications which can influence the bronchial responsiveness and these medications should be withheld before performing the BPT. These medications include short-acting (salbutamol and terbutaline), medium-acting (ipratropium and theophylline) and long-acting (formoterol, salmeterol and tiotropium) bronchodilators and should be withheld for 8, 24 and 48 hours respectively (13). The absolute and relative contraindications for bronchial challenge tests are listed in Table 1 (13).

Table 1 :

Absolute and relative contra-indications of BPT

Absolute contra-indications:

1. Severe airway obstruction at base line (FEV1< 50% predicted or <1.0 litre in adults).
2. Recent myocardial infarction (< 3months),
3. Recent cerebrovascular accident (< 3 months),
4. Uncontrolled hypertension (systolic BP >200 mm Hg or diastolic BP >100 mm Hg).
5. Known aortic aneurysm

Relative contra-indications:

1. Spirometry induced airway obstruction,
2. Moderate airflow limitation (FEV1 < 60% predicted value or <1.5 L)
3. Inability to perform acceptable quality spirometry
4. Recent upper respiratory tract infections (< 2 weeks),
5. During exacerbations of asthma,
6. Pregnancy
7. Nursing mothers
8. Epilepsy requiring drug treatment
9. Current use of cholinesterase inhibitors for myasthenia gravis

Informed consent should be obtained from each patient prior to carrying out BPT. Even though challenge tests done in carefully standardized manner are safe, the tests should be performed in a laboratory manned by trained medical personnel and technologists who have experience in treating acute bronchoconstriction and equipped with appropriate cardiopulmonary resuscitation equipment to treat severe bronchoconstriction. The important medications that should be available in the laboratory include epinephrine and atropine for subcutaneous injection and salbutamol and ipratropium for inhalation using metered dose inhalers. Uninterrupted supply of oxygen should be available. The laboratory should also be equipped with a stethoscope, sphygmomanometer, pulse oximeter and a small volume nebulizer. The patient should not be left unattended till the entire procedure including observation period following the test.

Bronchial challenge can be done with stimuli that are classified as direct and indirect stimuli. Pharmacological agents (e.g. methacholine and histamine) are direct stimuli acting directly on the bronchial smooth muscle (BSM) receptors causing it to contract. Indirect stimuli (e.g. exercise) cause the release of mediators such as prostaglandins, leukotriene and histamine locally in the airways and these mediators act on BSM receptors to cause contraction (14). The important direct and indirect stimuli that can be used for bronchial challenge tests are listed in Table 2 (12).

Table 2 :

Direct and indirect stimuli used for bronchial challenge tests

Direct stimuli

1. Methacholine
2. Histamine
3. Acetyl choline
4. Carbachol
5. Prostaglandin D2
6. Leukotriene C4/D4/E4

Indirect stimuli

1. Hypertonic aerosols (Hypertonic saline and Mannitol)
2. Hypotonic saline
3. Exercise
4. Eucapneic Voluntary Hypopnea (EVH)
5. Bradykinin
6. Adenosine
7. Propranolol
8. Metabisulfite
9. Tachykinins

Bronchial challenge tests with direct stimuli such as methacholine and histamine are very sensitive, but the specificity is low. As a result a positive test by direct stimuli does not confirm a diagnosis of asthma and a negative test rules out asthma (12). The indirect stimuli have a higher specificity for identifying patients with active asthma. The main indications for a BPT are to confirm the diagnosis of asthma, exercise-induced bronchoconstriction, to investigate cough-variant asthma and occupational asthma. The indications for BCT are given in Table 3 (12, 13).

Table 3:

Indications for bronchial challenge tests

1. Confirmation of the diagnosis of bronchial asthma
2. Confirmation of the diagnosis of exercise-induced bronchoconstriction
3. Investigation of cough-variant asthma
4. Identification and evaluation of the response and efficacy of drugs like anti-inflammatory drugs
5. Collection of sputum
6. Identification of those who may experience bronchospasm while diving with self-contained underwater breathing apparatus (SCUBA)
7. Clearance of unwanted secretions
8. Differentiation of asthma from chronic airflow limitation
9. Evaluation of elite level asthma

Certain medications/items have to be withheld prior to challenge testing. These medication/items and the time period for which each should be withheld are listed in Table 4 (13).

Table 4:

Medicines/Items that decrease bronchial responsiveness

Medicines/Items	Withdrawal period
Inhaled medications	
1. Short acting bronchodilators	8 hrs.
2. Medium acting bronchodilators	24 hrs.
3. Long acting bronchodilators	48 hrs.
Oral bronchodilators	
1.Theophylline	12 hrs.
2. Intermediate acting theophylline	24 hrs.
3. Long acting theophylline	48 hrs.

4. Standard α_2 agonists	12 hrs.
5. Long-acting α_2 agonists	24 hrs.
Cromolyn sodium	8 hrs.
Cetrizine	3 days
Leukotriene modifiers	24 hrs.
Coffee, tea, cola drinks	On the day of the study

I. Methacholine challenge test

BPT can be done either with methacholine or histamine. Methacholine is usually used for challenge testing and it is a dry crystalline powder. Since the pH of methyl choline is stable, there is no need for a buffered diluent. Sterile normal saline (0.9% sodium chloride) with or without 0.4% phenol can be used as the diluent (13). As methacholine is highly hygroscopic, it must be stored in a dry container in a freezer. Methacholine solutions should be labeled with the concentration of methacholine. Standardized solutions of histamine are made from histamine triphosphate powder and phosphate-buffered saline (PBS). PBS is used as a diluent because buffered solution of histamine becomes acid at higher concentrations and this may alter the response of the airways (13). Both histamine and methacholine solutions should be stored in dark at -4° C and both are stable at this temperature for three months.

a. Methacholine challenge protocols

Two dosing protocols are commonly used for bronchial challenge testing. These are the 2-minute tidal breathing method and the five-breath dosimeter method (13, 15).

i. 2-minute tidal breathing method

Ten doubling concentrations of methacholine in sterile vials are prepared and kept in a refrigerator. Solutions of methacholine should be warmed to room temperature before testing begins. The concentrations of methacholine for test are as given below. Diluent, 0.03, 0.06, 0.15, 0.25, 0.50, 1.00, 2.00, 4.00, 8.00, 16.0 mg/ml. The vials stored in the refrigerator are taken out 30 minute prior to testing to warm the solution to room temperature. 3 ml of fresh diluent or the lowest concentration of methacholine is put into the nebulizer using a sterile syringe. Then perform the baseline spirometry to calculate a target FEV1 using the formula: baseline FEV1 x 0.8 to indicate the 20% fall in FEV1. The nebulizer is powered by using dry compressed air and the pressure of the regulator is set at 50 lb/m². After putting the next higher concentration of the methacholine in the nebulizer, start the timer and begin nebulization instructing the patient to relax and breathe slowly at tidal breathing applying a nose clip for 2 minutes. The FEV1 is measured about 30 and 90 seconds after the nebulization is completed. The spirometry is repeated to obtain a good quality FEV1. At the end of the spirometry, the highest FEV1 from an acceptable maneuver is calculated. If the fall in FEV1 is less than 20%, empty the nebulizer and repeat the test with the next higher concentration of methacholine.

Spirometry should not be performed more than three or four times after each dose. The cumulative effect of methacholine can be kept constant by beeping the time interval between the concentrations of two subsequent concentrations to 5 minutes. If the FEV1 falls more than 20% from the baseline value or the highest concentration is given, terminate the test. Patient should then be observed for any symptoms or signs due to bronchoconstriction. If symptoms are observed, treat with inhaled bronchodilators, wait for 10 minutes and then repeat the spirometry.

ii. **Five-breath dosimeter method**
Five concentrations of methacholine is prepared and stored in a refrigerator. The concentrations of methacholine for dosimeter method are as given below.

Diluent, 0.0625, 0.25, 1, 4, 16 mg/ml.

2 ml of the first concentration is put into the nebulizer using a sterile syringe. Perform the baseline spirometry. Patient is instructed to hold the nebulizer upright with a mouth piece and wearing a nose clip. At the end of exhalation during the tidal breathing at functional residual capacity, the patient is instructed to inhale slowly and deeply from the nebulizer. The dosimeter may trigger it automatically soon after the inhalation begins. The patient is encouraged to continue inhalation slowly taking about 5 seconds to complete the inhalation and hold the breath at total lung capacity for another 5 seconds.

Measure the FEV1 about 30 and 90 seconds after the fifth inhalation from the nebulizer. The cumulative effect of methacholine can be kept constant by beeping the time interval between the concentrations of two subsequent concentrations to 5 minutes. At each dose, record the highest FEV1 from acceptable maneuvers. If the FEV1 falls more than 20% from the baseline value or the highest concentration is given, terminate the test. Patient should be observed for any symptoms or signs due to bronchoconstriction. If symptoms are observed, treat with inhaled bronchodilators, wait for 10 minutes and then repeat the spirometry.

b. **Calculation of response**
The % fall in FEV1 can be calculated in two ways by taking either the post – diluent or baseline value as the reference value (7). The lowest technically satisfactory FEV1 measured at 30 or 90 second after inhalation of diluents is taken as the pretest value. The % fall in FEV1 is calculated from the following equation:

$$\frac{(\text{Lowest FEV1 post diluent - lowest FEV1 post challenge}) \times 100}{\text{Lowest FEV1 post diluent}}$$

c. **Calculation of PC20 or PD 20**

PC 20 is used for tidal breathing method and PD 20 is the preferred index for dosimeter method. Calculation of PC20 or PD 20 is similar. The % fall in FEV1 is plotted against the concentration or dose of methacholine / histamine on a log scale. The PC 20 or PD 20 is obtained by linear interpolation between the last two points based on the following formula (16):

PC 20 =antilog [(log C1 + (log C2 – log C1) 20 – R1)] R2 – R1)

Where:

C1 = second last concentration

C2 = last concentration (> 20% FEV1 fall),

R1 = % fall FEV1 after C1,

R2 = % fall FEV1 after C2

Normal PC 20 for histamine and methacholine in adults is > 8 mg /ml and normal PD 20 is > 7.8umol at the recommended nebulizer output (17). There is a good agreement between the tidal breathing and dosimeter methods.

II. **Exercise induced Bronchoconstriction**
Exercise provokes an attack of asthma in 70 to 80 % of the population with clinically recognized asthma. It has been suggested that transient hyper osmolarity of the airway surface fluid as a result of evaporative water loss is a stimulus for exercise induced asthma (EIA) (18, 19). It has been reported that vascular engorgement and oedema of bronchial circulation are responsible for airways narrowing during exercise

though there is no direct evidence for these hypothesis (20). Airway cooling and drying during exercise stimulate the release of inflammatory mediators, such as histamine and the cysteinyl leukotrienes (21) thereby causing bronchoconstriction.

Monitoring the ventilation and controlling the inspired water content are important factors to control the water loss from the airways during exercise challenge tests (22). Exercise can be carried out on either a cycle ergometer or a motor driven treadmill. The time of exercise should be 6 to 8 minutes. Treadmill is started at a low speed and grade and both are progressively advanced during the first 2-3 minutes of exercise (13). The exercise is continued till the heart rate is achieved at 80-90% of the predicted maximum heart rate. The predicted maximum heart rate is calculated from the equation, 220-age in years.

In addition ventilation should reach 40-60% of the predicted maximum voluntary ventilation (MVV). Maximum Voluntary Ventilation is calculated from the formula FEV1x35. For cycle ergometer testing, a target work rate is calculated to achieve the target ventilation. The target work rate in watts is obtained from the equation (53.76 x measured FEV1)-11.07 (13). Spirometry should be performed in the seated position before exercise and then serially after exercise. FEV1 is measured in duplicate after exercise at 5, 10, 15, 20, and 30 min after cessation of exercise (13).The fall in FEV1 is noted. Since healthy individuals generally show an increase in FEV1 after exercise a fall of 10% or more is considered as abnormal. However a fall of 15% or more is more diagnostic of exercise induced bronchoconstriction.

III. Bronchial allergen provocation tests

The airway response to allergen can be assessed by allergen inhalation tests which may produce two types of responses; the early asthmatic response (EAR) and the late asthmatic response (LAR) (23). The EAR is an episode of airflow obstruction that occurs between 10 and 20 minutes after inhalation and resolves within 90 to 120 minutes. The LAR occurs between 3 and 8 hour after inhalation. The EAR is defined as the maximum percent reduction in FEV1 (% fall from base line) occurring in the first hour after challenge and the LAR is defined as the maximum % reduction in FEV1 occurring between 3 and 7 hrs after challenge.

The allergen extract for inhalation is selected based on the skin prick test (SPT) or the serum-specific IgE level. The largest skin wheal produced by the SPT or the highest serum-specific IgE level is to be recorded and these values should be in agreement with the symptoms that may occur on exposure to the allergen. The allergen for challenge test with proper dilutions can be prepared from standardized allergen extracts and these solutions should not be contaminated with endotoxin. Allergen challenge testing can be done either as segmental or total lung challenge. Total lung challenge can be done with high-dose or with low-dose allergen challenge (24, 25).

Allergen provocation is usually done in the morning to allow the measurement of LAR in addition to EAR. The patients are to be observed for at least 10 hrs after challenge to assess the LAR. The response to allergen challenge test is calculated from the maximal decrease in FEV1 compared to baseline during the EAR and LAR. A positive response for EAR is defined as a decrease in FEV1 → 20% from baseline. The LAR is usually characterized by a decrease in FEV1 of e"15% from baseline. Bronchial allergen provocation test is safe, including in children provided the test is done in a dedicated laboratory with experienced staff (25, 26. General reactions are rare, but asthma exacerbations can occur

Specific bronchial provocation tests are the gold standard for the confirmation of occupational asthma. Agents soluble in water or safe diluents, dust or vapours can be used for inhalation challenge testing with occupational agents. For all occupational agents, the levels should not exceed the threshold limit value for short term exposure limit (TLV-STEL) recommended by the American Conference for Governmental Industrial hygienists (ACGH) (27). Immediate, late and dual reactions may develop after a specific bronchial provocation test with occupational agents. The response is detected by measuring FEV1 at the time of immediate reaction is considered as positive response. FEV1 is usually assessed for at least 8 hours.

IV. Eucapnic voluntary hyperventilation

The eucapnic voluntary hyperventilation (EVH) was developed and standardized as a surrogate for an exercise test to identify EIB (28). The test is performed by the subject hyperventilating voluntarily a dry gas at room temperature. The gas contains 21% oxygen, 5% carbon dioxide, and 74% nitrogen. 5% carbon dioxide is required to maintain the arterial carbon dioxide level within the range during the exercise. The target ventilation is equivalent to 85% of the maximal voluntary ventilation with the duration of the test for 6 minutes (29). The target ventilation rate is calculated by multiplying the forced expiratory volume in one second (FEV1) by 30 and is expressed in litres corrected to body temperature, pressure, and fully saturated (BTPS).

The FEV1 is measured three times before the challenge test and the highest measured value is used to calculate the response. The FEV1 is measured in duplicate immediately after the challenge and at five, 10, 15, and 20 minutes after EVH. An additional measurement can be made at three minutes. The Airway narrowing is assessed by calculating the changes in FEV1. The percentage fall in FEV1 is calculated as follows:

100 x [FEV1 (before the test) "lowest value for FEV1 measured in the 20 minutes after the test]/ FEV1 before the test.

When the FEV1 declines by 10% or more at 5 or 10 min after EVH, it is considered as diagnostic of asthma (30).

V. Other inhalation challenge methods

Nebulized hypertonic saline can also be used as an indirect challenge method. Hypertonic saline increases the airway surface liquid osmolarity and this triggers the sensitized cells including mast cells to release inflammatory mediators (31) The results obtained from the hypertonic saline challenge is similar to the results obtained from the exercise and EVH tests. , The nebulized hypertonic saline challenge test is more economical and easier to administer (32). Dry powder mannitol can be used for challenge testing (33, 34). Encapsulated mannitol powder can be through a dry powder inhaler device and is delivered in progressive doubling doses of 5 mg, 10 mg, 20 mg, 40 mg, 80 mg, 160 mg, 160 mg, and 160 mg and the maximal total cumulative dose administered is 635 mg (33). 65 One minute after each dose, the FEV1 is measured in duplicate one minute after challenge. The challenge is terminated on reaching a 15% fall in FEV1 from baseline.

Adenosine 5'- monophosphate (AMP) is another agent that has been used for indirect provocation. AMP acts by stimulating the bronchial mast cells to degranulate and release histamine, leukotrienes, and other inflammatory mediators. AMP for inhalation is prepared by mixing AMP with phosphate-buffered solution (35). AMP is administered in progressively doubling concentrations within the range of 0.09 to 800 mg/mL (35). The AMP is administered to the subjects via a nebulizer for 2 minutes until a $\geq$20% fall in FEV1 is recorded.

REFERENCES

1. Grootendorst DC, Rabe KF. Mechanisms of Bronchial Hyperreactivity in Asthma and Chronic Obstructive Pulmonary Disease. Proc Am Thorac Soc 2004; 1: 77–87
2. Barnes PI. New concepts in the pathogenesis of bronchial hyperresponsiveness and asthma. J Allergy Clin Immonol 1989; 83:1013-1026 .
3. Postma DS, Koeter GH Klaas de vries, Clinical expression of airway hyperreactivity in adults. Clin Rev Allergy 1989;7: 321- 343
4. Paoletti P, Viegi G and Carrozzi L. Bronchial hyperresponsiveness, genetic predisposition environmental factors: importance of epidemiological research. Eur Respir J 1992; 5: 910- 912
5. Clough JB Holgate ST. The natural history of bronchial hyperresponsiveness. Clin Rev Allergy 1989; 9: 257-278
6. Woolcock AJ Peat JK: Epidemiology of bronchial hyperresponsiveness. Clin Rev Allergy 1989; 7; 245-256
7. Sterk PJ, Fabbri LM, Quanjer Ph H, Cockcroft DW, O' Byme PM, Anderson SD, Janiper EF Malo JL. Airway hyper-responsiveness: Standardized challenge testing with pharmacological, physical and sensitising stimuli in adults. Eur Respir J 1993; 6(Suppl 16) 53-83
8. Britton J. Airway hyperresponsiveness and the clinical diagnosis of asthma; histamine or history. J Allergy Clin Immunol 1992; 89 : 19- 22
9. Brand PLP, Postma DS, Kerstjens AAM, Koeter GH and the Dutch CNSLA Study Group. Am Rev Respir Dis 1991; 143; 916-921.
10. Woolcolck AJ Henkins Ch R. Assessment of bronchial responsiveness as a guide to prognosis and therapy in asthma. Med Clin North Am 1990;74; 753-765
11. Woolocock DW Hargreave FE. Airway responsiveness. Relevance of random population data to clinical usefulness. Am Rev Respir Dis 1990.494-500
12. Borges MC, Ferraz E, Vianna EO. Bronchial provocation tests in clinical practice. Sao Paulo Med J. 2011; 129:243-249
13. Crapo RO, Casaburi R, Coates AL, et al. Guidelines for methacholine and exercise challenge testing-1999. This official statement of the American Thoracic Society was adopted by the ATS Board of Directors, July 1999. Am J Respir Crit Care Med. 2000; 161:309-329.
14. Anderson SD, Brannan JD. Methods for «indirect» challenge tests including exercise, Eeucapnic voluntary hyperpnea, and hypertonic aerosols. Clin Rev Allergy Immunol. 2003; 24:27-54.

15. Ryan G, Dolovich MB, Roberts RS, Frith PA Juniper EF, Hargreave FF and Newhouse MT. Standardization of inhalation provocation tests: two techniques of aerosol generation and inhalation compared. Am Rev Respir Dis 1981; 123: 195-199

16. Juniper EF, Cockcroft DW, Hargreave FE. Histamine and methacholine inhalation tests: tidal breathing method. Laboratory procedure and standardization. AB Draco, Lund, Sweden, 1991.

17. Peat JK, Salome CM, Bauman A, Toelle BG, Wachilnger SL, Woolcock AJ. Reapeatability of histamine bronchial challenge and comparability with methacholine bronchial challenge in a population of Australian school children. Am Rev respire Dis 1991; 144;338-343

18. Anderson SD. Is there a unifying hypothesis for exercise - induced asthma? J Allergy Clin Immunol 1984; 73:660-665

19. Gilbert, 1A, and McFadden ER. Airway cooling and rewarming: the second reaction sequence in exercise-induced asthma. J. Clin. Invest. 1992; 90:699-704.

20. Anderson SD and Deviskas E. The airway microvasculature and exercise induced asthma. Thorax 1992; 47:748 -752

21. Finnerty, J. P., and S. T. Holgate. 1990. Evidence for the roles of histamine and prostaglandins as mediators in exercise-induced asthma: the inhibitory effect of terfenadine and flurbiprofen alone and in combination. Eur. Respir. J. 1990; 3:540-547.

22. Randolph, C. 1997. Exercise-induced asthma: update on pathophyiology. Clinical diagnosis and treatment. Curr. Prohl. Pediatr. 27:53-77.

23. Agache L, Bilo M, Braunstahl G-L, et al. In vivo diagnosis of allergic diseases—allergen provocation Tests. Allergy 2015;70: 355–365

24. Diamant Z, Gauvreau GM, Cockcroft W et al. Inhaled allergen bronchoprovocation tests. J Allergy Clin Immunol 2013; 132:1045–1055.

25. Taylor DA, Harris JG, O'Connor BJ. Comparison of incremental and bolus dose inhaled allergen challenge in asthmatic patients. Clin Exp Allergy 2000; 30:56–63.

26. Schulze J, Reinmuller W, Herrmann E, Rosewich M, Rose MA, Zielen S. Bronchial allergen challenges in children—safety and predictors. Pediatr Allergy Immunol 2013; 24:19–27.

27. American conference of governmental Industrial hygienists (ACGIH). Threshold limit values of chemical substances and biological exposure inducers. ACGIH.6500 Cincinnati, OH, USA 1992.

28. Argyros GJ, Roach JM, Hurwitz KM, *et al.* Eucapnic voluntary hyperventilation as a bronchoprovocation technique. Development of a standardized dosing schedule in asthmatics. Chest 1996; 109:1520–524.

29. Anderson SD, Argyros GJ, Magnussen H, Holzer K. Provocation by eucapnic voluntary hyperpnoea to identify exercise induced bronchoconstriction. Br J Sports Med 2001;35:344–347

30. Hurwitz KM, Argyros GJ, Roach JM, *et al.* Interpretation of eucapnic voluntary hyperventilation in the diagnosis of asthma. Chest 1995;108:1240–1245

31. Finnerty JP, Wilmot C, Holgate ST. Inhibition of hypertonic saline-induced bronchoconstriction by terfenadine and flurbiprofen: evidence for the predominant role of histamine. Am Rev Respir Dis 1989; 140:593-597.

32. Riedler J, Reade T, Dalton M, Holst D, Robertson C. Hypertonic saline challenge in an epidemiologic survey of asthma in children. Am J Respir Crit Care Med 1994; 150:1632-1639.

INDEX